Expert Guide to
Sports Medicine

OTHER TITLES IN THE ACP EXPERT GUIDE SERIES

ALLERGY AND IMMUNOLOGY
Edited by Raymond G. Slavin and Robert E. Reisman

INFECTIOUS DISEASES
Edited by James S. Tan

ONCOLOGY
Edited by Jacob D. Bitran

OTOLARYNGOLOGY
Edited by Karen H. Calhoun
Associate Editors: David E. Eibling and Mark K. Wax

PAIN MANAGEMENT
Edited by Bill McCarberg and Steven D. Passik

RHEUMATOLOGY
Edited by Arthur M. F. Yee and Stephen A. Paget

For a catalogue of publications available from ACP, contact:

Customer Service Center
American College of Physicians
190 N. Independence Mall West
Philadelphia, PA 19106-1572
215-351-2600
800-523-1546, ext. 2600

Visit our Web site at www.acponline.org

Expert Guide to
Sports Medicine

Matthew F. Davis, MD

Peter F. Davis, MD

David S. Ross, MD

EDITORS

American College of Physicians

Philadelphia

Clinical Consultant: David R. Goldmann, MD, FACP
Manager, Book Publishing: Diane McCabe
Developmental Editor: Victoria Hoenigke
Production Supervisor: Allan S. Kleinberg
Senior Production Editor: Karen C. Nolan
Interior Design: Kate Nichols
Cover Design: Elizabeth Swartz

Manufactured in the United States of America
Printed by Sheridan Books
Composition by Scribe

Library of Congress Cataloging-in-Publication Data

Expert guide to sports medicine / edited by Peter Davis, Matt Davis, David Ross.
    p. ; cm.
  Includes bibliographical references and index.
  ISBN 1-930513-64-X
    1. Sports medicine—handbooks, manuals, etc. I. Davis, Peter, 1968– II. Davis,
Matthew, 1968– III. Ross, David, MD. IV. American College of Physicians.
    [DNLM: 1. Sports medicine—methods. 2. Athletic injuries—therapy. QT 261 E96 2005]
  RC1211E974 2005
  617.1'027—dc22

                                        2005047430

05 06 07 08 09 / 9 8 7 6 5 4 3 2 1

Contributors

T. Ross Bailey, MEd, ATC, LAT
Associate Athletics Director
Texas Christian University
Fort Worth, Texas

**George C. Baker, MD, MBA,
  FAAD**
Mid Cities Dermatology
Bedford, Texas

**Kyle J. Cassas, MD, CAQ (Sports
  Medicine)**
Primary Care Sports Medicine
Steadman Hawkins Clinic of the
  Carolinas
Greenville, South Carolina

**Donald M. Christie Jr, MD, CAQ
  (Sports Medicine), FACP,
  FACSM**
Sports Physician and Internal
  Medicine Consultant
Lewiston, Maine

**Philip H. Cohen, MD, CAQ
  (Sports Medicine)**
Assistant Team Physician
Rutgers University Sports Medicine
Clinical Assistant Professor of
  Medicine and Family Medicine
UMDNJ-Robert Wood Johnson
  Medical School
New Brunswick, New Jersey

Gary R. Cooper, MD, FACC
Clinical Associate Professor
Division of Cardiovascular
  Medicine
Department of Internal Medicine
University of Florida
Gainesville, Florida

Stephanie M. Cooper, MD
Swedish Hospital
Seattle, Washington

**Matthew F. Davis, MD, CAQ
  (Sports Medicine)**
Internal Medicine—Sports
  Medicine
Dallas, Texas

**Peter F. Davis, MD, CAQ (Sports
  Medicine)**
Staff Physician and Medical
  Director
Southern Methodist University
  Health Center
Associate Professor
University of Texas Southwestern
  Medical Center
Dallas, Texas

**Kevin Eerkes, MD, CAQ (Sports
  Medicine)**
Clinical Assistant Professor
Department of Medicine
New York University School of
  Medicine
New York, New York

**Kimberly M. Fagan, MD, CAQ
  (Sports Medicine), FACP**
Birmingham, Alabama

**David M. Harsha, MD, CAQ
  (Sports Medicine)**
Director, Sports Medicine
St. Vincent Family Medicine
  Residency Program
Indianapolis, Indiana

John P. Jamison, MD
Orthopedic Surgeon
Faculty—Methodist Health System
  Primary Care Sports Medicine
  Fellowship
Dallas, Texas

Michael Lucido, PT, OCS, COMT
HealthSouth
Dallas, Texas

Melvin R. Manning, MD
Texas Sports Medicine and
  Orthopedic Group
Dallas, Texas

Michael J. Milne, MD
Orthopedic Surgeon
St. Louis, Missouri

**Balakrishnan (Balu) Natarajan,
  MD, CAQ (Sports Medicine)**
Private Practice
Associate Medical Director,
  Chicago Marathon
Chicago, Illinois

**Mark W. Niedfeldt, MD, CAQ
  (Sports Medicine)**
Associate Professor of Family and
  Community Medicine
Medical College of Wisconsin
Milwaukee, Wisconsin

Phil Page, PT, MS, ATC, CSCS
Baton Rouge, Louisiana

**Luis Palacios, MD, CAQ (Sports
  Medicine)**
Associate Professor
Department of Family and
  Community Medicine
University of Texas Southwestern
  Medical Center
Dallas, Texas

Scott E. Rojas, MD
Tarrant County—Infectious
  Disease
Fort Worth, Texas

**David S. Ross, MD, CAQ (Sports
  Medicine)**
Director
Methodist Health System
Primary Care Sports Medicine
  Fellowship
Associate Professor
University of Texas Southwestern
  Medical Center
Dallas, Texas

**S. Craig Veatch, MD, CAQ
  (Sports Medicine)**
St. Vincent Sports Medicine
St. Vincent Internal Medicine
  Residency Program Faculty
Indianapolis, Indiana

■ ■ ■

Preface

Because at least 10% of a primary care practice involves the evaluation of musculoskeletal disorders, internists must have a good foundation in musculoskeletal assessment. This is all the more necessary when the physician has many physically active patients.

Active patients include those who regularly participate in a sport or exercise routine and those who engage in frequent physical activity that is not strictly organized or scheduled. Therefore active patients not only include the high school cross-country runner, the college football player, the teacher who jogs every morning, and the real-estate agent who goes to the gym five days a week but also the housewife who periodically does yard work, the construction laborer, and the businessman who plays softball every weekend.

Sports Medicine is an essential resource for the primary care physician. Because a significant portion of the text addresses musculoskeletal injuries commonly seen in athletes, the title is accurate. However, this latest volume in the ACP Expert Guide series also discusses nutrition, the pre-participation screening examination, cardiovascular conditions, exercise-induced asthma, drugs and supplements, psychological issues, and other important areas in the diagnosis and treatment of *all* physically active patients.

The primary care practitioner, in fact, is often well suited to serve as team physician at the high school or college level because of the variety of medical issues that may be encountered. We encourage you to consider volunteering for such a position in your community. Treating athletes is a rewarding and valuable experience, one different in kind from treating the general population.

We have selected authors who themselves are internists, family practitioners, or orthopedic specialists. All understand the importance of the role of the primary care physician in treating sports-related injuries and conditions. Moreover, because physicians who are knowledgeable about sports medicine are in great demand, we suggest that you explore the valuable on-line and print resources available from the American College of Physicians, the American Medical Society of Sports Medicine, and the American College of Sports Medicine.

We would like to express our thanks to the individuals who have helped make *Sports Medicine* possible: Dominique Lemire-Ross, MT-BC, who provided some of the artwork for the musculoskeletal chapters; Lennard A. Nadalo, MD, who provided some of the radiographs for the same chapters; Julie Timms, of Methodist Health System, who also helped us acquire radiographs; and Mark Lavallee, MD, Amy Powell, MD, and Alishia Ferguson, PhD, who reviewed the manuscript. We also take pleasure in acknowledging Methodist Health System, Dallas, for its support of this project.

We are grateful to the American College of Physicians for making the commitment to publish *Sports Medicine* and their implicit acknowledgement of the importance of this subject to the primary care physician and internist. We extend special thanks to McGraw-Hill and Companies for their permission to reproduce the Preparticipation Physical Evaluation forms that can be found at the back of this volume.

Matthew F. Davis, MD
Peter F. Davis, MD
David S. Ross, MD

Contents

SECTION I

OVERVIEW

1

The Preparticipation Screening Examination

Matthew F. Davis, MD

Athletes at most levels of organized sports, from the high school to the professional level, require some type of preparticipation screening examination (PPSE). Like the annual physical examination for general patients, the PPSE is used to assess general health. Goals of the PPSE that are specific to athletes, however, are 1) identifying health issues that would limit or disqualify an athlete from participation, and 2) meeting the legal requirements for states and school districts for sports participation. For athletes and team physicians alike, the preparticipation exam signals the beginning of a new season. The PPSE gives the team physician the opportunity to meet new players and to become reacquainted with returning players. The PPSE allows the athlete to meet those individuals (athletic trainer, physician) who will be responsible for ensuring that training and participation will be safe.

Physicians engaged in preparticipation exams may have various motivating factors for their involvement, ranging from practice marketing and strict financial gain to a sense of duty and obligation to the community. Whatever that motivation, the physician engaged in the examination process has a responsibility to understand the purpose of the exam and his or her responsibility to the athlete. Physicians engaged in PPSEs who have limited knowledge or interest in cardiovascular and musculoskeletal systems can be useful for certain parts of the exam, but the final determination about clearance for participation is best done by a physician with some level of understanding of what problems in these areas constitute disqualification from certain sports.

The cost-effectiveness of preparticipation exams has been debated. According to estimates, greater than one million physicians' hours are invested in examining more than six million participants. Of these exams, less than 2% of those undergoing exams are disqualified. The addition of ancillary tests to the history and physical is also a debatable issue in terms of cost-effectiveness (1).

Timing and Format

The timing and frequency of the preparticipation exam may vary depending on the situation. Many states and school districts require that these exams be performed annually. Most exams should be performed 4 to 6 weeks before participation, so that problems can be addressed (1).

Office-based exams probably are ideal. In the office-based exam, the practitioner can address any problems discovered in the exam. The cost-effectiveness of this format is somewhat debatable, however. Additionally, if the examining physician has no affiliation with the school or organizing body, communication problems can arise. Physicians performing office-based PPSEs must make certain to communicate with the athletic trainer or parent(s) if limiting issues are discovered.

Station-based exams typically are conducted within or in conjunction with the school, and therefore communication problems are limited. Station-based or mass-screening exams are organized such that the athlete passes from one station to the next, where specific areas of the exam are conducted. Other advantages to station-based exams are that they may be more cost effective and time efficient. However, this is true only if there is good coordination with the ancillary personnel involved in the coordination of the exam (that is, the athletic training staff). A successful group screening is accomplished through careful planning and coordination between the facility, the physicians involved, and all ancillary personnel. A sample breakdown of stations is listed in Table 1-1. Some of these stations may be combined, depending on the available space and personnel.

The addition of stations to assess performance, flexibility, and other traits can also be considered, and the use of ancillary personnel at some stations is acceptable. It is also important to consider the location of each

---

Table 1-1   Preparticipation Examination Stations for Station-Based Exams

- Check-in
- Vital signs/height/weight
- HEENT (Head, Eyes, Ears, Nose, Throat) exam
- Cardiovascular exam
- Lung exam
- Abdomen/GU exam
- Musculoskeletal exam
- Skin exam

examining station when organizing a station-based exam. For instance, the cardiovascular exam should be performed in a location relatively free from noise, so that the examiner can appropriately auscultate the heart. Additionally, privacy considerations play a role in the location of the genitourinary portion of the exam (1).

For many athletes, the preparticipation exam is their only annual encounter with a health care provider. For these athletes, assessment of general health may be more important than determining clearance for sports participation. It is important to remember, however, that preparticipation exams conducted in a mass-screening format do not lend themselves to disease treatment. The exam is just a screening tool and should not be used as a substitute for a visit to a physician. The actual treatment of disease is better suited to an office-based exam or a specific visit with a physician to address the problem identified by the screening (1).

History

The preparticipation screening evaluation comprises a thorough history and physical examination.* The majority of patients whose athletic participation may be restricted or disallowed can be identified through their medical history. Several history questions are related to cardiac conditions. "Have you ever passed out or fainted during exercise?" is a question that can be asked by an examiner at every station in a group screening exam. Questions about familial sudden cardiac death are also extremely important. Such inquiries are used to help identify athletes at risk for sudden cardiac death due to conditions such as hypertrophic cardiomyopathy or prolonged QT syndrome (see Chapter 13). A history of exertional syncope generally warrants further evaluation before clearance. A careful review of the history form will generally alert the examiner to most conditions that may limit participation (2-4). Minors should complete the form in conjunction with their parents.

Physical Examination

The physical exam, used in conjunction with the history, provides an additional tool for identifying athletes who may need further evaluation before clearance:

- *Head, Eyes, Ears, Nose, Throat (HEENT)*—Note visual acuity. Athletes whose best corrected vision is less than 20/40 need protective eyewear. Vision must be correctable. Also note anisocoria for future reference.

---

*Sample history and physical examination forms can be found inside the back cover of this book.

- *Cardiovascular*—Examine the patient in static and dynamic positions. The murmur of hypertrophic cardiomyopathy decreases with squatting, whereas Valsalva's maneuver increases the obstruction and therefore increases the murmur. The murmur of aortic stenosis, however, decreases with Valsalva, yet increases with squatting. Any murmur greater than 3/6 in intensity or a diastolic murmur generally warrants further evaluation. Arrythmias found during the exam also warrant further evaluation with an EKG.
- *Lungs*—Note the presence of wheezes.
- *Genitourinary/Abdomen*—Note the possible presence of inguinal hernia. This is not necessarily a contraindication to participation, however. A solitary testicle may warrant counseling if participating in a contact sport. An undescended testicle warrants further evaluation.
- *Skin*—Note possible presence of zoster, moluscum, or other contagious skin conditions (see Chapter 7 for restrictions on return to play).
- *Musculoskeletal*—Perform a general screening musculoskeletal exam for those athletes without symptoms. For those athletes with symptoms or those who have a history of injury, a joint-specific examination may be necessary (Figures 1-1 to 1-14).
- Diagnostic tests such as complete blood count (CBC), HCT, EKG, echocardiogram, UA, and sickle cell screen are generally *not* recommended for asymptomatic athletes.

MUSCULOSKELETAL EXAMINATION (Figures 1-1 to 1-14)

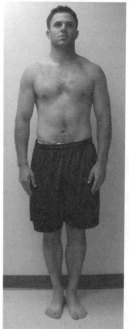

Figure 1-1   General inspection of athlete. The athlete stands facing the examiner (symmetry of trunk, upper extremities).

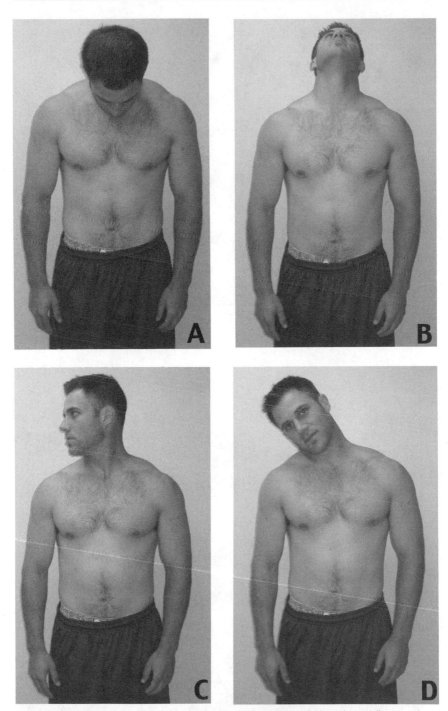

Figure 1-2 (A) Forward flexion, (B) extension. (C) rotation, and (D) lateral flexion of neck (range of motion: cervical spine).

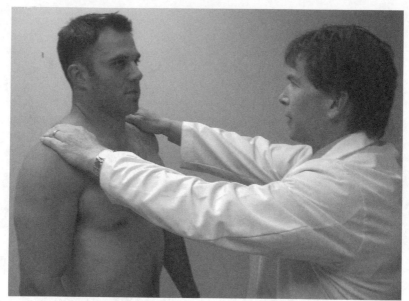

Figure 1-3   Resisted shoulder shrug (strength, trapezius).

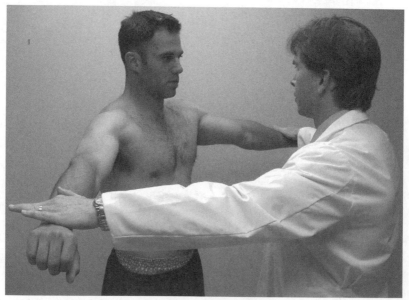

Figure 1-4   Resisted shoulder abduction (strength, deltoid).

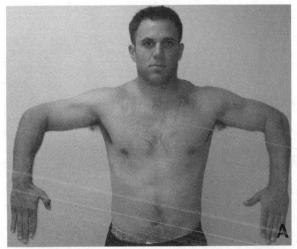

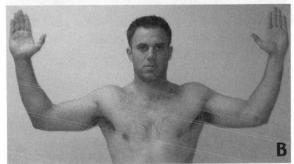

Figure 1-5   (A) Internal and (B) external rotation of shoulder (range of motion: glenohumeral joint).

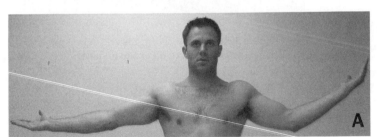

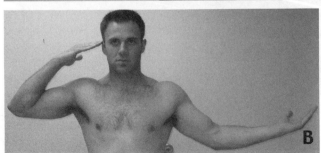

Figure 1-6   (A) Extension and (B) flexion of arm at the elbow (range of motion: elbow).

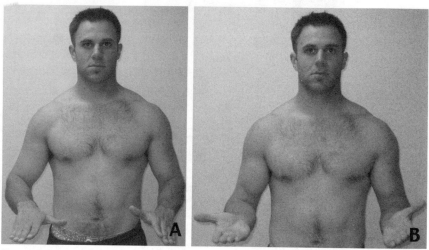

Figure 1-7   (A) Pronation and (B) supination of palm (range of motion: elbow and wrist).

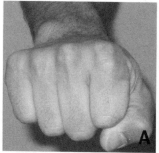

Figure 1-8   (A) Clench fist, then (B) slowly spread fingers (range of motion: hand and fingers).

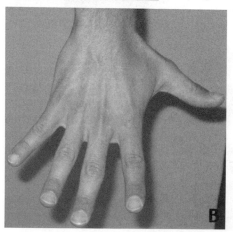

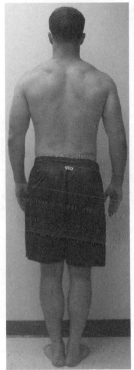

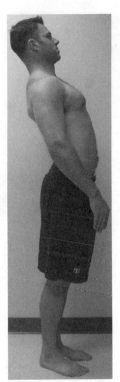

Figure 1-9 Inspect from behind to check for symmetry of trunk and upper extremities.

Figure 1-10 Back extension with knees straight (spondylosis/spondylolisthesis).

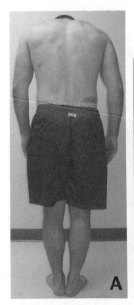

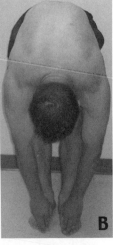

Figure 1-11 Back flexion with knees straight, facing (A) away and (B) toward examiner (range of motion: thoracic and lumbosacral spine; spine curvature, hamstring flexibility).

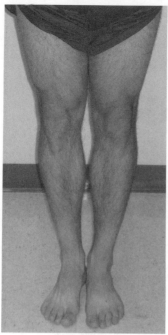

Figure 1-12   Inspect lower extremity alignment and symmetry.

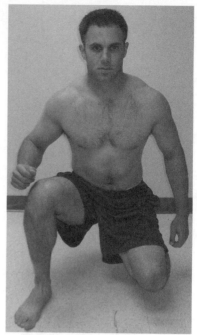

Figure 1-13   "Duck walk" three or four steps to check for motion of hip, knees, and ankle; balance; strength).

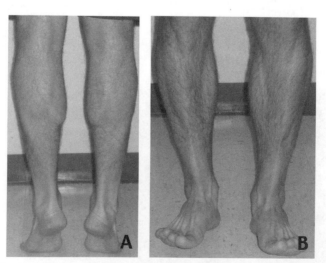

Figure 1-14   Standing on (A) toes and (B) heels to test balance and calf strength.

Clearance

Clearance is the final step in determining if an athlete can safely participate in the desired sport (5). Clearance is best determined by a physician familiar with the demands of the athlete's sport and the consensus guidelines published by 26th Bethesda Conference and the American Academy of Pediatrics (AAP). Clearance can be divided into three categories: 1) unrestricted sports activity (for a given sport); 2) clearance (that is, unrestricted activity for a given sport) after completion of further evaluation or treatment for the identified problem; and 3) participation in a given sport is not permitted. When determining whether or not to grant clearance to an athlete with a specific problem, the physician must decide if participation in the desired activity will pose a risk to the athlete or others. If the patient does have a health problem that would limit his or her participation in a particular sport, the physician should consider if clearance could be gained by completing treatment for the condition. Finally, if clearance cannot be granted for a particular sport or sports category, the physician should identify in what other sports the athlete might be allowed to participate.

The most common health problems preventing clearance that are found during a preparticipation exam are hypertension, ophthalmologic abnormalities, and genitourinary and musculoskeletal problems. Guidelines for clearance have been developed for many conditions, as seen in Table 1-2.

Table 1-2   Conditions to Consider When Making Clearance Decisions

Condition	May Participate?
Kidney (absence of)	QUALIFIED YES
Explanation: Athlete needs individual assessment for contact/collision and limited-contact sports.	
Liver (enlarged)	QUALIFIED YES
Explanation: If the liver is actually enlarged, participation should be avoided because of risk of rupture. If the liver is chronically enlarged, individual assessment is needed before contact/collision or limited-contact sports are played.	
Malignancy	QUALIFIED YES
Explanation: Athlete needs individual assessment.	
Musculoskeletal disorders	QUALIFIED YES
Explanation: Athlete needs individual assessment.	
Neurologic conditions	
History of serious head or spine trauma, severe or repeated concussions, or craniotomy	QUALIFIED YES
Explanation: Athlete needs individual assessment for contact/collision or limited-contact sports, and also for noncontact sports if there are deficits in judgement or cognition. Recent research supports a conservative approach to management of concussion.	

Cont'd

**Table 1-2   Conditions to Consider When Making Clearance Decisions
(cont'd)**

Condition	May Participate?

Convulsive disorder (well controlled)   YES

Explanation: Risk of convulsion during participation is minimal.

Convulsive disorder (poorly controlled)   QUALIFIED YES

Explanation: Athlete needs individual assessment for contact/collision or limited-contact sports. Avoid the following noncontact sports: archery, riflery, swimming, weight or power lifting, strength training, or sports involving heights. In these sports, occurrence of a convulsion may be a risk to self or others.

Obesity   QUALIFIED YES

Explanation: Because of the risk of heat illness, obese persons need careful acclimatization and hydration.

Organ transplant recipient   QUALIFIED YES

Explanation: Athlete needs individual assessment.

Ovary (absence of)   YES

Explanation: Risk of severe injury to the remaining ovary is minimal.

Respiratory conditions

Pulmonary compromise including cystic fibrosis   QUALIFIED YES

Explanation: Athlete needs individual assessment, but generally all sports may be played if oxygenization remains satisfactory during a graded exercise test. Patients with cystic fibrosis need acclimatization and good hydration to reduce the risk of heat illness.

Asthma   YES

Explanation: With proper medication and education, only athletes with the most severe asthma will have to modify their participation.

Acute upper respiratory infection   QUALIFIED YES

Explanation: Upper respiratory obstruction may affect pulmonary function. Athlete needs individual assessment for all but mild disease.

Sickle cell disease   QUALIFIED YES

Explanation: Athlete needs individual assessment. In general, if status of the illness permits, all but high-exertion, contact/collision sports may be played. Overheating, dehydration, and chilling must be avoided.

Sickle cell trait   YES

Explanation: It is unlikely that individuals with sickle cell trait (AS) have an increased risk of sudden death or other medical problems during athletic participation except under the most extreme conditions of heat, humidity, and possibly increased altitude. These individuals, like all athletes, should be carefully conditioned, acclimatized, and hydrated to reduce any possible risk.

Skin (boils, herpes simplex, impetigo, scabies, molluscum contagiosum)   QUALIFIED YES

Explanation: While the patient is contagious, participation in gymnastics with mats, martial arts, wrestling, or other contact/collision or limited-contact sports is not allowed. Herpes simplex virus is probably not transmitted via mats.

Spleen (enlarged)   QUALIFIED YES

Explanation: Patients with acutely enlarged spleens should avoid all sports because of risk of rupture. Those with chronically enlarged spleens need individual assessment before playing contact/collision or limited-contact sports.

Cont'd

Table 1-2   Conditions to Consider When Making Clearance Decisions
(cont'd)

Condition	_May Participate?_
Testicle (absent or undescended)	YES

Explanation: Certain sports may require a protective cup.

Adapted from American Academy of Pediatrics, Committee on Sports Medicine and Fitness. Medical conditions affecting sports participation. Pediatrics. 1994;94:757-60.

Table 1-3   Classification of Sports by Contact

Contact or Collision	_Limited Contact_	_Noncontact_
• Basketball	• Baseball	• Archery
• Boxing	• Bicycling	• Badminton
• Diving	* Canoeing/kayaking	• Bodybuilding
• Field hockey	(white water)	• Bowling
• Football	• Cheerleading	• Canoeing/kayaking
• Ice hockey	• Fencing	(flat water)
• Lacrosse	• Field events	• Crew/rowing
• Martial arts	▫ High jump	• Curling
• Rodeo	▫ Pole vault	• Dancing
• Rugby	• Floor hockey	• Field events
• Ski jumping	• Gymnastics	▫ Discus
• Soccer	• Handball	▫ Javelin
	• Horseback riding	▫ Shot put
• Team handball	• Racquetball	• Golf
• Water polo	• Skating	• Orienteering
• Wrestling	▫ Ice	• Power-lifting
	▫ Inline	• Race walking
	▫ Roller	• Riflery
	• Skiing	• Rope jumping
	▫ Cross-country	• Running
	▫ Downhill	• Sailing
	▫ Water	• Scuba diving
	• Softball	• Strength training
	• Squash	• Swimming
	• Ultimate Frisbee	• Table tennis
	• Volleyball	• Tennis
	• Windsurfing/surfing	• Weightlifting

Adapted from American Academy of Pediatrics, Committee on Sports Medicine and Fitness. Medical conditions affecting sports participation. Pediatrics. 1994;94:757-60.

However, remember that these are only guidelines and that all decisions should be individualized. The contact categories listed in Table 1-3 can help identify those sports in which the risk of potential injury from collision is high. Likewise, classification of sports by strenuousness is important for athletes with cardiac or pulmonary disease (Table 1-4).

When determining clearance, take care to fully inform all involved parties of any follow-up needed if problems are identified. This also must be done in a way that respects the athlete's privacy (2).

Medicolegal Issues

The goal of the physician performing the PPSE is always to protect the athlete's health. A physician who allows an athlete to participate despite clearly defined risks may be liable for malpractice. Additionally, it is inappropriate to grant medical clearance merely because the athlete and his or her family offer to sign a liability waiver. If restricted participation is considered, then it is generally advisable that the physician consult with several

Table 1-4   Classification of Sports by Strenuousness

◄──────────── *High-to-Moderate Intensity* ────────────►

High-to-Moderate Dynamic and Static Demands	*High-to-Moderate Dynamic and Low Static Demands*	*High-to-Moderate Static and Low Dynamic Demands*
• Boxing*	• Badminton	• Archery
• Crew/rowing	• Baseball	• Auto racing
• Cross-country skiing	• Basketball	• Diving
• Cycling	• Field hockey	• Equestrian
• Downhill skiing	• Lacrosse	• Field events (jumping)
• Fencing	• Orienteering	• Field events (throwing)
• Football	• Ping-pong	• Gymnastics
• Ice hockey	• Race walking	• Karate or judo
• Rugby	• Racquetball	• Motorcycling
• Running (sprint)	• Soccer	• Rodeoing
• Speed skating	• Squash	• Sailing
• Water polo	• Swimming	• Ski jumping
• Wrestling	• Tennis	• Water skiing
	• Volleyball	• Weight lifting

Low Intensity (Low Dynamic and Low Static Demands)

• Bowling
• Cricket
• Curling
• Golf
• Riflery

*Participation not recommended.
Adapted from American Academy of Pediatrics, Committee on Sports Medicine and Fitness. Medical conditions affecting sports participation. Pediatrics. 1994;94:757-60.

other specialists before a final decision is made. It is important that the athlete be informed of these decisions and the reasons behind them (6).

The Americans with Disabilities Act and the Rehabilitation Act have been cited in several court cases involving team physicians' decision not to grant clearance. The courts have not been uniform in their decisions on the legal authority of physicians to disqualify an athlete; however, it must be stressed that neither of these acts makes the physician liable for determining medical ineligibility (6).

Finally, the issue of civil liability for those physicians performing PPSEs warrants discussion. "Good Samaritan" laws may apply for physicians performing these exams free of charge. However, a physician must know the laws of his or her particular state, because some states do not offer legal protection under these statutes even if the exam was provided at no cost (6).

REFERENCES

1. Preparticipation Physical Evaluation, 3rd ed. American Academy of Family Physicians, American Academy of Pediatrics, American Medical Society for Sports Medicine, American Orthopedic Society for Sports Medicine, and American Osteopathic Academy of Sports Medicine. The Physician and Sports Medicine, McGraw-Hill Healthcare, Minneapolis, MN; 2005.

2. **Maron BJ, Zipes DP.** 36th Bethesda Conference: Eligibility recommendations for competitive athletes with cardiovascular abnormalities. J Am Coll Cardiol. 2005;45:1311-75.

3. Medical conditions affecting sports participation. Pediatrics. 1994;94(5):757-60.

4. **Sallis RE.** The preparticipation exam. In: Sallis RE, ed. Essentials of Sports Medicine. Philadelphia: Mosby-Yearbook; 1996:151-60.

5. **Mitten M.** When is disqualification from sports justified? Medical judgement vs. patients' rights. Phys Sportsmed. 1996;24(10):75.

6. **Magnes S, Hernerson J, Hunter S.** What conditions limit sports participation? Experience with 10,540 athletes. Phys Sportsmed. 1992;20(5):143.

2

■ ■ ■

Nutrition and Sports

Matthew F. Davis, MD

The importance of nutrition as it relates to athletic performance cannot be overemphasized. Proper nutritional input and fluid balance play a vital role in optimizing peak performance. Many athletes, however, are susceptible to nutritional quackery due to their strong desire to gain a competitive advantage (1). Information on fad diets, along with nutritional supplements that may or may not have any scientific basis, is readily available in numerous lay publications and on the Internet. It therefore becomes the responsibility of the physician counseling the athlete to guide him or her in making the proper decisions with respect to diet. While there is no single diet that is "right" for every athlete, there are several principles that every athlete should follow. Many of these principles, especially those related to fluids, are extremely simple, yet vitally important to athletic performance. Perhaps the most important tenet that needs to be stressed to the athlete is that, although there are no magic diets that will boost performance, making the wrong diet choices can *hinder* performance.

Fluids

Proper fluid balance is essential for peak athletic performance. Inadequate hydration not only hinders an athlete's ability to perform but can result in potentially life-threatening injuries such as heat stroke (2). A fluid loss of 1% of body mass can result in an increased heart rate, perception of effort, and premature fatigue (3,4). Proper hydration is important in all climates; studies have demonstrated that up to 2 liters of fluid can be lost with 90 minutes of vigorous of exercise, even in temperatures as low as 50°F. Exercise conducted in extremely low temperatures is also complicated by the body's increased urine production in response to cold stress (3).

Proper preexercise hydration can help minimize the potential for dehydration in numerous ways. Athletes should consume at least 400–600 ml of fluid 20–60 minutes before exercise. Preexercise fluid intake not only serves to maintain plasma volume but boosts gastric volume (2). Gastric emptying plays a crucial role in maintaining adequate fluid balance, and gastric emptying is higher when gastric volume is high (2). Because it is not uncommon for some elite level athletes to be chronically dehydrated, some athletes use hyperhydration as a strategy to boost athletic performance (5). In elite soccer players, a systematic regimen of 4.5 L/day of fluid 1 week before competition resulted in greater water reserves, improved thermoregulation, and increased body fluid by 1.1 liters (3). Additionally, hyperhydration with 500 ml of a carbohydrate drink 2 hours before competition for events where drinking is impractical or where the event is less than 1 hour (for example, in soccer or field hockey) may be useful (5).

Athletes typically do not hydrate themselves adequately *during exercise*. Numerous factors influence this, including coaching pressures, the nature of the sport, and ignorance. Thirst is a poor indicator of hydration status; in fact, most individuals are already dehydrated by the time they become thirsty (1).

Table 2-1 summarizes the amount of fluid athletes should ingest during training or competition. For events lasting longer than 1 hour, it is important to include some sodium in rehydration beverages. Plain water ingestion may actually delay rehydration by several mechanisms, including delaying thirst drive and increasing free water clearance (2,5).

Adequacy of rehydration is measured by body weight; athletes exhibiting excessive weight loss due to fluid loss should be excluded from competition. Numerous studies have shown that a solution high in sodium content improves fluid restoration (5). Postexercise hydration is particularly important to help avoid the chronic mild dehydration seen in many athletes. Additionally, athletes must generally consume at least 150% of weight lost to restore preexercise weight. For instance, if an athlete loses 5 kg during a training session, he or she needs to consume 7.5 kg of fluid to restore preexercise weight. Therefore, large volume coupled with high

Table 2-1   Intervals Between Breaks and Amount of Fluid Per Break

Estimated Weight Loss over 90 Minutes	Interval Between Breaks	Amount of Fluid per Break
2.7-3.0 kg (6-6.5 lb)*	10 min	250 ml
1.8-2.7 kg (4-6 lb)	15 min	250-325 ml
1.1-1.8 kg (2.5-4 lb)	20 min	225-300 ml
0.7-1.1 kg (1.5-2.5 lb)	30 min	175-225 ml
0-0.7 kg (0-1.5 lb)	45 min	175 ml

* Athletes who lose ≥ 3.2 kg (≥7 lb) over 90 minutes should stop practice or participation immediately.

sodium (up to 2.9 g/L) are necessary for proper rehydration. Most commercial sports drinks do not contain this large amount of sodium and therefore it may be necessary to couple a meal high in sodium content with fluid intake (2).

The exact type of fluid required for hydration depends on many factors, including duration of event, type of event, and athlete's palate. A general recommendation is that the fluid contain some carbohydrate and some electrolyte; however, the exact quantities of each are debatable. Drinks with large amounts of carbohydrate, such as fruit juices and soft drinks, have been shown to cause some gastrointestinal upset in athletes during competition (5), and those with a lower concentration of carbohydrate may not be as beneficial for certain types of events.

However, there are some general guidelines to follow. For all exercise lasting 1 hour or longer, hydration should take place with fluids that contain between 5%–8% (1.3-2 g/oz) of carbohydrate. Additionally, adding some sodium (0.5-0.7 g/L) to any rehydration beverage appears to be beneficial (5). Table 2-2 illustrates these guidelines.

Food As Fuel

There are essentially two sources of energy for exercise: glycogen and fat. During periods of low to moderate exercise, fats make up most of the fuel used for energy. During periods of high intensity exercise, fat cannot supply adenosine triphosphate (ATP) quickly enough to be used as a fuel source (2). Therefore, adequate carbohydrate stores become paramount for peak athletic performance. Table 2-3 shows what types of substrates are used for fuel depending on the activity level (2).

During early stages of exercise, muscle glycogen is the major source of carbohydrate used for exercising muscle. As activity progresses from low

Table 2-2   Amount of Fluid Needed Per Hour to Replace Carbohydrate and Fluid Lost in One Hour of Strenuous Activity*

Percent Carbohydrate	To replace 30 g/hr	To replace 40 g/hr	To replace 50 g/hr	To replace 60 g/hr
4	750 ml	1000 ml	1250 ml	Not recommended
6	Not recommended	667 ml	833 ml	750 ml
8	Not recommended	Not recommended	625 ml	750 ml

* Volumes are based on adequate fluid replacement of 600-1200 ml/hr and carbohydrate losses of 30-60 g/hr. Sports drinks such as Gatorade typically have 6% carbohydrate; others, such as All-Sport and Powerade, have 8% carbohydrate.

Table 2-3   Substrates Used for Energy Versus Activity Level

Macronutrient	Rest	Light-to-Moderate Exercise	High-Intensity Sprint-Type Exercise	High-Intensity Endurance Exercise
Protein	2-5%	2-5%	2%	5-8%
Carbohydrate	35%	40%	95%	70%
Fat	60%	55%	3%	15%

to high intensity, the liver increases its release of glucose to fuel the muscle. Blood glucose can supply 30 percent of the total energy required by active muscle (2), but liver glycogen stores are reduced by half after 1 hour of strenuous activity and nearly gone within 2 hours. Trained muscle exhibits the ability to use less muscle glycogen and more fat during submaximal exercise. This "glycogen-sparing" effect increases endurance, beacuse the body generally has more fat stores than muscle glycogen (1,3).

Muscle glycogen also is used with low-to-moderate intensity exercise because it takes about 20 minutes for fat to be available as a fuel source. Fat can be used as a fuel source for 4 to 6 hours for low-to-moderate intensity exercise (see next section).

Because most athletic events are high-intensity endeavors, muscle glycogen is the primary fuel for most sports (1). For athletes to maintain adequate muscle glycogen, they must have a diet that is high in carbohydrate. Without adequate carbohydrate intake, the muscle rapidly uses its available glycogen, and exercise intensity is decreased to the level allowed by the oxidation of fat. General dietary guidelines for athletes state that at least 7-8 g/kg should be taken on a daily basis (2). The exact amount of carbohydrate depends on the level and duration of training.

During a preexercise or precompetition meal, athletes should focus on obtaining adequate carbohydrate. A meal consumed 2 to 4 hours before competition should have 1–4 g/kg of carbohydrate to ensure adequate muscle and liver glycogen for those athletes involved in events lasting 1 hour or longer. Carbohydrate "loading" has some theoretic benefit for endurance events lasting longer than 90 minutes, such as long distance cycling and marathon running (6). A 6-day regimen consisting of tapered training and intake of 5 g/kg carbohydrate for the first 3 days, followed by 10 g/kg carbohydrate for the final 3 days, may boost performance (2). Potential adverse side effect of carbohydrate loading include excessive weight gain and stiffness (7).

For those events lasting longer than 1 hour, carbohydrate ingestion during the event has been shown to improve performance. For continuous events, such as a running race, the most practical way to obtain carbohydrate is with a sports drink containing 5%–8% carbohydrate. Consider high carbohydrate snacks or meals for events lasting significantly longer or in situations where several events are held on the same day.

Replacement of carbohydrate after exhaustive exercise or training can help minimize fatigue and may play a role in reducing the likelihood of "overtraining syndrome" (2). Within 30 minutes after exhaustive exercise, 1.5 g/kg carbohydrate should be consumed to speed muscle glycogen resynthesis. High carbohydrate fluids, such as soft drinks and fruit juices, can be used for this purpose. An additional 1.5 g/kg of carbohydrate should then be consumed within 2 hours (2). It is also advisable that some protein be consumed with the carbohydrate because this can speed muscle glycogen recovery (8). Even with proper dietary intake, it takes at least 24 hours to replenish muscle glycogen after prolonged exercise (2). Most athletes typically require 1 to 2 days rest coupled with high-carbohydrate intake to replenish their muscle glycogen (2).

Lack of proper carbohydrate intake may be a contributor to overtraining syndrome, the features of which are listed in Table 2-4. Overtraining syndrome is characterized by lack of sufficient rest to allow muscle glycogen to be restored. Complete recovery may take weeks (2).

Fat

Although the average American consumes nearly 40% of total calories as fat, dietary fat should constitute no more than 30% of total calories. This is especially true for athletes who are dependent on carbohydrate as a main source for muscle glycogen. However, significant reductions in dietary fat can impair performance for endurance athletes (2). Fat is used as fuel by exercising muscle when carbohydrate stores are depleted. In addition, extremely low-fat diets may not be able to provide adequate calories or carbohydrate, especially during periods of intense training or in preparation for an endurance event. Also, the fat-soluble vitamins A, D, E, and K are

Table 2-4   Signs and Symptoms of Overtraining Syndrome

Workout Symptoms	Physical Symptoms	Nonphysical Symptoms
• Usual workouts feel more difficult	• Persistent fatigue	• Difficulty sleeping
• Early fatigue during workout	• Muscle soreness	• Lack of motivation
• Faster heart rate with less effort	• Increase in overuse injuries	• Depression
• Decreased coordination		
• Decreased performance on strength or endurance testing		

Data from Hawley C, Schoene R. Overtraining syndrome. Phys Sportsmed. 2003;31:47-8.

taken through diet, as are some essential fatty acids. Some studies have shown that on a diet consisting of less than 20% fat, the expected increase in testosterone levels seen after resistance training are blunted. Therefore, some dietary fat is needed to maintain hormone synthesis and to avoid vitamin deficiencies (2).

During low-to-moderate intensity exercise, fat is used as a significant fuel source. Hormones such as norepinephrine and glucagon stimulate lipolysis and mobilization of free fatty acids. When exercise becomes intense, however, release of these free fatty acids does not keep up with the muscles' demand, and there is a shift to use of muscle glycogen as fuel (2).

Regular aerobic exercise greatly increases the body's ability to use fat as a fuel source. Chronic exercise increases the proliferation of capillaries in trained muscle, increases the size and number of mitochondria, and facilitates the rate of lypolysis within fat cells (2). The fat stores themselves within endurance-trained muscle are also increased. Hormones such as norepinephrine and glucogon are released during exercise, which stimulates lipolysis. Endurance athletes are able to exercise at a higher level of submaximal exercise due to this adaptive response. Despite this training adaptation, near-maximal sustained effort requires the presence of adequate muscle glycogen or circulating blood glucose. Higher-fat diets typically do not increase performance in endurance events for this reason (2,9).

Protein

Although the recommended daily allowance of protein for the general population is 0.8 g/kg/day, the average American diet provides far more than this (1.4 g/kg/day) (1). A popular belief among athletes, especially those involved in static exercise such as weight training, is that a large amount of protein needs to be consumed to counteract the muscle "breakdown" resulting from training. In fact, a large market of dietary supplements has been developed on this basis. However, whereas the recommended daily allowance for athletes is, in fact, higher than for nonathletes (between 0.9 and 1.9 g/kg/day), the increased requirement is relatively minimal. Studies based on strict nitrogen balance suggest that 1.2 g/kg/day is adequate for endurance athletes, for instance, whereas those athletes involved in resistance training, such as weightlifters and bodybuilders, may require up to 1.7 g/kg/day of protein (2). Physicians should make athletes aware that increasing protein intake beyond these levels does not result in additional increase in lean tissue, because there is a limit to the rate at which protein tissue can be accrued.

Protein itself may be used as an energy source. When carbohydrate stores are depleted, muscle protein may supply 5%–10% of the fuel used for energy. Therefore, physicians should advise those individuals who desire additional muscle mass that a well-balanced diet should be maintained;

otherwise, protein may be used as an energy source during training, negating the effects of increased protein intake (2,3).

Amino acid supplementation is unnecessary for many of the reasons just discussed. Advocates of these supplements believe that they may increase endurance and strength by allowing the body to more easily absorb the building blocks of protein. This is not the case; the intestine absorbs amino acids just as well when they exist in a more complex form as when they are ingested as a supplement (3). In fact, a concentrated amino acid solution may draw water out of the intestinal wall and into its lumen, which may precipitate cramping and diarrhea. Others have advocated that the ingestion of simple amino acids may enhance endurance by serving as substrate for energy and by delaying central nervous system fatigue. No study has demonstrated that this is the case. The bottom line is that amino acid supplementation has not been shown to increase muscle mass, endurance, or strength (2,3).

Vitamins and Minerals

Micronutrients play an important role in many metabolic pathways, such as protein and bone synthesis, hemoglobin synthesis, and immune function. Exercise may place a stress on these systems and therefore increase the demand for these micronutrients. This demand is generally small, and vitamin and mineral supplementation is typically not needed in well-nourished athletes. Athletes at risk for these nutrient deficiencies are those who restrict caloric intake in an effort to alter body habitus or compete at a certain weight. Additionally, those athletes who engage in "fad" diets may be at risk of micronutrient deficiencies (2,10).

Vitamin B
B-complex vitamins have several functions related to exercise. Thiamin, riboflavin, vitamin B_6, niacin, pantothenic acid, and biotin play a role as coenzymes in the catabolism of carbohydrate, protein, and fat (2,3). Additionally, vitamin B_{12} and folate are involved in the synthesis of hemoglobin and protein. Some data suggest that regular exercise may slightly increase the need for these nutrients, but these needs can generally be met with the increased dietary volume seen in most athletes. No studies suggest that supplemental B-complex vitamins improve athletic performance (3).

Vitamins A, E, and C
The antioxidant vitamins A, E, and C play a role in protecting cells from oxidative damage. Exercise has been shown to increase the production of free radicals, which, in theory, could lead to severe cell damage due to oxidation. However, studies have demonstrated that the body's antioxidant defenses remain adequate during periods of exercise and, in fact, may even be up-regulated in the setting of routine aerobic exercise (2,3). No studies

have demonstrated any performance enhancement by supplemental antioxidant vitamins in athletes who have a well-balanced diet (3).

Vitamin D

Vitamin D plays a role in calcium homeostasis. The main sources of vitamin D are fortified foods and the intrinsic production of the vitamin itself through exposure to ultraviolet light. Athletes at risk for vitamin D deficiencies are those who restrict dietary intake of fortified foods such as milk and those who lack exposure to UV radiation (for example, figure skaters). These athletes may benefit from vitamin D supplementation, not as a performance enhancer, but for overall health reasons.

Calcium

Calcium is important for maintaining bone mineral density and blood calcium levels. Studies have shown that female athletes, in particular, are at risk for inadequate calcium intake (10). This is generally seen in sports where body habitus may be viewed as important (for example, figure skating and gymnastics). Because maximum bone density is not achieved until the age of 30 to 35, calcium supplementation should be considered for at-risk athletes to assure that adequate bone mineral density is attained and maintained. The Nation Institutes of Health recommend that female athletes ingest between 1,000–1,500 mg of calcium per day, depending on menstrual status. Amenorrheic females should have more calcium in their diet than those who are not (1).

Iron

Iron deficiency is the most common type of nutrient deficiency seen in athletes (3). In theory, exercise may increase the demand for iron. Iron may be lost from sweat or from the loss of hemoglobin in urine as a result of intravascular hemolysis. Occult GI bleeding, sometimes seen in long-distance runners, may also cause iron loss. Additionally, improper diets that generally avoid meat, fish, and poultry greatly contribute to iron deficiencies. Vegetarian diets also place athletes at risk for iron deficiency because these diets have poor iron bioavailability. Early iron depletion generally does not effect athletic performance; however, if the condition is left untreated and progresses to iron deficiency anemia, performance will decrease dramatically. Many athletes exhibit transient decreases in hemoglobin and hematocrit during the early stages of training (3). These changes generally are the result of increases in plasma volume and therefore represent a "dilutional" anemia. As training progresses, typically hemoglobin and hematocrit will return to baseline.

Measuring serum ferritin concentrations is the best way to accurately measure iron stores. In mild iron deficiency, serum iron levels may be normal but the deficiency is evident by the low serum ferritin. Studies have shown that in competitive skaters, serum ferritin concentrations may be reduced by one half (10). Decreases in circulating iron, as measured by serum iron concentration, typically signal significant iron deficiency. These deficiencies may take months to correct, and it is therefore better to begin nutritional intervention before actual deficiencies develop. Such interventions include, for example, education of at-risk athletes, such as those involved in endurance sports and in sports like gymnastics where "body image" may be an issue.

Overall, the frequency of iron deficiency in female athletes is no different than in the general female population (2). It is on this basis that iron supplements generally are not recommended for all athletes. Even with mild iron deficiency, supplementation may not improve performance (2). Additionally, the indiscriminate use of iron supplementation may cause iron levels to increase to toxic levels; this is especially true for the 1.5 million Americans who are genetically predisposed to hemochromatosis.

Zinc

Zinc is another trace mineral needed for energy production. Regular exercise may increase the need for dietary zinc. Some studies have shown a significant loss of zinc in the urine after exercise. Some zinc also is lost in sweat (2). Athletes who avoid animal products may not have sufficient zinc in their diets, so these individuals should be counseled on the importance of alternative sources of zinc, such as whole grains or wheat germ (2,3).

Selenium

Selenium is a trace mineral that works in concert with the antioxidant vitamins. It is thought that selenium works with these antioxidants to protect the cell membrane from damage by circulating free radicals. Most athletes ingest an adequate amount of selenium in their diet. "Megasupplementation" with amounts in excess of 1000 mg/day have been associated with toxicity, which manifests itself as gastrointestinal dysfunction and hair loss (2).

Supplements

Selling vitamin and mineral supplements to not only athletes but to the general public is a multibillion dollar industry (2). As mentioned previously, there is simply no scientific evidence that vitamin and mineral supplementation boost athletic performance in well-nourished athletes. While some athletes may take the stance that vitamin supplementation "can't hurt," those who take "megavitamins" that have up to 1000 times the RDA may actually be setting the stage for vitamin or mineral toxicity. Table 2-5 shows the various manifestations of vitamin toxicity.

It is extremely important for the clinician to ask questions about vitamin and mineral supplementation, because most athletes will not volunteer this information. This will generally open the door to discussion on proper

Table 2-5   Manifestations of Vitamin Toxicity

Vitamin	Signs and Symptoms of Toxicity
A	Headache, vomiting, swelling of the long bones
D	Vomiting and diarrhea
K	Jaundice
Niacin	Flushing
C	Possibility of kidney stones

nutrition and allow the clinician to counsel the athlete on the right foods for peak performance.

REFERENCES

1. **Sallis RE.** Essentials of Sports Medicine. Philadelphia: Mosby-Yearbook; 1996.
2. Position of the American Dietetic Association, Dietitians of Canada, and the American College of Sports Medicine. Nutrition and athletic performance. J Am Diet Assoc. 2000;100(12);1543-53.
3. **McArdle WD, Katch FI, Katch VL.** Sports and Exercise Nutrition. Philadelphia: Lippincott Williams & Wilkins; 1999.
4. **Rehrer N.** Fluid and electrolyte balance in ultra-endurance sport. Sports Med. 2001;31(10):701-15.
5. **Sparling P, Millare-Stafford M.** Keeping sports participants safe in hot weather. Phys Sportsmed. 1999;27(7):27.
6. **Burke L, Hawley J, Scharabort E, et al.** Carbohydrate loading failed to improve 100-km cycling performance in a placebo-controlled trial. J Appl Physiol. 2000; 88:1284-90.
7. **Mellion MB, Walsh WM, Madden C, et al., eds.** Team Physician's Handbook, 3rd ed. Philadelphia: Lippincott Williams & Wilkins; 2001.
8. **Ivy JL, Goforth HW Jr, Damon BM, et al.** Early postexercise muscle glycogen recovery is enhanced with carbohydrate-protein supplements. J Appl Physiol. 2002; 93(4):1337-44.
9. **Burke L, Angus D, Cox G, et al.** Effect of fat adaptation and carbohydrate restoration on metabolism and performance during prolonger cycling. J Appl Physiol. 2000;89:2413-21.
10. **Ziegler P, Sharp R, Hughes V, et al.** Nutritional status of teenage female competitive figure skaters. J Am Diet Assoc. 2002;102(3):374-9.

3

■ ■ ■

Mass-Participation Events

David S. Ross, MD

Today, many communities hold mass-participation events. Mass-participation events are defined as athletic events with numerous participants at one period of time (for example, marathons, one-half marathons, and other long-distance running events; bicycle rallies and races; Nordic events; multisport events such as triathlons; "iron-man" triathlons; and walking rallies). The injuries sustained during such events are similar to those one may encounter in other sporting events; however, some types of injuries may be a result of the large number of participants (for example, crowding increases frequency of collisions, falls, and so forth) or course obstacles/adverse road conditions such as spectators, cars, and potholes. Common injuries in mass-participation events are listed in Table 3-1. In addition, the potential number of casualties presenting to the medical tent at one given time is dramatically increased. With few economic resources to provide extensive and adequate medical support, communities that support these events ordinarily recruit medical personnel who will volunteer their time to make the event as injury-free as possible. Community physicians take on this responsibility because of a true interest in a particular sport and/or enjoyment of the action associated with the event. Of all these, it is the well-educated primary care physician who is best suited to serve as a health care provider for mass-participation events, because most event-related problems are medical-related issues.

There are few research-based data on medical coverage of such events. Most of the information in this chapter is therefore based on anecdotal experience from those who have provided coverage for marathons, bicycle rallies, triathlons, and extreme sports. This chapter discusses medical coverage planning and the personnel necessary to provide adequate coverage and reviews the most common types of injuries and illnesses encountered in mass-participation events.

Table 3-1   Common Injuries in Mass-Participation Events

Event Type	Injuries
Running	Blisters, shin splints, muscle strains, ligamentous sprains, dehydration, heat- or cold-related illness,[*] hypothermia,[†] overuse injuries
Bicycling	Trauma—road rash; contusions; lacerations; fractured clavicle, wrist, radius/ulna; AC joint sprain (separated shoulder); muscle strains; cold- or heat-related illness; hypothermia
Nordic events	Cold-related illness, dehydration, muscle strains, blisters
Triathlon	Similar to running and bicycling; hyponatremia; specific swimming injuries[‡]

[*] Risk of heat- or cold-related illness depends on the weather. Heat-related illness includes muscle cramps, heat exhaustion, and heat stroke. Cold-related illness includes frostbite and hypothermia.
[†] Typically occurs in hot-weather events but can be seen in cold-weather events.
[‡] Examples include corneal abrasions due to goggles dislodging after being inadvertently kicked, contusions, and hypothermia depending on water temperature and time spent in water.

Overview

The management of most injuries sustained during mass-participation events will not differ from those at any other sporting events; however, it requires a great deal of coordination among health care providers because of increased numbers of patients in a given time. Advance planning is the key to providing adequate medical coverage for any mass-participation event. Usually, 6 to 12 months are needed to implement proper medical support. One physician should be designated to serve as the medical director and oversee medical operations. He or she should develop a strategy for the implementation of coverage for the event, determining the number of health care providers necessary for the event, recruiting health care providers, developing knowledge of the event rules and how they pertain to the medical team, reviewing the course layout, and coordinating services with the local fire department, police department, EMS, and hospitals. The medical director must work with the event director to acquire services and supplies for the event. In addition, he or she will need to inquire about event liability insurance that specifically will cover health care providers; one cannot rely on the "Good Samaritan" law as adequate protection. For example, if a physician volunteers his or her time to an event and wears a shirt with a practice logo or hands out business cards, this can be construed as a vehicle for promoting his or her practice and would likely negate the provision of the "Good Samaritan" law. Health care personnel may want to check with their institution or private liability insurance providers to see if coverage provisions are made for such events.

To prepare for the event, the medical director should create a checklist including the type of event, the rules for the event, course layout, expected number of participants, resources, communications, protocols, and a timeline. In addition, a review of the weather forecast for the day of the event is important; weather is a major factor that determines the number of participants who will seek medical care (1).

Key Elements in Preparing Medical Coverage

Type of Event and Number of Participants

The type of event and an accurate estimate of the total number of participants will help the medical director plan the necessary number of health care providers and the number, size, and proper spacing of medical aid tents. Table 3-2 illustrates injury rates based on event. Also consider the age range, gender, athletic ability (recreational, amateur, professional, and so forth) of the participants, as this information will help to determine the potential prevalence of injury. The medical director may need to include coaches, officials, spectators, and support staff in the total number of participants if it is expected that these groups will be under the care of the health care team; this should be clarified with the event director in advance.

Rules Governing an Event

The medical director must be well-versed in the rules that govern an event and be able to educate other health care providers about these rules. For example, some competitive events may not allow medical intervention while the event is taking place. In recreational events, there are no strict rules. Health care providers should intervene if there is concern about the health of any participant.

The medical director also should review the rules governing course modification with the event director. If it is a sanctioned event, determine who can alter or cancel an event. Extreme weather or an unforeseen event could lead to alteration or cancellation.

Table 3-2   Injury Rates for Different Types of Endurance Events

Endurance Event	Distance	Injury Rate
Running	41 km (marathon)	1%-20%
Running	21 km	1%-5%
Triathlon	225 km ("iron man")	15%-30%
Triathlon	51 km	2%-5%
Cycling	Variable	5%
Nordic skiing	55 km	5%

Adapted with permission from Jones BH, Roberts W. Medical management of endurance events. In: Cantu RC, Micheli LJ, eds. ACSM Guidelines for the Team Physician. Philadelphia: Lea & Febiger; 1991: 266-86.

Course Layout and Starting Conditions

The medical director should review the course map with the (nonmedical) event director. In addition, he or she should physically review the course, noting any areas that may pose a danger to participants. Look for immovable objects, traffic patterns, and water from sprinkler systems, for example, that may endanger athletes. Select areas to place medical aid tents, rest stops, and security. If necessary, decide where to station volunteers to notify participants of hazardous areas.

The medical director should work with the event director to discuss starting conditions. A wide start area without declines is preferred. Also, consider a wave or sequential start, depending on the number of participants. These methods will decrease the number of start-related traumatic injuries.

Resources

Far in advance of the event, the medical director must determine if specific funds have been budgeted for medical support. He or she will need to lobby for medical volunteers, supplies, shelter, and EMS support. If funds are not available for all or some of these items, the medical director will need to work closely with the event director to acquire specified items or services. Resources include local hospitals for medical supplies and volunteers; a ham radio club for communications; police department, fire department, and National Guard for support services; and local companies/corporations to donate items such as ice, water, sport drinks, tents, and food. See Table 3-3 for suggested medical supplies. For details on the planning of proper medical aid stations, see the discussion later in this chapter.

Table 3-3   Suggested Medical Supplies for Mass-Participation Events

• Defibrillator	• Sunscreen	• Coolers with ice
• IV start kits	• Basins	• Nonsterile gloves
• Bottled soap	• Towels	• Tape
• CPR disposable mask	• 4 × 4 gauze	• Sharps containers
• Band-Aids	• Trash bags	• Biohazard disposal bags
• Cellular telephone	• Alcohol preps	• Clipboards
• Rectal thermometer	• Incident reports	• Immersion bath
• Pens	• Bleach solution/spray	• Antibiotic ointment
• Bed sheets	• Cots	• Cold or warm beverages
• Dryer	• Acetaminophen	• Ibuprofen
• Code kit	• Blankets	• Stethoscope
• Laundry bag	• BP cuff	• Cooling fans and/or A/C
• Normal saline and D$_5$NS solution		

Communications

The medical director may consider contacting a local ham radio club to assist with an event. These clubs usually have members who are more than willing to volunteer their time. Each medical aid station can be assigned a radio operator, with the main medical tent serving as the communication base. Additional radio operators may be posted along the course to serve as spotters. The medical director should work with a communications leader to devise a communications protocol for the event. The communications leader can then review protocol with other ham club members, assign an operator to each medical aid station, and work with local fire and police departments to coordinate communications when assistance is needed. Utilize cellular telephones as a secondary or back-up communication system.

Protocols

The medical director should write and distribute to the health care team a set of standard protocols based on current data used by similar endurance events. Such protocols also serve as way to standardize health care administered to participants. Typical protocols for endurance events include exercise-associated collapse, cardiac arrest, chest pain, reactive airway disease, head and neck injuries, road rash, heat-related illness, and hypothermia. See Figure 3-1 for an example of a typical protocol.

Weather

Weather conditions are usually a big factor in what types of injuries are seen in the medical tent. The American College of Sports Medicine recommends the use of an environmental stress scale for heat and cold injury risk in mass-participation events (Table 3-4). Summer events should be scheduled in the early morning or evening to minimize solar radiation and air temperature. Winter events should be scheduled at midday to minimize the risk of cold injury. Measure the heat stress index at the event site. Wet bulb globe temperature (WBGT) is commonly used to gauge environmental heat stress by conveying information about humidity (wet bulb temperature), solar radiation (globe temperature), and dry bulb (air) temperature. Portable electronic devices that measure the WBGT are available through commercial vendors. In addition, one needs to account for the wind chill index during winter events (2-4).

Dehydration is common during prolonged endurance events in both cold and hot weather conditions because the average participant loses 0.47-1.42 liters of sweat per hour and fluid replacement is usually insufficient (1-3).

The four most common heat- and cold-related illnesses occurring during distance endurance events are heat exhaustion, heat stroke, hypothermia, and frostbite (2). Chapter 4 gives more information on environmental injuries.

TITLE: Head and Neck Trauma Guidelines

PURPOSE: To outline responsibilities of Medical Personnel in the management of head and neck trauma.

PRIORITIES
1. Ensure patient survivial.
2. Preserve spinal cord function.
3. Provide the best possible opportunity for an injured cord to recover.

ASSESSMENT
1. First, do no harm!
2. Do not move the patient except from immediate danger or for basic trauma management.
3. Always assume the patient has an unstable neck injury if he or she is unconscious, has numbness and paralysis, has neck pain, or experiences neck pain with movement.
4. Assess consciousness and implement ABCDE's:
   - A: Airway
   - B: Breathing
   - C: Circulation
   - D: Disability
   - E: Exposure
5. The jaw thrust technique is the preferred method for opening the airway in patients with suspected neck injury.
6. If the patient is unconscious or has altered consciousness, immobilize the neck and transport the patient to an emergency facility.
7. If patient is alert and oriented, are *any* (one or more) of the signs/symptoms below present? If so, immobilize the neck and transport the patient to an emergency facility.
   a. Any numbness, tingling, or paralysis?
   b. Any neck pain?
   c. Any pain with active range of motion?
   d. Any apprehension?
   e. Is there pain with palpatation of the C-spine?
8. If the patient does not have symptoms suggestive of neck trauma but has suffered a concussion (see description of signs/symptoms below), do not allow him or her to resume riding. Refer the patient to an appropriate medical facility.

Concussion Signs and Symptoms
   a. Headache
   b. Loss of consciousness
   c. Confusion (amnesia), even if it resolves in a short period of time
   d. Nausea/vomiting
   e. Blurred vision

EDUCATION
1. All participants are required to wear an ANSI/SNELL-certified helmet.
2. Encourage participants to follow all traffic laws/regulations.

Figure 3-1. Protocol example for biking event.

Table 3-4   Wet Bulb Globe Temperature (WBGT) Heat Safety Cascade and Risk of Thermal Stress

Risk of Thermal Stress	WBGT	Notes
Very high	28°C	Cancel, postpone, or modify the event
High	23-28°C	Advise participants of risk
Moderate	18-23°C	
Low	Below 18°C	Watch for hypothermia and hyperthermia; risk exists for both
Lower	Below 10°C	Watch for hypothermia
Increased risk of hypothermia and frostbite	Ambient $T < 0°C$	Consider wind-chill
Severe	Ambient $T < -4°C$	Cancel the event

Data adapted from American College of Sports Medicine. Position stand: Heat and cold illness during distance running. Med Sci Sports Exerc. 1996;28:i-vii.

Participant Education

The medical director should facilitate participant education about the potential medical risks of competing in an event. Participants need to be aware that certain medical conditions such as obesity, dehydration, lack of heat acclimatization, previous history of heat stroke, sleep deprivation, certain medications, sweat gland dysfunction, sunburn, or history of recent illness may exacerbate heat illness. Children sweat less than adults and have a lower heat tolerance; therefore, they may be at risk for heat-related illness.

Heat acclimatization can reduce the risk of heat illness. It is suggested that athletes train in a similar type of environment 10-14 days before the event (1-3). Participants need to be educated on the proper amount and type of fluids they should consume before, during, and after an event. In addition, they need to be advised of the early symptoms of heat- or cold-related illness. It is suggested that the novice participant exercise with a partner.

Provide education before an event through clinics or seminars, by publicizing the event in the media, and by distributing materials in the preregistration packet. Encourage participants (and potential participants) to visit an educational Web site before the event and make educational materials available on event day.

Implementing Event Coverage

On the day of the event, it is estimated that 2%-12% of all entrants will enter the medical aid station, depending on weather conditions (2).

Just before the start of the event, the medical director should make an announcement through the public address system about

1. Weather conditions
2. Type of clothing participants should wear
3. Potential obstacles and hazardous areas along the course
4. Appropriate fluid intake
5. Proper pacing
6. Location of aid stations
7. Other relevant information

Medical Personnel

The American College of Sports Medicine (ACSM) recommends the following medical personnel per 1,000 runners for endurance running events. In general, these recommendations can be used to estimate the number of health care providers needed for other endurance type events, such as bicycle rallies, triathlons, and Nordic events.

- One to two physicians
- Four to six podiatrists
- One to four emergency medical technicians
- Two to four nurses
- Three to six physical therapists
- Three to six athletic trainers
- One to three assistants

The majority of personnel should be based at the finish area. Other volunteers should be on hand to assist with medical records, replenishing of medical supplies, food and beverage service for the medical volunteers, and other needs. Volunteers may serve as security for the main medical command center, but also consider having local police stationed there. It is a nuisance having unauthorized personnel in the main medical area.

Place the main medical command within close proximity of the finish area. The center should be at least 23-139 m^2 for each 1,000 participants (2). Most participants who seek medical care will be evaluated in the finish area (1,2).

Medical Aid Stations

All medical aid stations should provide protection from the elements. See Table 3-5 for medical aid station placement intervals. The size of each station depends on its location; for example, some stations may be used more than once for "out and back" courses. Each station should be well-marked and participants should be advised of location in preliminary educational materials, as well as just before the start of the race. Typically, medical aid stations and rest stations will be combined, offering fluid,

Table 3-5   Placement of Medical Aid Stations

Event Type	Distance Separation Early	Distance Separation Late
Running	3 km (1.8 miles)	2 km (1.2 miles)
Bicycling	25 km (15 miles)	15 km (9 miles)

food, rest, and medical services for participants. While this seems logical and the efficient use of space and personnel, combining the two can pose problems. At times, a combination tent presents too much clutter to provide adequate medical care for those in need. In addition, we find many participants will suspect they need medical assistance just after a fluid station. We recommend that aid stations be placed a few hundred yards beyond the fluid station. Never integrate the main medical area at the finish line with other activities.

Evaluation and Treatment

Documentation of all those who are evaluated in aid stations is essential. Several mass-participation events use a standard event form to document these encounters. It is suggested that at least one ambulance per 3,000 participants be posted at the finish area and that one or more mobile emergency response vehicles be located on the course (2).

Rapid assessment should include vital signs, cardiovascular status, and central nervous system function. Temperature should be taken with a rectal thermometer; therefore, a barrier to allow privacy should be available to medical personnel. Do not rely on oral, tympanic, and auxiliary temperature, as they do not represent the true body core temperature (1,2).

Provide means of treating heat-related illnesses. For events held in extremely warm environments, the medical director should consider having immersion baths available, as these have been proven to dramatically reduce body core temperature (2,5). In addition, ice trashcans filled with towels should be placed in all medical aid tents. Some disadvantages of immersion are that hypothermic vasoconstriction ultimately slows heat loss, and immersion limits electrocardiogram (ECG) monitoring and access if resuscitation is required. (Please refer to Chapter 4 for more on the advantages and disadvantages of various cooling methods.)

Establish intravenous fluid protocols. Intravenous fluids should only be used on for those who cannot be adequately hydrated and cooled with oral fluids. Determine exercise-associated collapse (EAC) versus collapse secondary to heat related illness before administering IV fluids. Hyponatremia is a prevalent disorder in ultra-endurance events and must be considered in the differential diagnosis. Both EAC and hyponatremia are discussed in detail later in this chapter.

Table 3-6   Fluid Amount Required Per Participant

Location	Fluid Amount
Start/finish	0.34-0.45 L (12-16 oz)
Aid stations along course	0.28-0.34 L (10-12 oz)

Hot-weather mass-participation events: A selection of cool water and carbohydrate-elecrolyte beverages should be made available.
Cool-weather mass-participation events: A selection of warm water and carbohydrate-elecrolyte beverages should be made available.

The medical director should estimate the amount of fluid needed for each participant (Table 3-6). Cool fluid should be supplied for warm-weather events, and warm fluid should be supplied for cold-weather events. Serve both water and a carbohydrate-electrolyte beverage. Disposable paper cups are the most efficient and hygienic way to serve these fluids (2,6).

Communications

The main communication base should be located at the main medical tent at the finish area. This base should have direct communication with all aid stations, spotters along the course, mobile vehicles, police/fire/EMS personnel, and event directors. Spotters should notify health care officials of any participant who may need medical assistance, as well as look for potential unexpected risks to participants (unofficial vehicles on the course, water on the course, weather change, and so on). A backup communication system should always be available. The medical communication should be separate from communications for event logistics.

Post-Event Meeting

Following the event, the medical director should meet with his or her medical team to analyze data on the number of participants evaluated by the medical team, the type of injuries, and the problems encountered. This information should be discussed with the event director and used to help implement care for future events.

Treatment of Specific Event-Related Illnesses

Hyponatremia

Hyponatremia is the most common disorder of ultra-endurance events and has been noted in both warm and cold weather events (7). Hyponatremia is defined as a serum Na^+ < 135 mmol/L. Two theories have been proposed as to the cause of exercise-associated hyponatremia. According to the first theory, the cause is large water and salt losses in the sweat during prolonged exercise; however, studies to substantiate this theory are lacking. The second theory notes that the cause may be related to over-hydration of an athlete with replacement drinks with low or no sodium. There are studies to substantiate this theory. An increased incidence has been noted in females with slow finishing times; however, these studies are based on estimates of fluid consumption during the event and do not account for confounding factors such as medications, congenital disorders, and so on.

Possible signs and symptoms of hyponatremia include lightheadedness, nausea, vomiting, malaise, exhaustion, changes in mental status, headache, and seizure, all of which can lead to death. Studies have shown an increased prevalence in ultra-endurance-type events; however, the cause is debated. The severity of hyponatremia will dictate treatment. Those with asymptomatic hyponatremia should not be treated. Because most symptomatic hyponatremia is associated with fluid overload, appropriate management includes close observation and monitoring of serum sodium while awaiting spontaneous diuresis of retained fluid (6). Intravenous fluid should not be routinely given, because these athletes are already overloaded with fluid.

Some athletes may have hyponatremia associated with dehydration. Judicious use of intravenous fluid might be considered; however, the GI tract is the preferred route if the athlete is able to tolerate oral hydration (7). Pre- and post-race body weights of athletes may help in the assessment of fluid overload or dehydration. If an athlete has signs and symptoms suggestive of significant cerebral or pulmonary edema or is unstable, they should be transferred to a health care facility. The use of hypertonic saline in the treatment of exercise-induced hyponatremia has not been studied, but it is the usual treatment in those with significant symptoms such as seizures, coma, and mental confusion. One may consider furosemide in those who are fluid-overloaded.

Prevention is the key to reducing the incidence of hyponatremia in ultra-endurance events. Athletes should be educated about this potential problem and review guidelines for these types of events. The United States Track and Field Association has found this new data concerning regardless of the debate over the cause, and has revised their fluid replacement guidelines for athletic events. The suggested fluid intake is no more than 400-800 ml per hour (6). Compare this with the American College of Sports Medicine guidelines, which recommend 600-1,200 ml per hour (8). Although the role of salt supplementation is unclear, limited studies do show a benefit to replacing sweat losses with a sport drink containing sodium versus plain water (7).

Case Study 3-1

After completing a marathon, a 34-year-old white female presented to the main medical tent with nausea, disorientation, and significant fatigue. She required assistance to get to the medical tent. Her running partner stated that she had no significant past medical history and took no regular medications. Both runners visited every rest stop, drinking water or a sport beverage. They completed the marathon in about 5 hours. Assessment showed the patient to be in mild distress with a heart rate of 95, blood pressure of 100/50, respiratory rate of 18, and temperature of 39°C. Her skin was moist, and no signs of trauma were apparent.

This likely represents hyponatremia, though one would want to consider heat-related illness, exercise-associated collapse (EAC), or another medical condition. The findings suggestive of hyponatremia are 1) female, 2) nausea, 3) disorientation, 4) frequent intake of fluid during the event, 5) long finish time to complete event, and 6) relatively unremarkable vital signs with temperature less than 40°C. Heat-related illness is not likely. Patients with EAC usually will complete the event and collapse at the finish area. They will have resolution of symptoms within a few minutes after they have been placed in the supine position with legs elevated above the heart. Patients who suffer heat exhaustion usually are not disoriented, and their temperature is greater than 40°C. Those with heat stroke typically have disorientation, dry skin, and a temperature less than 40°C. The past medical history does not suggest other medical problems as the cause of these symptoms. If available, a serum sodium measurement would help in the diagnosis.

The patient should be transferred to the nearest medical facility for further evaluation. Consider the use of furosemide, especially in cases of fluid overload. Treatment with hypertonic saline solution should be considered with significant symptoms such as seizures or mental confusion, such as in this case.

Exercise-Associated Collapse

Exercise-associated collapse is one of the most common clinical syndromes seen in marathon and triathlon events. The syndrome consists of an inability to stand or walk unaided as a result of lightheadedness, faintness, dizziness, or syncope excluding musculoskeletal etiologies (5). A diagnosis of exclusion, rapidly rule out other potential life threatening disorders such as heat stroke, cardiac arrest, and significant hyponatremia. Typically, those with heat stress are hypotensive and tachycardic, and those with EAC will have a normal return of heart rate and blood pressure when placed in the supine position. Lethargy may be seen for a period of time because of the prolonged recovery from an exhaustive effort at the end of the event. Refer to Table 3-7 for differential diagnosis associated with collapse of a mass-event participant.

The pathophysiology of this disorder has been hypothesized as the pooling of blood in the lower extremity during the abrupt cessation of exercise resulting in a brief decrease in perfusion to the brain and other critical

Table 3-7   **Exercise-Associated Collapse Differential Diagnosis**

• Exercise-associated collapse	• Hyponatremia	• Muscle cramps
• Cardiac arrest	• Heat stroke	• Hypoglycemia
• Hypothermia	• Orthopedic conditions	• Other

organs. During activity, blood flow is directed to the skin and away from critical organs in attempt to lower the core body temperature; this is a confounding factor that amplifies the syndrome related to EAC at the abrupt cessation of exercise. The mechanism of collapse is thought to be multifactorial, not simply a result of dehydration (5,9).

Initial evaluation should include basic life support assessment. Seizures can be seen in an array of disorders, including EAC. One of the most important historical elements is the location of the athlete's collapse. Those who collapse during the event likely have a significant, life-threatening condition. Other important historical items should include use of drugs, supplements, and over-the-counter medications, as well as family history of sudden death or coronary artery disease at a young age. Physical exam should include vitals with a rectal temperature; *oral, tympanic, and axillary temperatures are not reliable and should not be used.* If possible, obtain orthostatic blood pressure and pulse. One can assess hydration status by observing dry mouth, sweat status, and skin tugor. Electrolytes (serum sodium), blood sugar measurement, and cardiac monitoring are helpful if available (5). As noted earlier, one must rule out other potential causes of a collapsed athlete such as cardiac arrest, heat-related illness, hyponatremia, hypothermia, and hypoglycemia. Intravenous fluid therapy usually is not necessary in the treatment of EAC. Typical treatment is oral hydration and elevation of the lower extremity. Expect resolution of symptoms within 15 to 30 minutes. Intravenous fluid therapy may be useful in those patients who are unconscious, suffer heat related illness, have persistent emesis, or exhibit prolonged hypotension and tachycardia (4,5).

Case Study 3-2

A 40-year-old male collapsed at the finish line of a marathon during a hot summer day. Observers noted the patient to be unresponsive for about a minute. His running partner stated that the patient had no past medical history, but that he did take over-the-counter nonsteroidal anti-inflammatory medication as needed. The partner reported that both drank an appropriate amount of fluid during the event. They had been training sporadically over the last few months for the marathon. Assessment of the patient showed that he was alert and oriented, with a pulse of 100, blood pressure of 90/40, respiratory rate of 20, and a temperature of 39°C. He denied pain in his neck or head or any other trauma. In addition, he denied use of supplements or drugs. He noted a sensation of fatigue and "grogginess" but denied any other symptoms. His skin was moist, and a white hue was seen. No other physical findings were appreciated, including evaluation of the C-spine.

This case likely represents EAC; however, one would need to consider heat-related illness, hyponatremia, arrhythmia, or another medical condition. Findings that support EAC include 1) collapse after completing the event, 2) quick resolution of symptoms, 3) a temperature less than 40°C, and 4) no significant past medicial history. Heat-related illness is not as likely because the temperature is under 40°C. An arrhythmia or other medical problems are not likely based on the brief history and physical exam.

The patient should be transported to the main medical tent and placed in a supine position with the feet elevated above the heart. He should be monitored and observed until complete resolution of symptoms.

Race Day Triage

The medical team should devise and implement an effective triage system on the event day. Consider a protocol that distinguishes serious and nonserious orthopedic and primary medical patient issues. The medical aid station can be set to handle these certain circumstances. A lead nurse and/or physician can triage patients to the appropriate areas. Any athlete with a temperature greater than 41°C should be assumed to be suffering from heatstroke. If the temperature is less than 41°C and the patient has stable vital signs and no obvious medical conditions to explain a change in mental state, then strongly consider hyponatremia as the diagnosis (2,3,5). If possible, measurement of serum sodium and the observation of weight change will help guide the medical team in the appropriate diagnosis and the use of intravenous fluid.

Conclusion

Mass-participation events provide a unique and complex experience for health care providers. Careful and advance planning is essential in providing appropriate care for these types of events. The event organizers should assign a medical director to oversee the implementation and operation of the health care team for the event. It takes a tremendous team effort to coordinate health care for mass-participation events. The medical director and health care team should be knowledgeable in the rules governing the event and the type injuries they may expect.

Appropriate systems and protocols need to be in place to ensure the best medical care possible. The health care team should be prepared to handle the most common ailments associated with mass-participation events. A post-event meeting should be held to review race day operations, the number of participants evaluated by the health care team, and the outcomes of those participants in hopes of improving the delivery of health care for future events.

RESOURCES

- **American College of Sports Medicine** www.acsm.org/
- **Hotter'n Hell One Hundred Bicycle Rally** www.hh100.org/
- **Chicago Marathon** www.chicagomarathon.com/
- **Twin Cities Marathon** www.twincitiesmarathon.org/
- **New York Marathon** www.ingnycmarathon.org/
- **Boston Marathon** www.bostonmarathon.org/
- **Mora Vasaloppet Nordic Ski Race** www.vasaloppet.org/
- **American Birkebeiner Ski Race** www.blnkic.com/

REFERENCES

1. **Robertson JW.** Medical problems in mass participation runs: recommendations. Sports Med. 1988;6:261-70.
2. **American College of Sports Medicine.** Position Stand: Heat and cold illness during distance running. Med Sci Sports Exerc. 1996;28(12):i-vii.
3. **Cheuvront SN, Haymes EM.** Thermoregulation and marathon running: biological and environmental influences. Sport Med. 2001;31(10):743-62.
4. **Roberts WO.** A 12-yr profile of medical injury and illness for the Twin Cities Marathon. Med Sci Sports Exerc. 2000;32(9):1549-55.
5. **O'Connor FG, Pyne S, Brennan FH Jr, Adirim T.** Exercise-associated collapse: an algorithmic approach to race day management. AJSM. 2001;5(3):212-29.
6. **Noakes T.** IMMDA Advisory statement on guidelines for fluid replacement during marathon running. New Studies in Athletics. IAAF Tech Q. 2002;17(1):15-24.
7. **Speedy DB, Noakes TD, Scheneider C.** Exercise-associated hyponatremia: a review. Emerg Med. 2001;13(1):17-27.
8. **American College of Sports Medicine.** Position Stand: Exercise and fluid replacement. Med Sci Sports Exerc. 1996;28(1):i-vii.
9. **Lebrun C.** Mass Participation Events. American College of Sports Medicine Advanced Team Physician Course. Lake Buena Vista, FL; 2000.

4

■ ■ ■

Environmental Influences on Sports Participation

Kimberly M. Fagan, MD

Although sports participation and athletic performance are directly affected by genetics and training, environmental issues play a secondary role. The effect of heat, cold, and altitude can be detrimental to the performance and overall health of the athlete and, in some cases, may even result in severe illness, injury, or death. Lightning, of course, is an "environmental factor" that invariably results in injury and sometimes in death. Fortunately, with awareness and appropriate immediate response, the vast majority of environmentally related deaths can be avoided.

Heat-Related Illnesses

Prevalence

Heat-related deaths are listed as the third most common cause of death in high school athletes (1). Some of the sports more commonly associated with heat-related illness are football, endurance running, and cycling. Most sports physicians feel that heat-related deaths are grossly underreported. That such deaths occur at all is a travesty because, if detected in time, they are 100% preventable.

Pathophysiology

Thermal regulation is a matter of balancing heat production with heat dissipation. Average energy production at rest is 70 W (1 kcal) per minute. With exercise, this can increase to 1000 W (14.3 kcal) per minute. The majority of energy (70%) is converted to heat rather than work. Theoretically, this would raise body temperature by 1°C every 5 to 8 minutes and limit exercise to less than 20 minutes (2). Radiant heat from the environment also contributes to an increase in core body temperature.

The body has a sophisticated means of dissipating heat in order to maintain the body temperature in an acceptable range, thereby allowing prolonged exercise. Centrally, the bloodstream, with its high heat capacity, transports blood from the working muscle to the brain. The anterior hypothalamus and other thermal-sensitive detectors in the body sense this increase in temperature and respond in an attempt to keep the core temperature at 37+/-1°C. The warm blood is then dissipated to the periphery for cooling by vasodilatation and sweating. The rate of transfer is measured by the skin blood flow and the temperature difference between the core and the skin. Rate of transfer during exercise may increase by 20 times that at rest. Both ambient temperature and humidity play a role in how well these mechanisms work. Peripherally, heat is transferred from the body by radiation, convection, conduction, and evaporation. Radiation is responsible for 55%-65% of heat loss when ambient temperature does not exceed body temperature. As ambient temperature exceeds body temperature, heat gain can result. Convection (heat transferred between skin and air/water molecules as they circulate past) may account for up to 15% of heat loss. Both ambient temperature and wind velocity are determining factors in the effectiveness of this transfer. Conduction plays only a negligible role in heat transfer. Evaporation that occurs both with respiration and perspiration typically accounts for 20%-25% of heat loss. However, as ambient temperature approaches and exceeds body temperature, this becomes the primary means of heat dissipation. For every 1.7 ml of sweat evaporated, 1 kcal of heat is dissipated (3). A fit person can deliver up to 30 ml/min of sweat to the surface. The degree of effectiveness of evaporation for heat loss is greatly affected by the humidity level; the higher the humidity is, the lower the water vapor pressure gradient and the less effective is evaporation for heat dissipation. When heat production exceeds heat dissipation, heat-related illnesses may occur.

There are several distinct entities within the context of heat illness: heat edema, heat cramps, heat syncope, heat exhaustion, and (exertional) heat stroke. Although separate, there is a continuum between each.

Heat Edema

Edema is the mildest form of heat-related illness. Swelling occurs in dependent areas as a result of cutaneous vasodilatation and orthostatic pooling. Treatment involves leg elevation, use of support hose, and ambulation as soon as possible. No medications are required, specifically no diuretics. Full recovery is the norm.

Heat Cramps

Painful spasms of the skeletal muscles of the arms, legs, and abdomen may occur as an early sign of heat-related illness. The precise mechanism is not understood. Contributing factors include lack of acclimatization, negative sodium balance interfering with calcium-dependent muscle relaxation, dehydration, hypokalemia secondary to hyperventilation, and diuretic use. Valid treatment includes stretching and appropriate hydration. Various anecdotal remedies have been used in the field, including pickle juice, yellow mustard, and "pinching your upper lip." Electrolyte solutions such as GatorLyte are also felt to be useful.

Heat Syncope

Heat syncope is an orthostatic syncope that usually occurs with prolonged standing (especially if the knees are locked) or with sudden increase from the seated or supine position. Peripheral vasodilatation with resultant postural hypotension occurs. Inadequate cool-down period and dehydration are felt to contribute. Recovery is rapid once the patient is placed in a supine position. Leg elevation may help. It is important to consider other potential etiologies of syncope (including metabolic, neurological, and cardiovascular causes) if recovery is not rapid.

Heat Exhaustion

Excessive loss of fluid and/or electrolytes, in addition to an increase in core body temperature, results in heat exhaustion, a potentially serious condition. The athlete often presents with a myriad of symptoms, which may include profuse sweating, fatigue, weakness, myalgias, headache, dizziness, visual disturbances, irritability, nausea, vomiting, chills, cutaneous flushing, tachycardia, and hypotension. These symptoms can mimic a multitude of disease processes. Mental status is not significantly impaired. Core temperature is usually less that 39°C (102°F) and always less than 40.5°C (104.9°F).

As soon as symptoms are detected, move the athlete to a cool environment with occlusive clothing removed. Fluid replacement is essential, and electrolyte replacement may be required. Remember that the patient may be hypo-, hyper-, or normo-natremic. A balanced salt solution should be used until specific electrolyte abnormalities are noted. Oral administration is preferred if the patient is able to tolerate it. A minimal intake of at least 1 liter/hour for the first few hours is needed. If the patient is unable to meet these goals or if more serious symptoms are present, then IV hydration is required; dextrose in one-half NS or NS is most commonly used. If possible, measure electrolytes before administering IV fluids. Close monitoring of pulse, blood pressure, orthostatic changes, mental status, and symptomatic response to treatment is imperative. If the patient is not responding to treatment or if the condition begins to deteriorate, then treat as exertional heat stroke.

Exertional Heat Stroke

Heat stroke is a life-threatening condition; death occurs in 10%-75% of cases (4). For the purpose of this book, only exertional heat stroke will be addressed.

In the continuum of heat-related illness, heat stroke distinguishes itself by acute mental status changes and a core body temperature > 40.5°C (104.9°F). A rectal temperature is most accurate; oral, tympanic, and axillary measurements are unreliable for assessment of core temperature (5). Be cognizant of the fact that body temperature may fall before a complete exam. If there is delay in obtaining a core temperature, a falsely reassuring lower temperature may register; this does not safely rule out heat stroke. The presence of sweating, which is uncommon in classical heat stroke, may be present in exertional heat stroke.

Multi-organ failure occurs as a result of hyperthermia. The release of endotoxins and cytokines also play a role in the progression and severity of heat stroke (6). Neurological findings range from confusion and ataxia to seizures and coma. Both decorticate and decerebrate posturing have been noted. Cerebral edema and severe volume depletion are common. Blood pressure may be normal on presentation but invariably progresses to hypotension. Mild respiratory alkalosis, severe lactic acidosis, hyperuricemia, hypokalemia, hypophosphatemia, and hypoglycemia are common. Markedly elevated CPK and aldolase levels reflect rhabdomyolysis. Other life threatening processes associated with heat stroke are acute renal failure, DIC, ARDS, and myocardial infarction.

Time is of the essence in initiating treatment. Once heat stroke is recognized, rapid cooling to lower core body temperature to 38.8°C (101.8°F) is critical. Some controversy exists over the appropriate cooling method. Methods include cold (32°F) or cool (55-65°F) water immersion, evaporative cooling, and ice packing. Each method has its own advantages and disadvantages.

Immersion allows rapid conduction of heat from body to fluid, with the rate of cooling averaging approximately 8°C per hour (7). Immersion also improves hypotension. Concern is over hypothermic vasoconstriction that improves blood pressure but diminishes peripheral circulation and ultimately slows heat loss. Shivering can occur and increase body heat; diazepam can inhibit the shivering. Chlorpromazine is no longer recommended due to its potential anticholinergic properties such as decreased sweating, hypotension, confusion, and reduction of seizure threshold. Immersion also limits ECG monitoring and access if resuscitation is required. Finally, an immersion container may not be readily available at an event. Evaporative cooling by removal of occlusive clothing, spraying with water, or wrapping in wet sheets with the use of a fan for convective cooling are easier and cause less shivering. Accessibility for monitoring or resuscitation is not an issue with this method.

The athlete should be transported to an appropriate medical facility promptly. In the hospital, treatment can expand to include cold gastric or peritoneal lavage. Continuous monitoring of vital signs, cautious use of IV fluids, and repeated core temperature evaluations are required.

Indicators of poor prognosis are an initial temperature greater than 41°C, prolonged duration of hyperthermia, coma for more than 2 hours, coma persisting after the patient's temperature returns to normal, oliguric renal failure, hyperkalemia, and aspartate aminotransferase (AST) greater than 1,000 (4). Of those that survive exertional heat strokes, 10% are permanently heat intolerant (8).

Prevention of Heat-Related Illness

Recognition of high risk factors helps alert the physician to an athlete who might warrant closer observation. Certain physical conditions in athletes, such as fever, dehydration, and uncontrolled systemic diseases like diabetes, hypertension, and hyperthyroidism, should raise concern for potential heat-related illnesses. Athletes with eating disorders are intolerant of temperature extremes. Those with increased body mass index also are at risk as a result of increased heat generation for any given workload, inefficient heat dissipation, and less heat activated sweat glands in the skin overlying adipose tissue. Extremes of age tend to be at high risk. For example, the adolescent athlete has a decreased ability to sweat, greater core temperature required to initiate sweating, and more heat produced than adults for any given level of activity (9). In the geriatric population, decreased vasodilatory response and decreased maximal heart rate with resultant decreased maximal cardiac output are postulated causes for increased predisposition to heat-related illness (10,11). Alcohol use/abuse and various medications both prescribed (anticholinergics, stimulants, and so forth) and not prescribed (cocaine, amphetamines, and so forth) can place the athlete at risk. Sleep deprivation is another risk factor.

Awareness of weather conditions at the time of practice or play can also alert one to high-risk situations. Various devices can be used to assess this risk. For instance, the wet bulb globe temperature (WBGT) index takes into account the combined effect of air temperature, relative humidity, radiant heat, and air movement. The American College of Sports Medicine has developed guidelines based on the result of this test.

Athletic teams frequently use a sling psychometer measuring both wet and dry bulb temperatures. The newer digital models have made this a very simple mechanism for establishing environmental risk guidelines. Other risk guidelines have been established without any equipment by using known temperature and humidity for the area. A heat stress danger graph plotting temperature against humidity provides warning zones for heat stress. An athlete who has suffered from heat-related illness is predisposed to developing future problems while exercising in hot conditions. Summer events should be scheduled for the early morning or evening if possible.

Although temperature and humidity are out of the direct control of the athlete, fitness and acclimatization are not. The effects of poor physical fitness are magnified in hot and humid weather. In the context of heat-related illnesses, acclimatization refers to the physiologic changes that result in improved heat dissipation; for example, increases in sweat production for any given increase in core temperature occur more rapidly in a conditioned athlete. Other physiologic changes that occur with acclimatization include increased blood volume, decreased heart rate at any given work load, decreased Na^+ concentration of sweat, decreased core temperature at any given workload, or heat stress. There is also a reduced perception of exercise intensity. The process of acclimatization typically requires 10 to 14 days of exercise in the heat for duration of 1 to 4 hours each session. It is recommended that the athlete begin with 15-minute intervals and gradually increase exposure time. Heat acclimatization should begin 10 to 14 days before sports participation.

Cold-Related Illnesses and Injuries

Prevalence

The overall prevalence of cold-related injuries in the athletic population is unknown. Most of the data in this area are related to the U.S. Armed Forces. Even in this population, the condition likely is underreported due to the inability of standard thermometers to detect low temperatures. Lack of uniform reporting further compounds this problem.

Pathophysiology

Cold-related injuries may occur as local injuries with or without systemic hypothermia. Local injuries are more likely to occur in exposed areas or extremities with poor circulation. In systemic hypothermia, all organ systems are at risk. These conditions will be discussed separately.

Hypothermia

Hypothermia is a systemic condition generally defined as a core body temperature of less than 95°F (35°C). The body's response to cold occurs at two levels: the periphery and the core. As ambient temperature decreases, skin temperature is lowered. The initial physiologic response is release of catecholamines. Piloerection (goosebumps) occurs, followed by peripheral vasoconstriction. Increased peripheral vascular resistance, increased heart rate, increased respiratory rate, and increased basal metabolic rate ensue.

Shivering can increase basal metabolic rate by a factor of five; however, as the body's temperature continues to drop, the sympathetic response is ablated. Multiple organ system dysfunctions occur, and basal metabolic rate progressively decreases. At core temperature of 28°C (82°F), basal metabolic rate is approximately 50% of normal (12).

Effects on the cardiovascular system include decreased cardiac output with decreased blood pressure and heart rate. ECG findings include prolongation of PR, QRS, and QT intervals. The myocardium becomes irritable, and arrhythmias are common. Atrial fibrillation with slow ventricular response is common. Deterioration to ventricular fibrillation is a significant risk as the core temperature drops below 28°C (82.4°F). Asystole occurs below 22°C (72°F).

Respiratory rate and tidal volume progressively decrease by a centrally mediated mechanism. Cough reflex is lost and cold bronchorrhea with copious secretions increase the risk for aspiration. Noncardiogenic pulmonary edema may develop. Respiratory arrest is likely at < 24°C (75°F). In addition, hypothermia shifts the oxyhemoglobin curve to the left, making oxygen extraction more difficult. Tissue injury is attenuated to some degree by the decreased metabolic rate and oxygen requirements.

Renal perfusion is initially increased by peripheral vasoconstriction resulting in "cold diuresis," which can lead to hypovolemia. Shifting of intracellular fluid to extracellular space compounds this. As a result, peripheral edema, hemoconcentration, and decreased renal perfusion can occur. Acute tubular necrosis and disseminated intravascular coagulation have been reported in this setting.

Lactic acidosis results from shivering and tissue hypoxemia. Hyperkalemia may occur if tissue damage is severe. The hypothermic patient may be hypoglycemic or hyperglycemic. Hypoglycemia can occur if glycogen stores are depleted from severe shivering.

Hyperglycemia is more likely with initial increase in catecholamine release, decreased insulin secretion, and inactivation of insulin at decreasing temperatures (13).

Neurological deterioration is seen early with confusion and ataxia. As temperature drops, mental status progressively worsens. Cough reflex is diminished, pupils become fixed and dilated, and areflexia occurs. At < 28°C (< 82°F), coma occurs.

Spectrum of Hypothermia

Although signs and symptoms of hypothermia occur on a continuum, it is clinically helpful to categorize according to core body temperature classifications. Note that these values are not exact; there is mild generalized variability in the ranges noted in the literature. Both temperature ranges (Celsius and Fahrenheit) have been slightly modified for ease of reference without loss of clinical significance.

Mild hypothermia occurs when core body temperature is between 32-35°C (90-95°F). Shivering is present with a resultant increase in metabolic rate and heat production. Sympathetic response results in an increased heart rate and respiratory rate. Peripheral vasoconstriction is maximal. Increase in renal blood flow occurs and can lead to a "cold" diuresis. Diuresis results in volume depletion and hemoconcentration. The oxyhemoglobin curve shifts to the left, diminishing oxygen extraction from the blood. CNS changes are noted with amnesia, ataxia, and dysarthria.

As the core temperature drops to 28-32°C (82-90°F), the shivering reflex is lost and there is decreased metabolic heat production. Heart rate slows and cardiac arrhythmias are common. Respiratory rate diminishes, and respiratory acidosis occurs as a result of CO_2 retention. Progressive neurological deficits are noted with a loss of motor control, areflexia, dilated pupils, and obtundation.

Severe hypothermia is heralded by the body's inability to maintain core temperature. All measures of heat conservation fail, and core body temperature falls below 28°C (< 82°F), resulting in coma. Respiratory rate continues to slow to apnea (< 27°C/< 81°F), and heart rate slows to asystole (< 22°C/< 72°F). The patient appears dead. Flatline EEG is noted at temperatures < 20°C (< 68°F).

On-Site Evaluation and Treatment

If the patient is responsive and a pulse is detected, immediately begin passive rewarming. Removing wet clothing alone can decrease conductive heat loss by five times. Wrap the patient in dry blankets or clothes if available. Use another warm body if necessary; another healthy individual can generate heat when in close contact with the patient to provide heat transfer and thus warm the patient. Passive rewarming has no ill effects on the cardiovascular system.

Active rewarming with warm blankets, warm water immersion, hot packs, and heating lamps is controversial. Be aware of two possible complications: "after-drop" and "rewarming shock." An initial "after-drop" in core temperature may occur as a result of reversal of peripheral vasoconstriction and recooling of blood as it circulates through the cold extremities. In "rewarming shock," rapid peripheral vasodilatation may precipitate hypovolemic shock, especially if "cold diuresis" has occurred. Warm-water immersion is also complicated by difficulty in adequately monitoring and providing resuscitative measures to the patient. Active core rewarming is used in the severely hypothermic patient. Warm IV fluids; warm, humid oxygen; peritoneal lavage (KCl free); extracorporeal rewarming; and esophageal rewarming tubes are useful tools in the inpatient but not in the field setting.

The unresponsive patient may initially seem to be in cardiac arrest due to peripheral vasoconstriction, bradycardia, apnea, fixed dilated pupils, and areflexia. Do not start CPR until after evaluating for a pulse for one full minute. If pulse is detected, do not start CPR, because this may invoke a fatal arrhythmia in the irritable myocardium. If no pulse is detected, initiate CPR. For patients whose core body temperature remains below 32°C (90°F), chest compression is considered by some to be controversial unless clear documentation of asystole or ventricular fibrillation is noted; again, this is over the concern of inducing a fatal arrhythmia. Defibrillation and other standard ACLS interventions are often unsuccessful in a patient with core temperatures less than 30°C (86°F) (14-16). Defibrillation still may be attempted with a maximum of three shocks during the rewarming process. This should be repeated after the temperature has increased to 30°C (86°F). Bretylium is the antiarrhythmic drug of choice and is used by some physicians as prevention against ventricular fibrillation in severely hypothermic individuals (17). Airway and ventilatory support are necessary in patients without spontaneous breathing. Hyperventilation should be avoided to prevent respiratory alkalosis and further irritation to the myocardium. Continue resuscitative efforts until the patient responds or until the patient is completely rewarmed but shows no response.

Keep in mind that any patient who is unresponsive at presentation should be treated with thiamine, dextrose, naloxone, and IV fluid challenge (D5NS) to address other plausible etiologies of neurological dysfunction contributing to the presentation. Intravenous fluids containing lactate should be avoided, because the liver cannot metabolize this in the hypothermic state. Comorbid injuries such as intracranial hemorrhage or spinal injury should be considered. All hypothermic patients should be evacuated to a warmer environment and adequate medical support as soon as possible. Transport the patient in a supine position to avoid orthostatic hypotension. Gentle handling is imperative in order not to induce an arrhythmia.

Prognosis is based to some degree on duration and extent of hypothermia. Those presenting with core body temperatures less than 26°C (78°F) are at increased risk of poor prognosis due to frequently associated ventricular fibrillation and asystole. There have been exceptions; the lowest body temperature recorded in a survivor is 16°C (60.8°F) (18). Other poor prognostic indicators are older age, asystole on presentation, complications of pneumonia, and hyperkalemia.

Focal Cold Injuries

Vasoconstriction is one of the body's few physiological protective measures against heat loss. It is also one of the major features leading to frostbite.

Focal cold injuries occur as a result of tissue freezing, tissue hypoxia, and damage related to the release of inflammatory mediators. As the tissue freezes, ice crystals form extracellularly, extracting water from the cell and leading to intracellular freezing. The combination of dehydration and electrolyte imbalance within the cell leads to cell death. Tissue hypoxia occurs as a result of local vasoconstriction accentuated by vascular endothelium damage. Increased blood viscosity occurs, capillary blood flow slows, and venous and arterial thrombi form, ultimately causing irreversible damage to the tissue. Prostaglandin F_{2a} and thromboxane A_2-inflammatory mediators are released, leading to a cascade of events resulting in further tissue ischemia.

Frostbite

Vasoconstriction is a key to frostbite. As the skin cools, cutaneous blood flow drops dramatically. This is especially true in the apical structures. As a result, the hands, feet, ears, and nose are most susceptible to injury. In male joggers without adequate coverage, the scrotum and penis are also at risk.

Frostbite is traditionally divided into four categories based on findings after rewarming. First-degree injury results in no tissue loss. Numbness and erythema are common, and yellow or white plaques are noted. Second-degree injury differs only by the presence of superficial blisters filled with clear or cloudy fluid. Third-degree injuries are distinguished by deeper, blood-filled blisters denoting injury to the dermis. A black eschar may develop. Fourth-degree injuries extend through the dermis with necrosis and tissue loss. Mummification may occur. Some prefer the simpler system of dividing injury into either mild with no tissue loss or severe with resultant tissue loss. Keep in mind that the severity of the injury often is difficult, if not impossible, to gauge in the early stages. Therefore, initial treatment is the same regardless.

Treatment in the field should focus on padding and protecting the involved extremity. Remove wet or constricting clothing and treat the extremity gently. Avoid performing friction rubs, since this is potentially damaging to the tissue. Field warming should be attempted only if refreezing can be avoided, because thawing and refreezing results in a much more significant injury (19). Rewarming is not necessary if the victim is within 2 hours of medical care.

Initial in-hospital evaluation should determine if concomitant hypothermia is present. If it is, treatment of hypothermia takes priority over focal cold injury care. Check for other associated injuries, such as fractures. Treatment of frostbite focuses on rapid rewarming of the affected extremity in water heated to 40-42.2˚C (104-108°F). When maximal dilatation is achieved, the skin will seem reddish-purple and will be pliable to the touch. This initial rewarming is painful and usually requires 15 to 30 minutes. Analgesics should be used as needed, and aloe vera should be applied to the injured area to inhibit prostaglandin. Ibuprofen in dose of 400 mg every 12 hours will inhibit the arachidonic acid cascade. Tetanus prophylaxis should be updated and 500,000 units of penicillin G given intravenously every 6 hours for the first 48 to 72 hours. Elevate the affected extremity to minimize edema. Hyperbaric oxygen may improve outcome. Traditionally, surgical intervention is delayed as long as possible. Clear demarcation between viable and nonviable tissue is often delayed for several weeks. There is a trend toward earlier surgical intervention after identifying nonperfused tissue by technetium phosphate and bone scan or by MRI/MRA (20).

Regardless of early intervention, severe frostbite may lead to mummification, spontaneous amputation, and other less severe complications. Pain, excessive sweating, numbness, joint stiffness, skin and nail changes, and cool extremities may persist. Bone changes include early epiphyseal closure in the skeletally immature and punched out lesions in the subchondral bone in those of any age.

Chilblain

Cold environment and high humidity place one at risk for chilblain, a condition felt to be related to a neurocirculatory skin disturbance resulting in red, swollen, and tender lesions. The dermatitis is associated with itching, and blisters and ulcerations may occur. The lesions are generally superficial and heal quickly. Feet, fingers, and ears are most commonly involved. Keep the area warm and dry, and avoid constricting clothing and shoes. A more severe form of chilblain—pernio—may occur. Burning and pain are characteristic, and the lesions are more severe, with development of necrotic skin and sloughing. In pernio, lesions are slow to heal.

Trenchfoot

Trenchfoot develops in a cold, wet environment. Temperature ranges from 0-10°C, and exposure is typically greater than 12 hours. The areas of the foot most likely affected are those with the poorest circulation, including the dorsum of the foot, the first and fifth metatarsals, and the posterior aspect of the heel. Treatment involves prompt removal of the cold and damp shoes and sock. Keep the area dry and warm.

There are three phases to trenchfoot. The *prehyperemic phase* lasts hours to days. The extremity is cold, numb, swollen, and pulseless. The *hyperemic phase* follows, lasting 2 to 6 weeks. During this time, vasomotor disturbances and tingling pain are noted. The final phase of trenchfoot is referred to as the *posthyperemic phase*, which may last for months with pain, itching, numbness, and edema persisting.

Prevention of Cold-Related Illnesses and Injuries

Recognition of high-risk athletes and situations is important. Those at the extremes of age are more susceptible to the effects of hypothermia. Alcohol is a vasodilator, increasing heat loss. It also impairs judgment, making the intoxicated individual at increased risk of exposure. Certain medications, including barbiturates and phenothiazine derivatives, inhibit the body's regulatory response to cold. Environmental conditions, including lower temperatures, higher altitude, and increased wind exposure, place the athlete at higher risk. Water immersion may increase conductive heat loss by a factor of 25 to 30, placing the immersed individual at risk even with very limited exposure. Any person who has suffered from previous cold-related illness or injury is at increased risk for future problems.

Prevention focuses on recognition of the above factors. At-risk patients should be counseled that appropriate clothing, including a hat, is essential. Layering is recommended. Cotton is ill-advised, because it accelerates heat loss if it becomes wet. Keep extremities warm and dry, and avoid constrictive clothing and the use of alcohol.

Altitude-Related Illnesses

Prevalence

Altitude-related illnesses are common in the mountainous parts of the United States. It is estimated that 20% of tourists to Colorado ski resorts with elevations greater than 3,000 meters will experience some form of altitude-related illness (21). This value is tripled in climbers on Mount Rainier at an elevation above 4,500 meters (22). Cases are often unrecognized or misdiagnosed as a hangover, fatigue, or a viral illness.

Pathophysiology

Unavoidable hypobaric hypoxia occurs as one ascends to higher elevation. The body's response to these changes determines if one will experience altitude-related illness. Compensatory mechanisms are available. A shift in the oxygen-hemoglobin dissociation curve to the right occurs between 3000-4300 meters (10,000-14,000 feet), thus increasing delivery of oxygen to the tissues. Increase in alveolar ventilation begins immediately. A blunted ventilatory response to hypoxia is a common finding in those with altitude-related illnesses. In part this is genetically determined. Depressants such as alcohol, sleeping pills, and codeine can also play a role. Hypoxemia causes pulmonary vasoconstriction, peripheral vasoconstriction, fluid retention, and cerebral hypoxia.

Acute Mountain Sickness

Acute mountain sickness is the most common form of altitude-related illness. It begins within 4 to 6 hours of rapid ascent to 2,500 meters or more in susceptible individuals. Symptoms are nonspecific; headache, fatigue, malaise, irritability, insomnia, anorexia, nausea, and dyspnea are usual symptoms. Dry cough and decreased urine output may be noted in more severe cases. Ataxia is a more ominous sign of progression of disease.

Be alert for acute mountain sickness. The symptoms often mimic other conditions, such as viral illness, dehydration, exhaustion, and hangover. History and physical exam should be sufficient to rule these out. It is important to recognize the signs and symptoms of acute mountain sickness because of its potential to progress to the more serious altitude-related illnesses.

Treatment is primarily symptomatic. Cessation of further ascent and rest are the initial recommendations. Acetaminophen or nonsteroidal anti-inflammatory drugs are usually adequate for the associated headache. Avoid opiates, since they are ventilatory suppressants. Oxygen, if available, will help with more severe headaches. Use an anti-emetic for nausea and vomiting. Prochlorperazine is a good choice because it also boosts the hypoxic ventilation response. Acetazolamide may be beneficial. If started early enough, 4 mg of dexamethone every 6 hours may help with more pronounced symptoms. Avoid alcohol and other depressants. Symptoms may last up to 4 days.

High-Altitude Pulmonary Edema

High-altitude pulmonary edema is a noncardiogenic condition with normal pulmonary wedge pressures and a high pulmonary artery pressure (23). One proposed theory is that it is related to fluid retention with over-perfusion of pulmonary vasculature and fluid leak into the interstitial and alveolar spaces. It occurs in 1%-2 % of those who ascend more than 3720 meters (12,000 feet) and has the highest death rate of any altitude-related illness. Since onset of symptoms is subtle, a high index of suspicion must be maintained.

Symptoms usually begin 24 to 96 hours after arrival to the high altitude, most typically occurring on the second night of travel. Periodic breathing at night (24) may lead to decreased nighttime arterial oxygen saturation, resulting in these symptoms. Onset may be preceded by symptoms of acute mountain illness. Decreased exercise performance, shortness of breath with exercise, and increased recovery time are often the first indications of a problem. These are easily dismissed as lack of conditioning or fatigue. Dry cough and increased heart rate are other signs. As the process progresses, dyspnea at rest, tachypnea, productive cough with pink frothy sputum, and orthopnea develop. Lethargy, ataxia, confusion, combativeness, and coma ensue. Exam reveals fever, signs of cyanosis, tachypnea, tachycardia, and rales. CXR shows bilateral patchy infiltrates. Labs reveal leukocytosis, hypoxemia and hypocarbia.

The treatment of choice is descent. Transport in the seated position aids in distribution of fluid. Give oxygen as soon as it is available, but do not allow this to delay transport to lower elevation. A continuous positive airway pressure (CPAP) mask seems to improve ventilation-perfusion match and oxygenation. Keep the patient still and warm. The effectiveness of medications is unclear. Acetazolamide is usually given, whereas other drug choices include furosemide, morphine, and, in some cases, dexamethasone. Oral nifedipine 10 mg every 4 hours may reduce symptoms (25).

Without prompt treatment, death is likely. Prognosis is excellent if descent is achieved. The patient may reascend when high-altitude pulmonary edema has resolved.

High-Altitude Cerebral Edema

The pathophysiology of high-altitude cerebral adema is similar to that seen in high-altitude pulmonary edema. The symptoms are similar to that of acute mountain illness, only significantly more severe. Onset is usually 2 to 3 days after arrival. This condition rarely occurs at altitudes less than 3720 meters (12,000 feet).

Severe headache, ataxia, confusion, and fatigue are typical. Other signs and symptoms are visual changes, cranial nerve palsies, hemiplegia, hemiparesis, hallucinations, and seizures. A component of pulmonary edema is common but not critical to the diagnosis. Symptoms can progress rapidly over 12 to 72 hours to coma and death.

The only proven treatment is descent. Interventions used in the treatment of high-altitude pulmonary edema are typically instituted if available.

Prevention of Altitude-Related Illnesses

The major determinant of a patient's risk for altitude illness is rate of ascent and previous history of altitude illness. One's level of fitness is not a factor.

Gradual ascent is recommended. At-risk athletes should be counseled to avoid abrupt ascents to altitudes higher than 3,000 meters, if possible, and to maintain this altitude for 2 to 3 days before further ascent. Advise patients to sleep at a lower altitude if possible. (The impracticality of this method, however, is obvious for the ski vacationer.) A high-carbohydrate (> 70%) diet improves respiratory quotient and helps alleviate some of the symptoms of acute mountain sickness. Adequate hydration is essential, because dehydration possibly plays a role in the predisposition to altitude-related illness. Avoidance of respiratory depressants such as sleeping pills and opiates and limitation of alcohol decreases the risk. Prophylactic medication is recommended for those with a history of altitude-related illness or for those going to considerable elevations very quickly. Acetazolamide is recommended at 250 mg 3 to 4 times a day starting the day before ascent and continued for 2 to 3 days. As a carbonic anhydrase inhibitor, acetazolamide induces a metabolic acidosis, creating a compensatory increase in ventilation that may help prevent hypoxia associated with altitude illness. A salmeterol inhaler has also been shown to decrease risk of high-altitude pulmonary edema by approximately 50% in high-risk individuals. The mechanism is felt to be related to the beta-adrenergic agonist properties that up-regulate the clearance of alveolar fluid, as noted in animal models

(26). Additionally, nifedipine, which lowers the pulmonary artery pressure, may be used prophylactically at a dose of 20 mg of sustained-release formula given every 8 hours while ascending and for the next 3 days at altitude. Exaggerated pulmonary artery pressure due to hypoxic vasoconstriction is felt to play a significant role in the development of high-altitude pulmonary edema (27). If the patient continues to have problems with symptoms of acute mountain illness, the medication should be continued until relief is achieved. If insomnia persists, a single dose at bedtime is helpful. This is contraindicated in those with a sulfa allergy. Acetazolamide is not a guaranteed prohibitive; it also is associated with potential side effects of peripheral paresthesias, diuresis, nausea, vomiting, and lethargy, which can cause confusion in the diagnosis of acute mountain illness. Dexamethasone 4 mg every 8 hours starting the 24 hours before ascent is advocated by some, but its use remains controversial.

Lightning Injuries

Prevalence

Lightning is responsible for more deaths in the United States than any other natural phenomenon (28). Injury and death related to lightning are more common in the summer months from June to September, corresponding with the highest prevalence of thunderstorms. The greatest incidence of storms is in the South. High mountain areas are also associated with a high risk. Overall death related to lightning injury is 30% with an illness rate as high as 70% (29).

Pathophysiology

Lightning produces a current of 30 to 300 million volts. It produces a direct current rather than the more damaging alternating current. The pathway that lightning takes is a major determinant of the type and location of the injuries sustained. A direct strike discharges directly through the victim. When lightning strikes a nearby object and then discharges to the victim, it is referred to as a side flash. Lightning traveling up one leg and down the other is called a stride potential. The flashover phenomenon occurs when the majority of the energy flows over the skin surface. Vaporization of surface water and blast effect to clothing is seen. There is no danger in touching a lightning victim; the strike is instantaneous and the victim does not remain electrified.

Spectrum of Injuries

Electrical resistance in human tissue varies. Nerves and blood vessels are most susceptible to injury, because they pose the least resistance. The ascending order of resistance and injury potential is muscle, skin, tendon, fat, and bone.

Cardiac Injury

Cardiac arrest is the most common cause of death in the lightning victim. The direct current delivered initially causes asystole. This subsequently returns to spontaneous electrical activity due to the automaticity of the heart. Arrhythmias may occur. Direct damage to the heart muscle is possible depending on the strike pathway; however, this is rare. Transient hypertension and tachycardia have also been noted.

Respiratory Injury

Respiratory arrest occurs as a result of paralysis of the brainstem's respiratory system. This paralysis takes longer to recover from than that of the cardiac system. If artificial ventilation is not provided, hypoxemia occurs with resultant cardiac arrhythmias and cardiac arrest. This is likely the major determinant of death in the initial post-lightning-strike period.

Neurologic Injury

Injuries to the central nervous system are the second most common cause of death in the lightning victim. Direct passage of the electrical current through the central nervous system can result in coagulation of the cerebral cortex, intracranial hemorrhage, and paralysis of the respiratory center of the brainstem. Three-fourths of those injured lose consciousness; two-thirds experience at least temporary paralysis. The vast majority are confused or amnesic of the event. Chronic problems may develop, including seizures, motor disturbances, psychiatric symptoms, chronic pain syndromes, sleep disturbances, and headaches.

Cutaneous Injury

The location of burns is of clinical significance. Leg burns are associated with five-fold increase in death rate. Individuals with cranial burns are four times more likely to die (30).

Burns are not inevitable. Discrete entry and exit burns are rare in lightning victims, as opposed to those with electrical injuries. Burns follow distinct patterns.

Victims will likely have a combination of different types of burns. Feathering is pathognomonic of lightning injury. This is a transient finding that may not occur for several hours and resolves within 24 hours. It may be the result of electron showering rather than an actual burn. Linear burns occur over the areas of highest sweat concentration. Axillary and breast involvement are common. These are partial-thickness burns, 1 to 4 cm in width, which may not appear until several hours after the strike.

Punctate burns are small and circular, full- or partial-thickness, and often occur in clusters. Thermal burns are secondary burns that occur as the result of burning clothes or heating of metal objects next to the skin. Deep burns are rare in lightning victims.

Sensory Organ Injury

Rupture of the tympanic membrane occurs in approximately 50% of victims. Temporary sensorineural hearing loss is common and possibly related to the associated thunder. Cataracts may occur within a few days after a person is struck by lightning; in others, they may take months to years to develop. A fixed dilated pupil may be noted initially and, though alarming, is generally a transient finding due to autonomic disturbances. Other more serious findings have been reported, including optic nerve injury, retinal detachment, vitreous hemorrhage, iritis, and corneal abrasions.

Vascular Injury

Initial presentation with cold, mottled, pulseless extremities is common in vascular injury. This may mimic a compartment syndrome, and it is thought to be related to vasomotor instability and arterial spasm. Symptoms usually resolve over several hours. Fasciotomies are not indicated. Potential for deeper vascular injury that is not immediately present should nevertheless be kept in mind.

Musculoskeletal Injury

Musculoskeletal injuries are related to the explosive effect of lightning and should be considered during initial evaluation and transport of the lightning victim. These blunt injuries include fractures, dislocations, and spinal injuries.

Treatment

If conscious, the patient is likely to require little emergency intervention before transport. On the field, focus on the unresponsive first. The greatest risk is cardiorespiratory arrest. Follow standard emergency measures, assessing vital signs and instituting CPR as mandated. Keep in mind that ventilatory support typically is needed for a more prolonged period of time than cardiac support. Treat all unconscious patients as though they have spinal cord injuries. Deep tissue injuries with the associated risk of rhabdomyolysis are uncommon. Fluid loading and administration of mannitol and furosemide are not recommended.

In-hospital care is standard protocol for any severely injured patient. Special attention to cardiac and neurological status is important. Obtain a baseline ECG and cardiac enzymes. Serial neurological exams are important; any alteration in mental status prompts further diagnostic studies with computed tomography (CT) or MRI. Examine the spine and pelvis and view them radiographically. A drop in blood pressure mandates evaluation for intra-abdominal or pelvic bleed. Although rhabodomyolysis is rare in the lightning victim, administer lab tests to check the urine for myoglobin and renal function. Baseline visual acuity and auditory function should be established with special attention to the tympanic membrane for potential rupture. All patients should have a follow-up exam with an ophthalmologist after discharge.

Prevention of Lightning Injuries

At-risk athletes should take precautions to avoid sports performance during thunderstorms. Such athletes should be educated on how to calculate a storm's distance. (If you see lightning, count the seconds until you hear thunder. Divide this number by five to calculate the number of miles.) Keep in mind that lightning may travel more than 20 miles before touching down; it is therefore recommended that one take cover when the source of lightning is within 6 miles (a 30-second count). There are now portable lightning detectors available that can detect strikes from as far away as 40 miles. Experts recommend that one wait 30 minutes after the last lightning strike to resume outside activity.

If indoor shelter is not available, a hard-top car can provide reasonable protection. Do not touch metal. Convertibles, even with the top up, provide little, if any, protection. The rubber of the wheels offers no protection.

If no protective shelter is available, do not take refuge under a lone tree; it is more likely to attract lightning than a group of trees. If necessary, take cover under the lowest in a grouping of trees. Do not huddle with others; it is best to stay at least 15 feet apart. Clustering increases the likelihood that one bolt of lightning could injure more than one person. Do not sit or lay on the ground. Crouch or squat on the balls of the feet with knees together. Place hands between knees. Make yourself the smallest target possible.

Avoid water. Get out of boats and off bodies of water. Do not take a bath or shower during electrical storms. You can get shocked if you are near pipes or faucets.

Telephone lines, metal pipes, or objects such as umbrellas, aluminum bats, golf clubs, and bicycles can conduct electricity. Electrical shocks may be transmitted along any electrical cord. Avoid these objects when lightning is in the vicinity.

Remember when you are assisting a lightning victim that lightning *can* strike twice.

Conclusion

Illnesses and injuries caused by environmental factors are a frequent occurrence among persons who participate in sports. Heat- and cold-related illnesses and injuries, which are often life threatening, are believed to be underreported and therefore even more common than is generally accepted. However, environmentally related illnesses are highly preventable and, when they do occur, are usually associated with a good prognosis if treatment is prompt. Physician awareness of risk factors and patient education are important components of illness prevention.

REFERENCES

1. **Lee-Chiong TL Jr, Stitt JT.** Heatstroke and other heat-related illnesses: the maladies of summer. Postgrad Med. 1995;98:26-36.

2. **Saltin B, Gagge AP, Stolvijik JAJ.** Muscle temperature during submaximal exercise in man. J Appl Physiol. 1968;25:679-88.

3. **Nadel ER, Pandolf KB, Roberts MF, et al.** Mechanisms of thermal adaptation to exercise and heat. J Appl Physiol. 1974;37:679-88.

4. **Hassanein T, Tazack A, Gavaler J, et al.** Heatstroke: Its clinical and pathological presentation, with particular attention to the liver. Am J Gastroenterol. 1992;87: 1382-96.

5. **Hansen RD, Olds TS, Richards DA, et al.** Infrared thermometer in the diagnosis and treatment of heat exhaustion. Int J Sports Med. 1996;17(1):66-70.

6. **Hammami MM, Bouchama A, Al-Sedeirys, et al.** Concentration of soluble tumor necrosis factor and interleukin-6 receptors in heatstroke and heat stress. Crit Care Med. 1997;25:1314-19.

7. **Armstrong LE, Crago AE, Adams R, et al.** Whole body cooling of hyperthermic runners: comparison of two field therapies. Am J Emerg Med. 1996;14(4):355-8.

8. **Armstrong LE, DeLuca JP, Hubbard RW.** Time course of recovery and heat acclimation ability of prior exertional heatstroke patients. Med Sci Sports Exer. 1990; 22:36-48.

9. **Barr-Or O.** Temperature regulation during exercise in children and adolescents. In: Gisolf C, Lamb DR, eds. Perspective in Exercise Science and Sports Medicine. v. 2, Youth, Exercise and Sports. Indianapolis: Benchmark; 1989:335-67.

10. **Kenny WL, Hodgson JL.** Heat tolerance, thermoregulation and aging. Sports Med. 1987;4:446-56.

11. **Tankersley CG, Smolander J, Kenney WL, et al.** Sweating and skin blood flow during exercise: Effects of age and maximal oxygen uptake. J Appl Physiol. 1999;71:236-42.

12. **Chernow B, Lake CR, Zaritsky A, et al.** Sympathetic nervous system "switch off" with severe hypothermia. Crit Care Med. 1983;11(9):677-80.

13. **Fitzgerald FT.** Hypoglycemia and accidental hypothermia in an alcoholic population. West J Med. 1980;133(2):105-7.

14. **Nicodemus HF, Chaney RD, Herold R.** Hemodynamic effects of inotropes during hypothermia and rapid rewarming. Crit Care Med. 1981;9(4):325-8.

15. **Paton BC.** Accidental hypothermia. Pharmacol Ther. 1983;22(3):331-77.

16. **Reuler JB.** Hypothermia: pathophysiology, clinical setting and management. Ann Intern Med. 1978;89(4):519-27.

17. **Dronen S, Nowak RM, Tomlanovich MC.** Bretylium tosylate and hypothermic ventricular fibrillation. Ann Emerg Med. 1980;9(6):335.

18. **Southwick FS, Dalglish PH.** Recovery after prolonged asystolic cardiac arrest in profound hypothermia. JAMA. 1980;243:1250.

19. **Merryman HT.** General principles of freezing and refreezing injury in cellular materials. Ann N Y Acad Sci. 1960;85:503.

20. **Barker JR, Moore WD, Kucan JO, et al.** Magnetic resonance imaging of severe frostbite injuries. Ann Plast Surg. 1997;38(3):275-9.

21. **Honigman B, Theis MK, Kozlol-McLain J, et al.** Acute mountain sickness in a general tourist population at moderate altitudes. Ann Intern Med. 1993;118:587-92.

22. **Stuster JW.** Space Station Habitability Recommendations Based on a Systematic Comparative Analysis of Analogous Conditions. Washington, DC: National Aeronautics and Space Administration; 1986.

23. **Schoene RB.** Pulmonary edema at high altitude: Review, pathophysiology and update. Clin Chest Med. 1985;9:491-507.

24. **Khoo MC, Kronauer RE, Strohl KP, Slutsky AS.** Factors influencing periodic breathing in humans: a general model. J Appl Physiol. 1982;Sep(53):644-59.

25. **Bartsch P, Maggiorini M, Ritter M, et al.** Prevention of high-altitude pulmonary edema by nifedipine. N Engl J Med. 1991;325:1284-9.

26. **Sartori C, Allemann Y, Duplain H, et al.** Salmeterol for the prevention of high altitude pulmonary edema. N Engl J Med. 2002;346:1631-6.

27. **Bartsch P, Maggiorini, Retter M, et al.** Prevention of high altitude pulmonary edema by nifedipine. N Engl J Med. 1991;325(18):1284-9.

28. **Weigel E.** Lightning, the underrated killer. NOAA. 1986;6(4):2.

29. **Vigansky KN.** National summary of lightning 1986 storm data. 1986;28(12):1-9.

30. **Cooper MA.** Lightning injuries: prognostic signs for death. Ann Emerg Med. 1980; 9:134-8.

5

■ ■ ■

Psychology and Behavior in Sports Medicine

Peter F. Davis, MD

At every level of sport, the psychological well-being and behavior of the athlete influences his or her success. Psychological well-being may motivate a previously sedentary patient to begin an exercise program, and may help an elite athlete develop the coping skills needed to recover from a sports-related injury. However, when motivation becomes *pressure* to succeed, this can cause damage to both physical and emotional health. Athletes often may present with physical symptoms (as in eating disorders or overtraining) that cannot be fully treated without investigation of the patient's mental health. Some athletes even will imperil their health to gain a competitive advantage—for example, through the use of banned ergogenic agents—and therefore physicians need to be aware of such behaviors in order to identify and treat this type of substance abuse.

Exercise and Weight Management

The benefits of regular physical activity are well documented. Much illness and death could be reduced if the general population used exercise on a regular basis as part of their daily health regimen. Nevertheless, nonadherance to exercise programs is a common problem, and therefore helping patients change behavior patterns about exercise is an important challenge that clinicians face. Fortunately, primary care physicians can have great influence in helping patients modify behavior, especially when it comes to an exercise prescription. Simple physician counseling, for instance, has been shown to be effective in motivating patients to make lifestyle changes, including exercise. Behavior modification theory, such as that used in cardiac rehabilitation programs, can be applied to exercise; it involves setting short- and long-term goals, receiving feedback and modifying goals when appropriate, and encouraging such strategies through prompts (phone calls or mailed reminders) or diaries to maintain behavior. Some goals may include meeting goal weights and being vigilant about adhering to exercise; other goals may be more specific, such as "I will participate in a 5-kilometer run this spring." Diaries can provide feedback about compliance. Older or obese individuals may be faced with several psychosocial obstacles to beginning an exercise program, and the clinician must help the patient overcome these obstacles in order to begin and maintain healthy behavior. Individualization should help.

Most successful strategies for weight management involve caloric reduction and increased physical activity. A continued physical activity program appears to be a good predictor of long-term weight management. Factors that positively influence adherence to a physical conditioning program are listed in Table 5-1 (1).

Eating Disorders

Although the popular conception of the patient with an eating disorder is the young woman obsessed with her appearance, eating disorders may also be encountered in athletes. Among athletes, these disorders are more commonly found in women who participate in sports where pressures to be thin are great, particularly diving, swimming, dancing, and gymnastics. Anorexia nervosa and bulimia are two common eating disorders that may or may not coexist. Anorexia nervosa is primarily characterized by a refusal to maintain a minimal normal body weight and by a fear of obesity that persists even after significant weight loss. Bulimia nervosa, on the other hand, is characterized by episodes of binge eating and compensatory behavior to prevent weight gain, such as self-induced vomiting. The purging may be a result of the guilt that follows the binge. Unlike anorexia nervosa, bulimia is not accompanied by extreme weight loss; however, anorexics may also become bulimic or develop bulimic behavior. Depression and bipolar disorder can coexist with eating disorders. Both anorexia and bulimia can be life threatening, with a 2%-10% fatality rate for anorexia (2).

Table 5-1   Factors That Positively Influence Exercise Behavior

- Physician encouragement and counseling
- Realistic short-term and long-term goals
- Prompts (e.g., a diary)
- Exercising with others
- Variety of exercise
- Regularity of exercise
- Positive periodic feedback

Diagnostic criteria for anorexia and bulimia are given in Tables 5-2 and 5-3 respectively (3). Females encompass 95% of all patients with these disorders. Ages range from early adolescence to early thirties. The overall prevalence is 1:800 in the athletic population. The prevalence of anorexia is higher in those patients with first-degree relatives with the disorder. It is difficult to establish the exact prevalence of eating disorders in the athletic population; however, several studies have been done in college-level athletes involving small sample sizes. Up to 62% of female athletes admitted to some type of disordered eating. Most reported vomiting, using "diet pills," fasting, or using laxatives or diuretics.

Some eating disorders may fall outside the strict definitions set by the DSM, yet be pathologic. One example of such a behavior is caloric restriction accompanied by excessive exercise. With some binge-purge behavior, the purging may be characterized by a period of dietary restriction followed by binge eating. Purging can take many forms, including use of laxatives and diuretics or emetics and sometimes excessive exercise. While this type of behavior may not fully meet DSM criteria for an eating disorder, athletes exhibiting this behavior may be at an increased risk for developing an eating disorder.

Table 5-2   DSM-IV Diagnostic Criteria for Anorexia Nervosa

A. Refusal to maintain body weight at or above a minimally normal weight for age and height

B. Intense fear of gaining weight or becoming fat, even though underweight

C. Disturbance in the way in which one's body weight or shape is experienced, undue influence of body weight or shape on self-evaluation, or denial of the seriousness of the current low body weight

D. In post-menarcheal females: amenorrhea (i.e., the absence of at least three consecutive menstrual cycles)

Table 5-3   DSM-IV Diagnostic Criteria for Bulimia Nervosa

A. Recurrent episodes of binge eating. An episode of binge eating is characterized by both of the following:

   a. Eating, in a discrete time period, an amount of food that is definitely larger than most people would eat during a similar period of time and under similar circumstances

   b. A sense of lack of control over eating during the episode (e.g., a feeling that one cannot stop eating or control what or how much one is eating)

B. Recurrent inappropriate compensatory behavior in order to prevent weight gain, such as self-induced vomiting; misuse of laxative, diuretics, enemas, or other medication; fasting; or excessive exercise

C. The binge eating and inappropriate compensatory behavior both occur, on average, at least twice a week for 3 months

D. Self-evaluation is unduly influenced by body shape and weight

E. The disturbance does not occur exclusively during episodes of anorexia nervosa

Etiology and Clinical Manifestations

The cause of eating disorders is multifactorial. Athletes are influenced by societal pressures to appear thin. This cultural preoccupation, in combination with unhealthy coping mechanisms, leads the athlete to try to manage weight, which gives a sense of control. Of the other psychological factors that contribute to this disease, most are characterized by inadequate interpersonal relationships. The physician dealing with these patients should detail a history of any physical or sexual abuse. There is a high prevalence of alcohol and drug use in bulimics.

Several biologic factors have been implicated in the development of disordered eating. As mentioned, females are proportionally more likely than men to develop these problems. One theory suggests that imbalanced central serotonin metabolism is involved in the pathogenesis of this disease. Decreased cholecystokinin and disorders of melatonin have also been implicated.

The pathophysiology of anorexia is similar to starvation. Cardiac effects include muscle atrophy and decreased cardiac output. Valvular incompetencies also may be observed. The most potentially life-threatening problem with anorexia and bulimia is arrhythmias, which mostly are encountered in individuals who have electrolyte imbalances. Electrocardiograms may exhibit low voltages or a prolonged QT interval.

Clinical hypothyroidism may be present in anorexics, and because of hypothalamic dysfunction, amenorrhea may develop (see also the section "Female Athlete Triad" later in this chapter). Because of caloric restriction, particularly poor calcium intake, these individuals are at greater risk for developing osteoporosis. A central diabetes insipidus may also be seen due to impaired release of vasopressin.

Gastrointestinal effects of anorexia include gastric dilation, illeus, and fatty liver. Chronic induced emesis can lead to Mallory-Weiss tears, as well as tooth enamel erosion. A hypochloremic metabolic acidosis leading to hypokalemia may result. Volume depletion is common and is further enhanced by athletic activity. Elevated amylase levels may be seen as a result of parotid gland swelling in those individuals who induce vomiting frequently. Laxative abusers may present with edema, fluid retention, or chronic constipation.

The clinical presentation of those individuals with eating disorders varies. Most often a physician is consulted initially for a problem other than an eating disorder; however, a detailed history may reveal that the athlete is amenorrheic and restricting calories. In extreme cases of anorexia, the patient appears emaciated, yet is unconcerned or even defiant in the face of this grave health issue. The patient will not complain of hunger and will most often be concerned about when the usual exercise regimen can resume. Physical exam reveals a thin patient who may be bradycardic and hypothermic.

Evaluation and Treatment

The differential diagnosis should include analysis of malignancy, intestinal disorders such as inflammatory bowel disease, endocrinopathies, and psychiatric illness. The initial evaluation should include a history that documents the patient's attitude toward weight loss and eating habits. Encourage the patient to keep a food diary. It may be useful to question the patient about chronic constipation, compulsatory behavior, and reflux symptoms. The physical exam should include a through cardiac exam, which may indicate the need for echocardiography. Laboratory evaluation should document any electrolyte imbalances. Thyroid function tests help rule out any thyroid disorders.

No single treatment is best for disordered eating. A multidisciplinary approach must include the physician, mental health provider, nutritionist, coach, and athletic trainer, as well as family. Psychologic counseling in the form of cognitive behavior therapy can be useful. Fluoxetine has been shown to have some potential benefit for those individuals with bulimia. Weekly weigh-ins should be performed on each patient until 85% of ideal body weight is reached. Blood pressure and pulse should also be measured. Goal-setting should be a priority, with a weight gain goal of one pound per week. Be aware that conflicts often arise between patient and health care providers about goal-setting. Those individuals who are amenorrheic should be monitored for the resumption of menses.

Indications for inpatient admission include a weight loss greater than 40% of ideal body weight, arrhythmias, hypokalemia that is unresponsive to oral replacement therapy, altered metal status, and significant depression.

The natural history of these disorders varies. Seventy-five percent of anorexics eventually gain near-normal weight; however, nearly two-thirds continue to have issues with intermittent dieting and binge eating. Cardiac arrhythmia is the main reason for death, and poorer outcomes are found in individuals with both anorexia and bulimia, those who present at an older age, and patients who present with an extremely low body weight.

Female Athlete Triad

The female athlete triad is a syndrome that encompasses three medical problems: disordered eating, osteoporosis, and amenorrhea. It is unclear how many women have this disorder; however, between 15%-62% of female athletes have admitted to some type of disordered eating, and 3.4%-66% have amenorrhea. It is not necessary to meet the DSM criteria to be diagnosed with disordered eating. In some patients, the "eating disorder" may, in fact, merely represent a case in which caloric needs are not being met given the level of the patients' activity; strictly speaking, it is not an outright eating disorder (i.e., anorexia nervosa or bulimia) as defined by the DSM. Amenorrhea in this group is usually an exercise-induced amenorrhea, which is most closely linked with hypothalamic dysfunction. Amenorrhea is defined as primary (absence of menses by the age of 16 with or without secondary sex characteristics) or secondary (absence of three consecutive menstrual cycles or two fewer cycles per year). Osteoporosis is defined by the World Health Organization as a bone mineral density greater than 2.5 SD below the young adult mean.

Athletes who are at greatest risk are those participating at the elite level in sports emphasizing appearance and low body weight. The diagnosis of this triad should be considered in any female athlete presenting with symptoms associated with any of the three components (4).

Evaluation

Evaluation should include a history detailing cold intolerance, gastrointestinal symptoms, menstruation, and stress fractures. A physical exam may reveal some of the same findings seen in those individuals with an eating disorder. A pelvic exam is indicated in the presence of amenorrhea. Laboratory evaluation should explore for any electrolyte imbalances. Because many medical problems can cause amenorrhea, athletic amenorrhea should be a diagnosis of exclusion. A pregnancy test and endocrine evaluation should be done to explore other possible causes of amenorrhea. Besides a pregnancy test and pelvic exam, the clinician should evaluate thyroid-stimulating hormone, follicle-stimulating hormone, prolactin, and a complete blood count. An evaluation of bone mineral density might be indicated in those individuals for whom osteoporosis is suspected, such as a person with an eating disorder and a stress fracture.

Osteoporosis is of concern in the female athlete who is amenorrheic because of the risk of irreversible bone loss. Skeletal accretion occurs until the third decade in women, with weight-bearing exercise, calcium intake, and hormonal factors influencing bone build-up. Genetic factors also play a role. Inadequate estrogen, as is seen in amenorrheic athletes, leads to decreased bone mass. This is of particular concern in young women who should be building bone mass because this loss of bone mass at an early age may be irreversible. Female athletes who present with a stress fracture should be questioned about their menstrual and diet history, and a proper evaluation for bone mineral density should be obtained if osteoporosis is suspected.

Treatment

Once the diagnosis is made, treatment of the female athlete triad should be individualized. Interventions should be made to address proper nutrition. Contracts can be helpful to establish goals and guidelines about when it is acceptable to return to athletic activity. A reduction in intensity and volume of training by 5%-20% may be all that is necessary to allow necessary weight gain and resumption of normal menses. Proper nutrition and caloric intake should be emphasized, including adequate calcium intake. Calcium intake should be 1,500 mg/day for those athletes who may have low levels of estrogen. However, calcium intake alone will not prevent estrogen-related bone loss. There is some controversy surrounding hormone replacement therapy (HRT) and the female athlete triad; no data currently supports it. Most evidence for the use of HRT in this disorder has been derived from amenorrheic postmenopausal women (4). Most clinicians would agree that HRT should be considered for women who have athletic amenorrhea and do not respond to conservative therapy of weight gain and training reduction. HRT can be prescribed as oral contraceptive pills or in transdermal patch preparations. The level of estrogen in these preparations is adequate to provide bone protection. When designing a treatment strategy, often it is helpful to develop a team approach involving patient, physician, mental health provider, nutritionist, coach, and athletic trainer

---

Case Study 5-1

A 21-year-old female college student presents to her physician with worsening bilateral lower leg pain, left greater than right. She reports no previous episodes of this type of pain but notes that it seems to be getting worse, especially since she changed her exercise routine four months ago. Physical exam reveals a thin female with bilateral anterior tibial pain to palpation; the remainder of the exam is normal. Plain film radiographs are unrevealing.

Further questioning reveals that the patient runs for one hour daily. She has had only two menstrual periods in the last year, the most recent three months ago. She usually skips breakfast; she mostly eats salads. A nuclear bone scan reveals increased uptake in the left tibia, consistent with a stress fracture. Urine pregnancy testing is normal as are TSH and electrolytes.

The patient is eventually diagnosed with disordered eating and is referred to a nutritionist and a psychologist who specializes in eating disorders. She is started on oral contraceptives, and her exercise program is restricted until the stress fracture heals. Further management will be coordinated with the patient's family.

Psychological Aspects of Injury and Overtraining

Most athletes will face injury at some point, and many suffer some type of emotional distress when an acute injury takes them out of their sport; however, this distress diminishes once an athlete perceives that progress towards recovery is being made. Factors influencing emotional recovery include the patient's attributional style, types of supports structures available, secondary gain, and stressors outside of athletics. Attribution styles include one's general outlook on life (that is, pessimistic or optimistic). Those individuals with an adaptive attribution style are more likely to have a positive emotional recovery. Support structures are important to ensuring that the patient does not feel isolated and maintains a positive mental attitude. The more support the patient receives, from coaches, teammates, significant others, family, and friends, the better is the prognosis. Each person plays a different role in the patient's life. Support can include anything from verbal reinforcement to the mere presence of another to motivate and encourage progress. Arguably, the most influential factor in a patient's recovery is secondary gain: money, prestige, status, power, anything the patient uses to motivate himself or herself either to improve or to remain out of the sport (personal communication, Derrick Blanton, Psy.D., Southern Methodist University). Secondary gain can work both for and against a patient.

Often athletes will present with vague muscle pain, fatigue with training, or shortness of breath with exercise—signs of overtraining syndrome (OTS). OTS is a complex condition that involves intense exercise, inadequate recovery, and subsequent mood disturbances and decreases in athletic performance. Synonyms for OTS include *burnout, staleness,* and *chronic fatigue.*

There is considerable overlap between the signs and symptoms of overtraining syndrome and major depression (Table 5-4). The exact cause of OTS is unknown, but most agree that it is difficult to find one single cause and there are few biological markers to identify those individuals with the syndrome. Studies have linked a decrease in adrenocorticotropic hormone (ACTH), growth hormone, prolactin, and catecholamines to OTS; however, none of these tests is equivocal. Nutritional deficiencies may play a role; theories have implicated inadequate carbohydrate stores or caloric deficiencies. Such deficiencies may also result in OTS when combined with maladaptive response to stress and, in addition, some types of altered neuroendocrine response (5).

Table 5-4   Signs and Symptoms of Overtraining Syndrome and Depression

- General fatigue and/or malaise
- Insomnia
- Change in appetite
- Loss of motivation
- Lack of mental concentration

If overtraining syndrome is suspected, evaluate for endocrinopathies (such as thyroid disorders), hematologic problems (such as anemia or mononucleosis), and electrolyte disturbances.

Treatment of OTS consists of relative rest. The clinician should keep in mind that total inactivity may itself be stressful; therefore, treatment must be individualized. Even though few data exist about effectiveness of antidepressants and OTS, consider pursuing pharmacologic therapy, such as a serotonin reuptake inhibitor. There is no definitive marker for recovery and, as a result, resumption of full training should be based on symptomatology. If the symptoms are not severe, one might expect complete recovery in a month's time.

Psychiatric Disease in the Athletic Population

A wide variety of psychiatric diseases are encountered in the athletic population. Most literature has focused on the beneficial effects of exercise on mental health. Studies indicate that college athletes score higher on tests for vigor and extroversion and lower in depression, fatigue, and total mood disturbance than nonathletic controls. Nevertheless, athletes are susceptible to the same mental health issues as the general population (for example, depression, personality disorders, substance-related disorders, anxiety, and eating disorders). Several case reports have documented diseases such as Tourette syndrome, panic disorder, and bipolar disorder in high-level athletes. Dementia pugilistica is a phenomenon where boxers may demonstrate various neurocognitive deficits.

Depression may be encountered in athletes who may present with typical depressed mood, anhedonia, sleep disturbances, and loss of appetite. It is useful to differentiate situational post-injury depression from true endogenous depression. As previously mentioned, endogenous depression may be difficult to distinguish from overtraining syndrome (see Table 5-4). Allowing the athlete to understand the steps toward recovery is usually all that is necessary in situational depression. Endogenous depression, however, requires a different therapeutic approach, including appropriate psychotherapy and antidepressant medications.

Drugs and Supplements in Sports

Many athletes turn to drugs and supplements to help them gain a competitive advantage, sometimes even willingly risking their health in doing so. Because of these health risks, the National Collegiate Athletic Association (NCAA) and the International Olympic Committee (IOC) have banned many ergogenic aids, particularly in the last decade. Recreational drugs may also be abused by athletes, generally for the same reasons that nonathletes abuse them. Substance use and abuse is found in all levels of athletes, and NCAA statistics have revealed substance use at all levels of competition (6). Physicians should be aware of these types of behaviors and understand the unique goals of athletic patients in order to identify substance use problems and to help redirect patients toward more healthy means of achieving their goals.

Recreational Drugs

Recreational drug use may be seen in athletes both in and out of competition. Alcohol has a prominent place in sports marketing. While college athletes express more negative attitudes towards alcohol, they are just as likely to engage in alcohol misuse as nonathletes. Of concern in athletics are the reduced muscle glycogen levels, diuresis, and impaired thermoregulation caused by alcohol use. Alcohol is banned by the NCAA in riflery and pentathlon, and in fencing and shooting for international competition.

Marijuana produces increased reaction time and increased heart rate. Maximal heart rate is reached earlier in exercise, resulting in decreased exercise capacity. There is no known beneficial effect on athletic performance. Marijuana is illegal and banned by the NCAA.

Cocaine is a stimulant that increases synaptic concentration of dopamine. There have been several well-publicized deaths related to cocaine use in athletes. The drug induces a negative effect on glycogenolysis. Other adverse reactions include hypertension, tachycardia and myocardial hypersensitivity, coronary artery vasospasm, and psychosis. Its use is banned by both the NCAA and the IOC (7).

Ergogenic Drugs

Ergogenic aids are supplements or drugs that athletes use to enhance performance. Locker rooms and gyms perpetuate misinformation and myth about these substances. The physician who is involved in caring for athletes at an elite level should be aware of those substances that are restricted by the NCAA and IOC (Table 5-5).

Beta-adrenergic agonists (clenbuterol, terbutaline, albuterol, salmeterol) are commonly used in the treatment of reactive pulmonary disease but are also used by athletes to enhance performance. These agents have anabolic properties; animal studies have shown these agents to result in an increase

---

Table 5-5   Drugs and Supplements Used by Athletes to Enhance Performance

• Beta-agonists	• Creatine
• Beta-blockers	• Anabolic steroids
• Amphetamines	• Human growth hormone (HGH)
• Caffeine	• Blood doping

in muscle mass, and human studies have shown an increase in muscle strength. An increase in the use of albuterol among American Olympians was seen between 1984 and 1994, as these drugs were unrestricted in Olympic competition until 1992, when their anabolic properties were elucidated. Studies have found that the incidence of asthma (and presumed beta-agonist use) was as high as 50% in the 1988 winter Olympics (8,9). Clenbuterol is considered to be the drug with the most potent anabolic properties. Large doses usually are required for these medications to be anabolic. Excessive beta-adrenergic agonists stimulation may precipitate angina, seizure, hypertension, and excessive tachycardia.

Other inhaled and oral beta-adrenergic medications warrant special consideration, and the physician prescribing these medications should check with the sanctioning body to determine if they are allowed.

Beta-adrenergic antagonists are commonly used to treat hypertension, heart failure, arrhythmias, and migraine headache. The negative ionotropic effects of and decreased cardiac output associated with these drugs are obviously not beneficial to most athletes, especially the endurance athlete. However, because of the reduction in heart rate, tremor, and palpitations that they induce, these drugs have been found useful in several sports. Metoprolol has been associated with an improvement in shooting because these effects allow more accurate aim. The IOC bans these medications in sports where the drug may enhance performance (archery, shooting, fencing, biathlon, modern pentathlon, and others). The NCAA bans these drugs for shooting (riflery).

Amphetamines have been shown to increase physical energy and motivation on a short-term basis. Methylphenidate hydrochloride is an amphetamine used in the treatment of attention deficit hyperactivity disorder (ADHD). Its commonality, particularly among high school and college students, has made it a popular drug to use as an athletic aid. However, amphetamines have not been shown to enhance athletic performance but may enhance aggressive behavior. Of concern are the adverse effects of these drugs, such as shunting blood from the skin, which may lead to heat illness. The IOC bans the use of these drugs, and the NCAA permits their use in therapeutic doses for athletes with documented ADHD. Detailed urine testing can distinguish between the different types of amphetamines.

Caffeine can be ergogenic at high levels. It produces diuresis, gastric acid release, and increased heart rate and blood pressure. At the cellular level, it has been discovered that caffeine increases plasma free fatty acid levels and muscle triglyceride use and spares muscle glycogen stores early in exercise. A small increase in plasma epinephrine may occur. Endurance running and cycling have been studied in subjects using caffeine with enhanced performance. CNS stimulation may also produce an enhancement of exercise. The NCAA and IOC allow caffeine use up to a urine level of 12 mcg/ml (8 cups of coffee in 2 to 3 hours). Adverse effects of caffeine include hypertension, tachycardia, and restlessness.

Case Study 5-2

A 38-year-old male recreational basketball player presents to his physician with anterior knee pain. He had been seen for various acute problems in the past but had no significant medical history. Office records detailed a history of "vitamin" use. The patient's blood pressure is 140/96, which is much higher than readings on previous visits. The patient states that he has been using a "stimulant free" supplement in order to gain energy in his church basketball league. He last used the supplement the morning of the previous day.

The physician diagnoses and treats patellofemoral syndrome. Additionally, because of the blood pressure concern, the patient is requested to bring the supplement on his follow-up visit. He returns two weeks later and, after careful review, the physician notes that the "stimulant free" supplement contains caffeine at unknown levels. The patient stops taking the supplement, and his blood pressure returns to normal levels.

Athletes and others have used supplements such as ma huang (ephedra) in an attempt to increase energy and lose weight. Other supplements, such as caffeine (guarana), have been combined with ephedra alkaloids to enhance their effect. Several highly publicized deaths possibly linked to these thermogenic supplements have raised awareness of the adverse effects of dietary supplements. Athletes should be discouraged from using thermogenic supplements. Ephedra alkaloids (including ephedrine and pseudoephedrine) are commonly found in over-the-counter cold remedies and should be used with caution in athletes. High-level athletes should be aware that some sanctioning bodies ban their use (10,11).

Creatine is a natural substance found in raw meat and fish and is used in energy synthesis within the myofibrils. Athletes in the 1992 Olympic games first used this supplement, and now its use is widespread. In vivo, creatine monophospate (phosphocreatine) acts as an immediate source of phosphate groups to rephosphorylate ADP to ATP, which is necessary in muscle activation and myosin chain activity. The goal of creatine supplementation is to provide abundant phospate to quickly regenerate ATP from ADP and thus delay muscle fatigue. Creatine is normally supplied in quantities of about 1 g/d in the usual American diet. Endogenous creatine is also produced in the liver, kidney, and pancreas using amino acid precursors. Commercially available creatine is sold as a supplement, not as a drug, and its exact content is difficult to quantify. Small amounts of weight gain may be seen in users of this supplement. Evidence suggests that creatine may improve exercise involving short-term, high-energy strength tasks (that is, short sprints) but does not help endurance athletes. Questions remain about the long-term safety of this supplement. Adverse effects of creatine include cramping, dehydration, diarrhea, and possible adverse renal effects (12).

Human growth hormone first came onto the market in 1986 in a biosynthetic form. Clinical applications include treating children who have a human growth hormone (HGH) deficiency and have short stature. It has received attention as a "rejuvenator." HGH does not seem to have any intrinsic anabolic properties; however, it may be lipolytic, which may appeal to body builders. Its adverse effects are weight gain, peripheral edema, carpal tunnel symptoms, and hyperinsulinemia. This substance is banned by the NCAA and IOC.

Testosterone and its synthetic derivatives have both anabolic and androgenic properties. They act to promote protein synthesis, mainly through the activation of RNA polymerase, thus leading to increased muscle and strength. To achieve ergogenic effects, doses must be increased to 10 to 100 times what would be used for standard medical purposes. Steroids may be administered orally or through injection. These drugs have been used by and in athletes since the 1950s, when eastern Europeans began using them. The corresponding widespread use of these drugs prompted the IOC to develop a banned-substance list in the late 1960s, and it started routine testing for these substances at the 1976 Olympic games in Montreal. There may be a significant placebo effect involved in performance gains in those who abuse this drug.

Adverse effects are many. Acne and changes in hair pattern are cosmetic issues that may readily identify users. Gynecomastia can occur and may be irreversible. Anabolic steroids may be hepatotoxic, which occurs more commonly with oral preparations. Peliosis hepatitis has been reported after chronic intermittent use. Low-density lipoprotein (LDL) may increase and high-density lipoprotein (HDL) may decrease; blood pressure increases may be a result of increased vascular volume. Oligospermia and axoospermia have been reported, along with testicular atrophy. Tendon ruptures may occur as a result of increased muscle strength without an increase in tendon strength. An athlete with sudden increase in size and a tendon tear should be questioned about anabolic steroid use.

Adverse psychological consequences have been noted in users. Studies have indicated that increased aggression may be seen in users of anabolic steroids. Hypomania and post-use depression has also been associated with steroid use in athletes.

Blood doping is a technique wherein one's hematocrit is artificially raised. Endurance athletes have used this to gain competitive advantages by theoretically increasing oxygen uptake and delivery to exercising muscle. This may be done using erythrocyte transfusions or by the administration of recombinant human erythropoietin (rhEPO). Blood doping was initially done through transfusion; however, currently rhEPO has been used more frequently. Use of testosterone in women may be considered a form of blood doping because it may increase the action of endogenous erythropoeitin. Studies have shown an increase in speed in those individuals whose hematocrit is increased. Of concern is the fact that rhEPO can increase hematocrit to levels which would increase blood viscosity and predispose one to venous or arterial thrombosis. This effect may be accentuated in individuals starting an exercise session with a hematocrit of 55% and ending with a hematocrit of 60%-65% due to dehydration. Other adverse effects of blood doping are possible infections from homologous transfusions (HIV, cytomegalovirus [CMV], hepatitis) and transfusion reactions. Although blood doping is banned, testing for exogenous rhEPO has proved difficult, and athletes have used clever techniques to avoid detection. Many athletes have admitted to using doping to gain a competitive advantage.

Performance Enhancement Through Psychology

An often-overlooked aspect of sport is performance enhancement through psychology. Several techniques have been used and studied to enhance athletic performance. A simple technique is using goal-setting to help athletes achieve higher levels of performance. Long-range goals are established and broken down into realistic, manageable, observable, and measurable steps. It is important that these steps be attainable to promote self-efficacy, self-esteem, and motivation toward the long-range goal. It is equally important that performance is measurable to ensure progress towards the intended goal, to isolate areas requiring more attention, and to demonstrate effectiveness. To help achieve an athlete's goal, various other techniques have been implemented, including imagery or visualization, cognitive-behavioral therapy (that is, self-talk), and biofeedback. *Imagery and visualization* is just as it sounds—using one's mind to imagine and visualize the desired positive outcome. The image should be as specific as possible, including the sights, sounds, smells, and feel of the situation. *Cognitive-behavioral therapy* is used to identify the maladaptive, negative thoughts an athlete may be experiencing before, during, and/or after a performance. Often these thoughts are outside of conscious awareness and, at other times, the thoughts are clearly visible and apparent to all. *Biofeedback* is a term describing the process of recording the body's physiological responses to provide information about an individual's state of mind and being. It provides information about the body's temperature, heart rate, muscle tension, respiratory rate, and physiologic responses. The data are monitored, recorded, and "fed back" as events occur. Interpretation of this information allows users to see how internal and external events affect physiologic reactions. Professional counseling is integrated to allow the athlete to adapt their responses (personal communication, Derrick Blanton, Psy.D., Southern Methodist University).

REFERENCES

1. **American College of Sports Medicine.** ACSM's Guidelines for Exercise Testing and Prescription, 6th ed. Baltimore: American College of Sports Medicine;2000: 243-5.

2. **Korndorfer SR, et al.** Long-term survival of patients with anorexia nervosa: a population-based study in Rochester, Minn. Mayo Clin Proc. 2003;78:278-84.

3. **American Psychiatric Association.** Diagnostic and Statistical Manual of Mental Disorders, 4th ed. Washington, DC: American Psychiatric Association; 1994:544-50.

4. **Hobart JA, Smucker DR.** The female athlete triad. Am Fam Physician. 2000; 61:3357-64, 67.

4. **Johnson MD.** Disordered eating in active and athletic women. Clin in Sports Med. 1994;13(2):355-68.

5. **Armstrong LE, VanHeest JL.** The unknown mechanism of the overtraining syndrome. Sports Med. 2002;32(3):185-209.

6. **Green GA, Uryasz FD, Petr TA, Bray CD.** NCAA study of substance use and abuse habits of college student-athletes. Clin J Sport Med. 2001;11(1):51-6.

7. **Schwenk TL.** Psychoactive drugs and athletic performance. Phys Sportsmed. 1997;24(1):32-53.

8. **Wilber RL, Rundell KW, Szmedra L, et al.** Incidence of exercise-induced brochospasm in Olympic winter sport athletes. Med Sci Sports Exerc. 2000;32(4):732-7.

9. **Weiler JM, Ryan EJ III.** Asthma in United States Olympic athletes who participated in the 1988 winter Olympic Games. J Allergy Clin Immunol. 2000;106(2):267-71.

10. **Haller CA, Benowitz NL.** Adverse cardiovascular and central nervous system events associated with dietary supplements containing ephedra alkaloids. N Engl J Med. 2000;343(25):1833-8.

11. **Haller CA, Jacob P, Benowitz NL.** Pharmacology of ephedra alkaloids and caffeine after single-dose dietary supplement use. Clin Pharmacol Ther. 2002;71:421-32.

12. **Graham AS, Hatton RC.** Creatine: a review of efficacy and safety. J Am Pharm Assoc (Wash). 1999;39(6):803-10.

SUGGESTED READINGS

Almada AL, Kreider RB, Rerriera M, et al. Effects of creatine supplementation on body composition, strength, and sprint performance. Med Sci Sport Exercise. 1998; 30:73-82.

Eichner RE. Ergogenic aids: what athletes are using—and why. Phys Sportsmed. 1997;25(4):70-83.

Fuentes RJ, Rosenberg JM. Athletic Drug Reference 1999. Durham, NC: Glaxo Wellcome; 1999:.

Smith AD. The female athlete triad: causes, diagnosis, and treatment. Phys Sportsmed. 1996;24(7):67-87.

Van Raalte JL, Brewer BW. Exploring Sport and Exercise Psychology. Washington, DC: American Psychological Association; 1998.

Wee CC, McMarthy EP, Davis RB, Phillips RS. Physician counseling about exercise. JAMA. 1999;282:1583-8.

Woolsey MM, ed. Eating Disorders: A Clinical Guide to Counseling and Treatment. Chicago: American Dietetic Association; 2002.

6

The Exercise Prescription

Luis Palacios, MD

The benefits of exercise on health outcomes have been well defined (1-4). Technology, although making life easier, has also reduced the daily caloric expenditure; people can now shop online and therefore are not required to leave the house to obtain many basic goods. A more sedentary lifestyle in combination with easy access to high-calorie foods has created widespread concern over the increasing number of children and adults who are both inactive and obese. For these reasons, professional medical associations have appealed to the public to make exercise part of regular daily activities (4-6). In addition, they are advised to obtain information on exercise from their physicians. Unfortunately, rather than receiving specific guidelines on an exercise plan, patients may receive general, nonspecific information, which may cause disillusionment and lead the patient not to initiate an exercise program or to terminate an exercise program early (7-11). Therefore, it is essential that the primary care physician become skilled at dispensing appropriate instructions on how to start an exercise program and be able to monitor the patient's progress at intervals to track success.

Benefits of Exercise

The promotion of exercise to alter life-attenuating illnesses has been well-accepted in the medical community (1-6,12-14). Much effort has been placed on promoting healthy lifestyles, including habitual exercise for adults, as well as children (8-11,15,16). As the percentage of obese children who carry that burden into adulthood increases, it is crucial that patients adopt a regular exercise routine (11). Differences with respect to quality and quantity of habitual exercise have been noted among ethnic groups, especially African- and Mexican-American children. Such differences have

---

Table 6-1   Benefits of Exercise in Older Adults

Cardiovascular
- Improves physiologic parameters (Vo_{2max}, cardiac output, submaximal rate-pressure product)
- Improves blood pressure
- Decreases risk of coronary artery disease
- Improves congestive heart failure symptoms and decreases hospitalization rate
- Improves lipid profile

Osteoporosis
- Decreases bone density loss in post-menopausal women
- Decreases hip and vertebral fractures
- Decreases risk of falling

Cancer
- Potential decreased risk of colon, breast, prostate, and rectum cancer
- Improves quality of life and decreases fatigue

Diabetes mellitus (type 2)
- Decreases incidence of DM
- Improves glycemic control
- Decreases hemoglobin A_{1C} levels
- Improves insulin sensitivity

Osteoarthritis
- Improves function
- Decreases pain

Neuropsychologic health
- Improves quality of sleep
- Improves cognitive function
- Decreases rates of depression and improves Beck scores
- Improves short-term memory

Other
- Decreases all-cause mortality
- Decreases all-cause morbidity
- Decreases risk of obesity
- Improves symptoms in peripheral vascular occlusive disease

---

been offered as a cause for the greater disease burden in these populations (17).

The benefits of regular exercise include improvements in cardiovascular and pulmonary physiology, endocrine and metabolic stability, and mental state (Table 6-1) (12,13,18-20). Attenuation or maintenance of appropriate weight is an additional benefit that can decrease illness and death by decreasing the development of cardiovascular and/or endocrine diseases. The greatest benefit is seen in those previously sedentary individuals who become physically active; patients who are already active will continue to benefit, but in smaller increments.

Biologic and Physiologic Changes with Aging

Biologic and physiologic differences that affect a patient's ability to perform exercise can be seen at extremes of age (21-24). For example, vestibular function and muscle mass decrease with age and may lead to gait instability (14,24). Skeletal immaturity in adolescents may lead to apophyseal injury due to the increase in muscle and tendon strength overcoming the weak apophysis. The primary care physician involved in the care of adolescents, "masters" athletes, or older adults must understand these differences in order to provide advice about safe participation in activities.

Children and Adolescents

Rather than viewing children and adolescents as "smaller adults," it is important to understand the basic physiologic concepts to adequately care for these patients. Before puberty, girls and boys have similar strength potential. There is no difference in muscle fiber type or ability to metabolize fat, and responses to endurance load stresses are similar (25,26).

In preadolescents, heat tolerance is decreased due to greater surface area to weight ratio, reduced sweating capacity, reduced sweat rate/sweat gland, increased sweat threshold, decreased cardiac output, and increased Na^+ and Cl^- in the sweat (23,24).

Older Adults

Similar to children and adolescents, changes in the physiologic responses to physical stress have an effect on the ability of older adults to respond to exercise (13,14,21-24). Every organ system is involved in the changes associated with aging. Neurologic changes include total neuronal volume loss and function loss, producing a decrease in nerve conduction velocities, which has an effect on balance and reaction times. Cardiopulmonary system changes include decreased vascular compliance, leading to increases in blood pressure, which, in turn, can lead to left ventricular hypertrophy and decreased cardiac output. Lung changes leading to decreased exercise tolerance include intrinsic factors, such as decreased elasticity of pulmonary tissue, and extrinsic factors, such as decreased chest wall muscle mass, producing lower respiratory excursion. Decreased cardiac output in combination with loss of sweat production due to senile skin changes produce a lower heat tolerance and an increased risk of heat-induced injury.

Dangers and Hazards of Exercise

When giving recommendations or dispensing treatment, physicians should be cognizant of the risks associated with participation in exercise. The media regularly reports on deaths of participants in mass-start events such as "fun runs" or marathons. Such stories of the deaths of these unfortunate participants result in a sense of bewilderment about how such seemingly healthy individuals could be struck down participating in what we would assume to be healthy activity. The most common cause of catastrophic events during or immediately after exercise, in all age groups combined, is atherosclerotic coronary artery disease (13,27,28). It is estimated that the relative risk of an acute coronary event is approximately two to six times higher during exercise, the precipitating cause being greater cardiac muscle oxygen demands during exercise that are not met in diseased tissue. The resultant effect is alteration in depolarization, repolarization, or conduction velocity, leading to increased ventricular ectopy and, eventually, a ventricular arrhythmia. Increased cardiac muscle contractility during exercise produces a constrictive effect on the coronary arteries that may lead to disruption of an atherosclerotic plaque. This disruption, combined with platelet activation or hyperactivity, may produce thrombosis of a significant vessel. This effect seems to be greater in individuals who exercise at irregular intervals as compared to those who exercise regularly.

Vigorous exercise, whether as an isolated event or cumulatively, can also produce acute physical trauma including strains, sprains, and fractures, depending on the requirements of the activity. Chronically, vigorous exercise may lead to overuse syndromes that have an effect on the ability, motivation, and desire of the patient to continue participation in regular exercise (24,29).

Screening Patients

The role of the physician in screening patients before vigorous exercise is vital in ensuring safe involvement. Although not an absolute guarantee against death or injury, physician health screening validates the patient's desires and motivation and also promotes the patient-physician relationship (7-11,15,16).

Screening should be performed after a discussion with the patient that allows the physician to understand the reasons for instituting an exercise program and to dispel any unrealistic expectations. The physician can also identify those patients who should not participate in strenuous physical activity or should do so only under medical supervision (Tables 6-2 and 6-3). Physicians can set apart any medical or physical condition that, with correction, will allow the patient to participate. The first step is either to review an already-established history and recent physical exam or to perform a preparticipation exam for new or unfamiliar patients.

The American Heart Association has published recommendations for preparticipation screening of competitive and recreational athletes.

Table 6-2   Coronary Artery Disease Risk Factor Thresholds for Use with ACSM Risk Stratification

Risk Factors	Defining Criteria
Positive	
Family history	MI, coronary revascularization, or sudden death before age 55 in father or other male first-degree relative (i.e., brother or son); before age 65 in mother or other female first-degree relative (i.e., sister or daughter)
Cigarette smoking	Current smoker or former smoker who has quit only within the previous 6 months
Hypertension	SBP ≥ 140 mm Hg or DBP ≥ 90 mm Hg, confirmed by measurements on at least 2 separate occasions, or those on antihypertensive medications
Hypercholesterolemia	Total serum cholesterol of > 200 mg/dL or HDL < 35 mg/dL or on lipid lowering medication (If LDL is available, use > 130 mg/dL rather than total cholesterol > 200 mg/dL)
Impaired fasting glucose	Fasting blood glucose of ≥ 110 mg/dL, confirmed by measurements on at least 2 separate occasions
Obesity	BMI ≥ 30 kg/m^2 or waist girth > 100 cm
Sedentary lifestyle	Those neither participating in a regular exercise program nor meeting the minimal physical activity recommendations* in the Surgeon General's report
Negative	
High-density lipoprotein (HDL)	> 60 mg/dL (It is common to sum risk factors in making clinical judgments; if HDL is high, subtract one risk factor from the sum of positive risk factors because high HDL decreases CAD risk)

* 30 minutes or more of moderate physical activity on most days of the week.
Adapted with permission from American College of Sports Medicine Guidelines for Exercise Testing and Prescription, 6th ed. Philadelphia: Lippincott Williams & Wilkins; 2000; 22-32.

Table 6-3   Initial ACSM Risk Stratification

Low risk	Younger individuals (men < 45; women < 55) who are asymptomatic and meet no more than one risk factor threshold from Table 6-2
Moderate risk	Older individuals (men ≥ 45; women ≥ 55) or those who meet the threshold for two or more risk factors from Table 6-2
High risk	Individuals with one or more signs/symptoms* suggestive of cardiovascular or pulmonary disease or known cardiovascular†, pulmonary‡, or metabolic§ disease

* Pain or discomfort (or other anginal equivalent) in the chest, neck, jaw, arms, or other areas that may be due to ischemia; shortness of breath at rest or with mild exertion; dizziness or syncope; orthopnea or paroxysmal nocturnal dyspnea; ankle edema; palpitations or tachycardia; intermittent claudication; known heart murmur; unusual fatigue or shortness of breath with usual activities.
† Cardiac, peripheral vascular, or cerebrovascular disease.
‡ COPD, asthma, interstitial lung disease, cystic fibrosis.
§ Diabetes mellitus (type 1 and 2), thyroid disorders, renal or liver disease.
Adapted with permission from American College of Sports Medicine Guidelines for Exercise Testing and Prescription, 6th ed. Philadelphia: Lippincott Williams & Wilkins; 2000; 22-32.

History

A personal history of symptoms consistent with coronary artery disease should be collected. Utilization of a standardized questionnaire can facilitate and streamline the process of evaluation (see below). Ask the patient about a history of chest pain (with or without radiation), shortness of breath, palpitations, or syncope during exertion. These symptoms, even in adolescents and young adults, have been found to be associated with the risk of sudden death. Questions about a history of smoking may assist the physician in introducing the prospect of smoking cessation to prevent long-term consequences. Inform patients that smoking decreases exercise tolerance and that it is best to start with a lower level of activity with gradual increases in duration and/or intensity. Patients with a history of cough after strenuous activity may have exercise-induced asthma that may be ameliorated with the use of bronchodilators. Patients with asthma may need modification of their medication so that they can participate in exercise effectively and safely.

Data collection should include medications the patient may be taking for acute or chronic medical problems, because these may affect participation in an exercise program. For example, patients on diuretics or decongestants may be at risk for dehydration. Patients on oral hypoglycemics or insulin may need to monitor their blood sugar more frequently and modify or change their regimen to avoid hypoglycemic episodes (see Chapter 12). Many patients who decide to take on an exercise regimen may also be influenced by the intense marketing of over-the-counter supplements that purport to enhance or improve health. Unfortunately, many of these "natural" compounds contain the stimulants caffeine or ephedra (30). Healthy patients may be able to tolerate these substances, but they may be deleterious in a patient with coronary, renal, or endocrine disease.

Physical Examination

A general physical examination should be undertaken to identify any potential risk factors (15,16), including unidentified medical problems, such as undiagnosed diabetes mellitus or hypertension, and any musculoskeletal problems. In the HEENT portion of the examination, poor visual or hearing acuity may not disqualify a patient from participating in exercise, but correction will decrease the risk of injury. The pulmonary exam is best used to confirm the current health status of patients with underlying pulmonary problems. A patient with asthma or chronic obstructive pulmonary disease with clinical evidence of wheezing or rhonchi may benefit from treatment initiation or modification. Cardiac examination may elicit problems that may necessitate further testing before beginning an exercise program (see section on Risk Stratification below). Abdominal examination may reveal findings of organomegaly. The physician may counsel the patient with a recent infectious mononucleosis infection against strenuous exercise or activity that may lead to blunt trauma to the abdomen until the spleen has returned to normal. In women, a genitourinary examination may reveal urethrocele or cystococele causing stress incontinence. Uterine prolapse, depending on the severity, may be a cause of discomfort while performing strenuous activity. Although these problems are not life threatening, they may be socially embarrassing to the patient and lead to premature termination of an active lifestyle.

Musculoskeletal assessment in a health screening examination should be directed at identifying disorders that may lead to acute or chronic overuse injury. For example, although patients with osteoarthritis of the knees benefit from increasing muscle tone and strength of the supporting muscles of the joints, jarring physical activity may exacerbate the arthralgias. Therefore, instruct patients to limit the activity to cushioned surfaces. Patients with foot problems that may cause a gait with overpronation (for example, bunions, hallux valgus, and hammertoes) may benefit from obtaining good walking/running shoes and inserts or orthotics.

Laboratory Tests

In otherwise healthy patients, regular use of blood work to assess readiness for exercise is not necessary or cost effective. Instead, use blood work only for those patients identified at high risk or those with chronic medical conditions. In patients with hypertension or diabetes mellitus, electrolyte levels rule out renal disease or allow for correction of any anomaly before proceeding with vigorous exercise. A complete blood count (CBC) identifies patients with anemia and may be useful in women with irregular menses or poor dietary habits. These patients may benefit from correction before initiation of exercise, as the anemia may cause poor exercise tolerance. An ECG may be reserved for patients identified by history to be at risk (for example, those with a history of chest pain, palpitations, or unexplained syncope) or those whose clinical examination warrants additional study (for example, auscultatory abnormalities, including murmurs or irregular heart beat).

Pulmonary Function

In patients with pulmonary disease, a formal pulmonary function test may help in management of disease before exercise (24). In addition, patients with a history of poor exercise tolerance or symptoms consistent with exercise-induced asthma may benefit from such tests.

Risk Stratification

Before an exercise program is initiated and after the physician has identified the reasons why a patient may want to undertake an exercise program, a decision must be made about whether additional investigations need to be performed, including a general medical examination and any ancillary studies.

There are established guidelines with respect to the classification of individuals based on risk factors (see Tables 6-2 and 6-3). Patients can de divided into three groups: low, moderate, or high-risk (24).

Low-risk patients include asymptomatic younger or middle-aged individuals (men < 45 and women < 55) with no more than one of the following risk factors: diabetes mellitus (or impaired glucose tolerance), hypertension, hypercholesterolemia, and obesity. They also must not be smokers, or must have quit smoking over 6 months ago, and must not lead a sedentary lifestyle.

Moderate-risk patients include older individuals (men ≥ 45 and women ≥ 55) or who have two or more of the risk factors listed under low risk patients.

High-risk patients include individuals who have known cardiovascular, pulmonary, or endocrine disease, or those who have symptoms consistent with cardiac, pulmonary, or peripheral artery disease. These symptoms include typical anginal chest pain, fatigue or shortness of breath that is out of the ordinary with usual activities, palpitations or tachycardia, peripheral edema, dizziness or syncope with activity, orthopnea, paroxysmal nocturnal dyspnea, and intermittent claudication.

Once a patient has been placed into a particular classification, the physician can determine whether a diagnostic examination is necessary to detect illnesses that would place the patient at risk for injury, illness, or loss of life if he or she were to undertake an exercise program. An exercise stress test may be an attractive enhancement to a diagnostic examination and should be considered for moderate- to high-risk patients. In general, patients who are at low risk do not require a diagnostic preparticipation examination or an exercise stress test for performing moderate or vigorous exercise. High-risk category patients who wish to participate in moderate or vigorous exercise should not only have an examination but also should be considered for exercise stress testing. Screening patients before exercise allows for the identification of certain characteristics that may be associated with cardiovascular complications during exercise (Table 6-4) (13,24). For example, an adult male with poor exercise tolerance and a history of exceeding recommendations may be at higher risk and therefore require additional counseling about limitations.

Fitness Testing

Physical fitness is a term with many meanings, depending on the individual or the situation. An athlete may determine fitness as being able to contend in his sport at the highest and most competitive level. A woman who is now 3 years past delivery of her last child may define fitness as returning to

Table 6-4   Characteristics Associated with Exercise-Related Cardiovascular Complications

Clinical status	Multiple myocardial infarctions, impaired LV function (EF < 30%), rest or unstable angina, serious arrhythmias at rest, high-grade left anterior descending lesions and/or significant (≥ 70% occlusion) multivessel atherosclerosis on angiography
Exercise training Participation	Disregard for appropriate warm-up and cool-down, consistently exceeds prescribed training heart rate (i.e., intensity violators)
Exercise test data	Low or high exercise tolerance (≤ 4 METs or ≥ 10 METs), chronotropic impairment of drugs (< 120 beats/min), inotropic impairment (exertional hypotension with increasing workloads), myocardial ischemia (angina and/or ST-depression of ≥ 0.2 mV), malignant cardiac arrhythmias (especially inpatients with impaired left ventricle function)
Other	Cigarette smoker, male gender

Adapted with permission from American College of Sports Medicine. Guidelines for Exercise Testing and Prescription, 6th ed. Philadelphia. Lippincott Williams & Wilkins, 2000.

prepregnancy weight and activity level. An elderly patient may define fitness as maintaining adequate strength and endurance to perform the activities of daily living. Our perception of what defines or determines fitness depends on our personal experiences, cultural influences, and future goals (11,17). For example, a patient who, in his teenage and young adult years, was a competitive athlete may feel he is not fit because he can no longer perform at the same level, although he still functions at a level above his peers. Another patient may feel he can never attain fitness due to the cultural perception presented to us by the media. These influences affect the patient's willingness and desire not only to initiate an exercise program but also to stay motivated until his goals are attained. Because of this, the physician may want to perform fitness testing, which allows the determination of current physical and physiologic status and provides a baseline to measure progress in the exercise program (1,24). It also assists in keeping the patient motivated by providing sensible and realistic exercise goals.

Because physical fitness can be defined in broad terms depending on the individual or situation, an established definition of "health-related physical fitness" has been assembled to assist physicians in helping patients reduce health-related risk factors. Health-related physical fitness incorporates five distinct and independent factors: cardiorespiratory endurance, muscle strength and endurance, flexibility, and body composition (1,16). The aim of health-related physical fitness is to promote prevention of chronic disease and debility and/or alter the course of established disease or infirmity.

Used before beginning an exercise program, health-related fitness testing helps establish a patient's current fitness baseline and provides a way for the physician to stratify risk for disease or injury (24). It also provides the patient tangible data of where he is currently and can provide motivation by generating specific, realistic, and sensible fitness objectives. The data obtained during health-related fitness testing also assists in the exercise prescription by identifying areas of weakness when addressing all the fitness components. By establishing a baseline during fitness testing, periodic evaluations can measure progress and therefore act as a stimulus to patients.

For fitness testing to be of any practical use to the primary care physician, it must be valid, reliable, easy to administer, and reasonably priced (1,24). With respect to cost, there are many options depending on the amount of money the patient may be willing to spend if these services are not covered by insurance—and in many cases they will not be. Many of these tests are easy to administer and would be reasonable for a primary care physician to provide in his office.

Patient willingness and readiness to participate in an exercise program is the first step. It would be reasonable to require consent from the patient before testing. Risk assessment should include risk of injury while performing fitness testing. An established questionnaire such as the PAR-Q (The Canadian Society for Exercise Physiology, Physical Activity Readiness Questionnaire; Figure 6-1) can be used to determine readiness. Prior to the test, patients should be given specific instructions, including avoidance of substances such as nicotine, caffeine, alcohol, tobacco, or food at least 3 hours beforehand so that patients are able to maximize their effort and give a better picture of their current fitness state. Patients should be instructed to wear loose, comfortable clothing and good walking/running shoes. Patients should avoid other strenuous activity or exercise on the day of testing and have sufficient sleep the night before (24).

The testing environment should be adequate for the tests being performed and have a friendly and relaxed atmosphere. It should include facilities for the patient to change into exercise clothing. The patient should receive clear explanations of the tests being performed.

Body Composition

The importance of obesity as a risk factor for coronary artery disease, diabetes mellitus, and osteoarthritis is well established (1-6,12). Unfortunately, the incidence of obesity in the United States is increasing and is disproportionately higher in Hispanics and blacks. *Body composition* refers to the percentage of fat versus fat-free weight and can be measured by different techniques of varying complexity and expense.

Densitometry is considered the gold standard and can be performed utilizing hydrostatic (underwater) weighing or by plethysmography. These methods are well-studied and are standards by which all other methods are compared. Hydrostatic weighing is the oldest method available, but it is expensive, time-consuming, and may be difficult for some patients to tolerate (24).

Anthropometric measurements are obtained by measuring skinfolds and utilizing standard conversion tables to arrive at a percent of body fat. This is an inexpensive procedure that can be performed in the office once the physician or staff member has become a proficient technician in this

Physical Activity Readiness
Questionnaire - PAR-Q
(revised 2002)

PAR-Q & YOU

(A Questionnaire for People Aged 15 to 69)

Regular physical activity is fun and healthy, and increasingly more people are starting to become more active every day. Being more active is very safe for most people. However, some people should check with their doctor before they start becoming much more physically active.

If you are planning to become much more physically active than you are now, start by answering the seven questions in the box below. If you are between the ages of 15 and 69, the PAR-Q will tell you if you should check with your doctor before you start. If you are over 69 years of age, and you are not used to being very active, check with your doctor.

Common sense is your best guide when you answer these questions. Please read the questions carefully and answer each one honestly: check YES or NO.

YES	NO	
☐	☐	**1. Has your doctor ever said that you have a heart condition and that you should only do physical activity recommended by a doctor?**
☐	☐	**2. Do you feel pain in your chest when you do physical activity?**
☐	☐	**3. In the past month, have you had chest pain when you were not doing physical activity?**
☐	☐	**4. Do you lose your balance because of dizziness or do you ever lose consciousness?**
☐	☐	**5. Do you have a bone or joint problem (for example, back, knee or hip) that could be made worse by a change in your physical activity?**
☐	☐	**6. Is your doctor currently prescribing drugs (for example, water pills) for your blood pressure or heart condition?**
☐	☐	**7. Do you know of any other reason why you should not do physical activity?**

If you answered

YES to one or more questions

Talk with your doctor by phone or in person BEFORE you start becoming much more physically active or BEFORE you have a fitness appraisal. Tell your doctor about the PAR-Q and which questions you answered YES.

- You may be able to do any activity you want — as long as you start slowly and build up gradually. Or, you may need to restrict your activities to those which are safe for you. Talk with your doctor about the kinds of activities you wish to participate in and follow his/her advice.
- Find out which community programs are safe and helpful for you.

NO to all questions

If you answered NO honestly to all PAR-Q questions, you can be reasonably sure that you can:

- start becoming much more physically active – begin slowly and build up gradually. This is the safest and easiest way to go.
- take part in a fitness appraisal – this is an excellent way to determine your basic fitness so that you can plan the best way for you to live actively. It is also highly recommended that you have your blood pressure evaluated. If your reading is over 144/94, talk with your doctor before you start becoming much more physically active.

DELAY BECOMING MUCH MORE ACTIVE:

- if you are not feeling well because of a temporary illness such as a cold or a fever – wait until you feel better; or
- if you are or may be pregnant – talk to your doctor before you start becoming more active.

PLEASE NOTE: If your health changes so that you then answer YES to any of the above questions, tell your fitness or health professional. Ask whether you should change your physical activity plan.

Informed Use of the PAR-Q: The Canadian Society for Exercise Physiology, Health Canada, and their agents assume no liability for persons who undertake physical activity, and if in doubt after completing this questionnaire, consult your doctor prior to physical activity.

No changes permitted. You are encouraged to photocopy the PAR-Q but only if you use the entire form.

NOTE: If the PAR-Q is being given to a person before he or she participates in a physical activity program or a fitness appraisal, this section may be used for legal or administrative purposes.

"I have read, understood and completed this questionnaire. Any questions I had were answered to my full satisfaction."

NAME ________________________________

SIGNATURE ________________________________ DATE ________________________

SIGNATURE OF PARENT ________________________________ WITNESS ________________________
or GUARDIAN (for participants under the age of majority)

Note: This physical activity clearance is valid for a maximum of 12 months from the date it is completed and becomes invalid if your condition changes so that you would answer YES to any of the seven questions.

 Supported by: Health Canada Santé Canada continued on other side...

Figure 6-1 PAR-Q form. (*continues on page 92*)

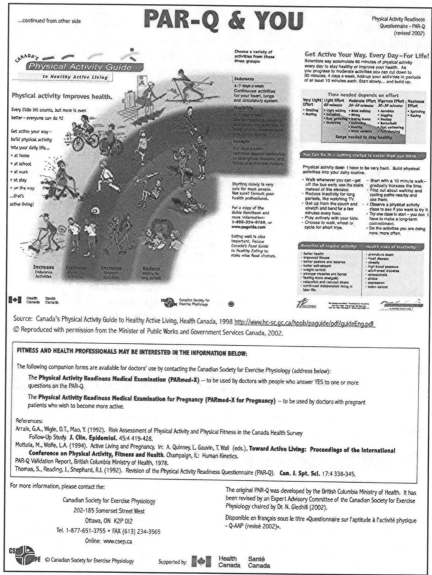

Figure 6-1   PAR-Q form *(cont'd)*.

method. The sum of the subcutaneous fat measured is then used to calculate total body fat. This method correlates well with hydrostatic measurements once the technique is mastered and population-specific formulas are used to convert the data.

Bioelectrical impedance is a newer method of determining the percentage of body fat. It has enjoyed popularity because of its ease of use, portability, affordability, quick availability of results, safety, and ability to measure large numbers of patients in a short period of time. It is commonly seen in fitness centers or in health care fairs for this reason. As its name implies, bioelectrical impedance involves transmitting a small electrical current through a portion of the body and measuring the resistance. Because fat is not a good conductor of electrical current and fat-free mass is, this resistance can be used to calculate body fat. Measurements utilizing this device can be as accurate as skinfold measurements, as long as appropriate procedures are used before measurement. It is affected by hydration status, so the patient must refrain from eating or drinking within 4 hours of the study, avoid moderate or vigorous activity 12 hours before, and avoid alcohol, diuretic agents, and caffeine 48 hours before.

Cardiorespiratory Fitness

When discussing fitness goals with patients, it is not unusual for them to describe their vision of fitness as being able to jog or run a desirable amount. For example, a postpartum mother might state that she wants to get in shape so as to be able to complete a tennis match with her friends.

Exercise involves the coordination of multiple organ systems to perform desirable body movement and therefore biomechanical work. Maximizing the capacity of each system and improving the neuromuscular facilitation between the organ systems is an outcome of fitness. By definition, *cardiopulmonary fitness* is the measure of cardiovascular functional capacity or, simply put, the ability of the heart and lungs to provide blood and oxygen to the musculoskeletal system. It is the ability to perform dynamic activity utilizing the large muscle groups in the body in moderate- to high-intensity exercise for prolonged periods (1,24).

For the clinician, the best way to assess this type of fitness is by measuring maximal oxygen uptake (Vo_{2max}) by using the equation Vo_{2max} = maximal cardiac output (L/min) (arterial-venous oxygen difference). Because there can be very little change in arterial-venous oxygen difference, this is truly a measure of cardiac output.

There are two ways to measure cardiopulmonary fitness; one is by performing a maximal test, and the other is by performing a submaximal test. Maximal testing, as the name implies, is carried out to exhaustion, whereas submaximal testing is carried out to a predetermined intensity. Maximal testing may be appropriate for athletes or patients who are capable physically of tolerating the potential stress of an "all-out" effort. It can be performed in the office or in field tests. Common field tests include the 1.5 mile test, where the patient tries to get the best time for that distance, or the Cooper 12-minute test, where the patient sees how far a distance they can achieve in that time limit. Maximal tests are inappropriate for patients who are physically frail, have a history of prolonged sedentary habits, or have a known cardiac history.

Submaximal testing is ideal because it limits the risk of injury that may be caused by maximal exertion. The cutoff typically used is 85% of the heart rate maximum based on age (heart rate maximum = 220 – age). In the office, a treadmill test is the most commonly employed method. After a brief warm-up, the test is begun and speed and intensity are increased, usually in 2-3 minute increments, until the patient achieves 85% of his heart rate maximum.

Muscular Fitness

The wide appeal of this health-related fitness category among the public has given rise to a mass-media barrage in the form of infomercials. The infomercial industries supply us with fantasized versions of individuals with hypertrophied, well-defined musculature, phenomenally attained through minimal labor and/or by miraculous technology. The definition of *muscular fitness* includes muscular strength and endurance. Strength is the maximal force generated by a muscle unit or group at a given velocity. Endurance is the ability of the muscle unit or group to perform repeated contractions with decreased muscle fatigue. Muscular strength is usually measured by performing a one-repetition maximum (1-RM). The 1-RM is then used in a ratio of weight pushed over body weight. Standardized tables based on age can be used to measure baseline and progression. The two most commonly used exercises in this test are the bench press and the leg press.

Flexibility

Probably one of the most undervalued components of health-related fitness, *flexibility* is the ability to move a joint through its complete range of motion (1,24). Its importance lies in its ability to affect movement by allowing the transfer of the energy produced by the specific muscle while utilizing as much of the muscle as possible. Flexibility is specific to the joint being tested. It is affected by intrinsic factors, including ligament and surrounding tissue compliance and muscle viscosity, as well as extrinsic factors, including an adequate warm-up and pre- and post-exercise stretching. Flexibility is tested by measuring range of motion in degrees of the joint being tested. A common test is the sit-and-reach test, which is performed while the patient sits on the floor. A yardstick is placed between the patient's legs and the amount of forward flexion is measured by the best of three attempts.

The Exercise Prescription

Recommendations for initiation of an exercise program may be given after identifying any risk factors that would make it unsafe for participation. The exercise prescription is designed to improve health by decreasing risk factors through improved physical fitness. Improved health is achieved not only by reducing the risk of chronic disease, such as hypertension or diabetes mellitus, but also by allowing the patient to preserve muscle strength to support an upright posture.

The recommendation for health-related physical fitness is for patients to accumulate a minimum of 30 minutes of moderate-intensity exercise utilizing large muscle groups on most days of the week (1-4,24). A visual instrument to assist patients with quality and quantity of exercise is the Activity Pyramid (Figure 6-2). A unit of measurement is the metabolic equivalent (MET). A MET is equivalent to 3.5 ml/kg/min O_2 consumed, with 1 MET being equivalent to resting metabolic rate. Activity is then measured in multiples of this. For example, walking at 4 miles per hour is equal to approximately 4 METS. Tables can be consulted for MET estimates for a multitude of activities (Tables are available in the American College of Sports Medicine's Guidelines for Exercise Testing and Prescription, 6th edition) Moderate-intensity exercise is defined as activity of 3 to 6 METS. Caloric expenditure can be used to determine exercise quality, although there is variability in where the ceiling is regarding benefit. One can see this in the equation used to calculate caloric expenditure: kcal/min = (METS × 3.5 × body weight in kg)/200. The recommendation is an expenditure of 150-400 kcal per day. The amount of expenditure depends on the patient's ability to exercise, as well as his or her fitness goals. It is reasonable to expect previously sedentary or debilitated patients initially to have caloric expenditure at the lower end, whereas other patients may have high caloric expenditures. Regardless, the goal should be for patients eventually

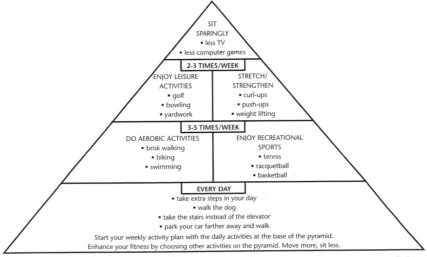

Figure 6-2   Activity Pyramid. (Adapted from American College of Sports Medicine. Guidelines for Exercise Testing and Prescription, 6th ed. Philadelphia: Lippincott Williams & Wilkins; 2000.)

to increase their caloric expenditure to a higher level. In most patients, health status is good and risk of injury or death is low, and supervision is not required. In patients who are debilitated, supervision may be necessary to teach any necessary skills to perform the exercise, to make sure they are capable of performing the desired exercise, and to monitor cardiopulmonary status as necessary.

To be effective, the exercise prescription should include the following five components: mode of exercise, frequency, intensity, duration, and progression (1,24).

Mode of Exercise

The importance of choosing the appropriate exercise mode for patients can not be overstated. An activity that is not enjoyable for the patient most likely will lead to early termination of that exercise mode. During the evaluation for an exercise prescription, the physician should question the patient about any previous modes of exercise the patient may have participated in, any limitations the patient may have in being able to perform certain activities, and any barriers (including economic) that may prohibit the patient from being able to participation. For example, patients with limited finances may not be able to join a fitness club or purchase expensive exercise equipment. To obtain health-related fitness benefit from exercise, the activity should incorporate the use of large muscle groups performing rhythmic aerobic activity. To maintain interest in an exercise program, a wide range of activities should be available that account for varying performance skills. In patients whose main interest is primarily health-related (to prevent chronic disease or to restore to a previous health status), activities that have little interindividual variation but are constant in intensity may be of benefit; examples of this are walking, running, or cycling. Patients may then progress to activities in which skill is required but the intensity is constant, such as swimming or skating. Finally, patients may progress to activities where both intensity and skill are more unpredictable, such as racket sports.

Frequency

For the patient to benefit from exercise, the activity needs to be performed often enough to affect cardiopulmonary as well as muscular adaptation. This has to be balanced by the patient's abilities, desires, and ultimate health fitness objectives. A recommended frequency of between 3 to 5 sessions per week seems to provide the best cardiopulmonary benefit. Individuals at a higher functional status who are mentally and physically capable of exercising at a higher workload, such as 70%-85% of their maximum heart rate (HR_{max}), may be able to achieve a desirable fitness at the lower frequency number, whereas debilitated patients may benefit from increased frequency (up to twice daily, if necessary) at a much lower intensity (40%-50% HR_{max}). Additional social constraints should be considered (for example, work, family, and economic issues) when recommending frequency of exercise to patients; telling a patient to exercise daily may be unrealistic and inappropriate.

Intensity

The assumption that exercise needs to be intense to achieve any cardiopulmonary benefit is without merit. It is well-established that deconditioned patients can receive significant benefit from low-intensity activity. The intensity for health-related fitness should be at a minimum-to-moderate quality—between 4 and 6 METS. Intensity may be monitored by patients utilizing a percentage of the heart rate or heart rate reserve (Table 6-5). The intensity can be at a minimum of 50%-65% HR_{max} to a maximum of 90% HR_{max}. An additional method to determine intensity is to use the heart rate reserve (HRR). The HRR for cardiopulmonary benefit is between 40%-85%. Utilizing intensity as a measure allows the physician to individualize the exercise to the patient's current status and needs. For example, it may be more acceptable and reasonable for a patient who is deconditioned to start at the 50% HR_{max}, therefore encouraging continued participation in that activity rather than developing frustration and/or injury. Patients who are already active and looking at improving their aerobic conditioning would be candidates for intensity levels of 85%-90%.

Duration

An equal part of the equation for exercise benefit is the length of time the activity is performed. Rhythmic activity must be of long enough duration to produce any benefit. The recommendation is for between 20-60 minutes of continuous or intermittent activity, excluding warm-up and cool-down. If the activity is intermittent, it should consist of a minimum of 10 minutes. Most organizations, such as the American Heart Association, Centers for Disease Control, and the Office of the Surgeon General, recommend an accumulation of at least 30 minutes of moderate intensity exercise 5 or more days of the week or at least 20 minutes of vigorous intensity exercise at least 3 days of the week. To decrease the potential for cardiovascular or

Table 6-5 Monitoring Exercise Intensity

Method of Calculation	Calculation
Percent of HR_{max}	$HR_{max} = 220 - Age \times Desired\%$
HR Reserve Method	Target HR Range = $([HR_{max} - HR_{rest}] \times [Desired\%]) + HR_{rest}$

musculoskeletal injury, consider the patient's health status, as well as his or her goals, when prescribing exercise bouts. A patient who has poor health status but who wants to exercise for 30 minutes daily will be better able to tolerate, enjoy, and benefit from a lower intensity bout of exercise, whereas a patient who is training for a 10 K run may need higher intensity and longer duration to be able to accomplish his or her goal. As the patient progresses, the duration can be increased to achieve a higher conditioning level.

Progression

One of the desirable outcomes of an exercise prescription is the establishment of lifelong physical activity and fitness maintenance. One way of doing this is by establishing sensible goals with a starting point and an end point, gradually building toward greater workloads to achieve that end point. Progression of exercise must be individualized for each patient. Considering the reasons for initiating an exercise program, as well as the overall goals and aspirations of the patient, is vital for success. Irrespective of the reasons for initiating an exercise program, there are three components in the progression of exercise: a conditioning stage, an improvement stage, and a maintenance stage (1,24).

The *conditioning phase* is an introduction to the exercise prescription that allows patients to familiarize themselves and become proficient in any specific skills that may be required to perform the exercise (for example, proper weight lifting technique). In addition, the introduction can be used as a way of promoting enjoyment in the exercise by limiting the strenuousness to 55%-70% HR_{max} and decreasing the potential risk of injury (muscle soreness or overuse syndromes). The length of this phase will vary, but in general, it is approximately 4 weeks in length if the recommended frequency is 3-4 times per week.

An *improvement stage* can follow once the patient is physically and mentally prepared. In this stage, which should last approximately 4-6 months, the exercise impulse is intensified to produce cardiopulmonary endurance conditioning, strength, and flexibility, depending on the goals. The intensity to produce overall improvements in fitness should be anywhere from 55%-90% HR_{max} with a frequency of 3-5 times per week and progression in intensity every 2-3 weeks. Progression should be dictated by the patient's age, current level of conditioning, and existing injuries. Older patients may benefit from a slower progression in the exercise regimen. Injuries that may halt or slow progression, although undesirable, will inevitably occur in some patients. If the exercise program has to be put off due to injury, deconditioning may occur, which will further slow progression.

The *maintenance stage* usually occurs after 6 months and is essential for the patient to be able to preserve any acquired health-related fitness. If the patient has been able to sustain an exercise program up to this point, one of the goals of this stage is to keep up interest in the health-related fitness. This can be achieved by reexamining the goals and objectives and possibly setting new ones. Factors that may affect goal-setting should be considered, and counseling should be provided as necessary. Patients may lose interest if they feel they have not achieved all or part of their goals. If not adequately addressed, nagging injuries may dishearten individuals.

Conclusion

The benefits of exercise in the prevention or modulation of chronic disease burden has been well described (1-5). Obesity, a factor in the development of many chronic diseases, is increasing to epidemic proportions in this country, especially in the Hispanic and black communities (11,14). In addition to poor dietary habits, the lack of regular exercise is a major contributor to this problem. Regular exercise is a health-related activity that can and should be undertaken to prevent these problems. Although there are some risks, the primary care physician can minimize these by performing a comprehensive evaluation of patients who desire to undertake an exercise program. The exercise prescription should include components to enhance cardiopulmonary adaptation, strength, and flexibility and should be individualized to take into account the patient's current health status. Progression should be measured to develop enjoyment of the activity and prevent injury. The exercise prescription as provided by the primary care physician should guide the patient toward a lifelong habit of regular exercise.

REFERENCES

1. **American College of Sports Medicine.** Position stand: The recommended quantity and quality of exercise for developing and maintaining cardiorespiratory and muscular fitness, and flexibility in healthy adults. Med Sci Sports Exerc. 1998;30(6): 975-91.
2. **National Heart, Lung and Blood Institute, Obesity Education Initiative Expert Panel.** The Practical Guide: Identification, Evaluation and Treatment of Overweight and Obesity in Adults. Publication No. 00-4084. Rockville, MD: National Institutes of Health; October 2000.
3. **Fletcher GF, Balady G, Blair SN, et al.** Statement on Exercise: Benefits and Recommendations for Physical Activity Programs for all Americans. A Statement for Health Professionals by the Committee on Exercise and Cardiac Rehabilitation of the Council on Clinical Cardiology, American Heart Association. Circulation. 1996;94:857-62.

4. **Department of Health and Human Services.** Physical Activity and Health: A Report of the Surgeon General. Atlanta: US Department of Health and Human Services, Centers for Disease Control and Prevention, National Center for Chronic Disease Prevention and Health Promotion; 1996.

5. **Pate RR, Pratt M, Blair SN, et al.** Physical activity and public health: a recommendation from the Centers for Disease Control and Prevention and the American College of Sports Medicine. JAMA. 1995;273(5):402-7.

6. **National Institutes of Health.** Physical activity and cardiovascular health: NIH Consensus Development Panel on Physical Activity and Cardiovascular Health. JAMA. 1996;276(3):241-6.

7. **Galuska DA, Will JC, Serdula MK, et al.** Are health care professionals advising obese patients to lose weight? JAMA.1999;282(16):1576-8.

8. **Orleans CT, George LK, Houpt JL, et al.** Health promotion in primary care: a survey of US family practitioners. Prev Med. 1985;14(5):636-47.

9. **Wechsler H, Levine S, Idelson RK, et al.** The physician's role in health promotion revisited: a survey of primary care practitioners. N Engl J Med. 1996;334(15); 996-8.

10. **Christmas C, Anderson RA.** Exercise and older patients: guidelines for the clinician. J Am Geriatr Soc. 2000;48:318-24.

11. **Anderson RE, Crespo CJ, Bartlett SJ, et al.** Relationship of physical activity and television watching with body weight and level of fatness among children: results from the Third National Health and Nutrition Examination Survey. JAMA. 1999; 279(12):938-42.

12. **American College of Sports Medicine.** Position stand: Physical activity, physical fitness, and hypertension. Med Sci Sports Exerc. 1993;25(10):i-x.

13. **American College of Sports Medicine.** Position stand: Exercise for patients with coronary artery disease. Med Sci Sports Exerc. 1994;26(3):i-v.

14. **Brennan FH.** Exercise prescription for active seniors: a team approach for maximizing adherence. Phys Sportsmed. 2002;30(2):19-29.

15. **Nied RJ, Franklin B.** Promoting and prescribing exercise for the elderly. Am Fam Phys. 2002;65(3):419-26.

16. **Kligman EW, Hewitt MJ, Crowell DL.** Recommending exercise to healthy older adults: the preparticipation evaluation and exercise prescription. Phys Sportmed. 1999;27(11):42.

17. **Crespo CJ.** Encouraging physical activity in minorities: eliminating disparities by 2010. Phys Sportsmed. 2000;28(10):36-51.

18. **American College of Sports Medicine.** Position stand: Exercise and type 2 diabetes. Med Sci Sports Exerc. 2000;32(7):1345-60.

19. **Colberg SR, Swain DP.** Exercise and diabetes control: a winning combination. Phys Sportsmed. 2000;28(4):63-81.

20. **Chintanadilok J, Lowenthal DT.** Exercise in treating hypertension: tailoring therapies for active patients. Phys Sportsmed. 2002;30(3):11-23.

21. **American College of Sports Medicine.** Position stand: Heat and cold illness during distance running. Med Sci Sports Exerc. 1996;28:i-x.

22. **Bar-Or O.** Nutrition for child and adolescent athletes. Gatorade Sports Sci Instit. 2000;13(2):SSE #77.

23. **Kenney LW.** The older athlete: exercise in hot environments. Gatorade Sports Sci Instit. 1993;6(3): SSE # 44.

24. **American College of Sports Medicine.** Guidelines for Exercise Testing and Prescription, 6th ed. Philadelphia: Lippincott Williams & Wilkins; 2000.

25. **American Academy of Pediatrics.** Policy statement: Strength training by children and adolescents. Pediatrics. 2001;107(6):1470-2.

26. **Benjamin HJ, Glow KM.** Strength training for children and adolescents: What can physicians recommend? Phys Sportsmed. 2003;31(9):9-26.

27. **Kestin AS, Ellis PA, Barnard MR, ct al.** Effect of strenuous exercise on platelet activation state and reactivity. Circulation. 1993;88(4 Pt 1):1502-11.

28. **Thompson, PD.** Cardiovascular risks of exercise: avoiding sudden death and myocardial infarction. Phys Sportsmed. 2001;29(4):

29. **O'Connor FG, Howard TM, Fieseler CM, Nirschl RP.** Managing overuse injuries: a systematic approach. Phys Sportsmed. 1997;25(5).88.

30. **Armsey TD, Green GA.** Nutrition supplements: science vs. hype. Phys Sportsmed. 1997;25(6):76.

SECTION II

MEDICAL CONDITIONS (NON-MUSCULOSKELETAL)

7

■ ■ ■

Infectious Diseases
in Sports Medicine

Scott E. Rojas, MD

hile infectious diseases clearly have an effect on our everyday lives, the role of sports participation in the transmission of such disease merits considerable attention. As sports generally involve differing levels of contact between competitors, the risk of communicable disease is inherent in participation. In general, the fitness of a person to compete precludes the presence of a significant medical illness and provides protection to those with whom he would come into contact in such a competition. Unfortunately, many illnesses, particularly viral infections, may be most contagious at or before the onset of significant symptoms.

This chapter will focus on those infections for which the athlete is at increased risk. Because infections involve the complex interaction between a host and a microorganism, one must consider the conditions that impair host defense or immune response, the characteristics of particular pathogens that allow them to cause disease, and the conditions that place the host in contact with such pathogens.

Host Defense

Risk of infection is related to multiple factors, including the susceptibility of the host, the size and route of the inoculum, and the virulence of the pathogen. Participation in sports may affect the physical barriers of defense, resulting in an increased risk for transmission of pathogens by direct contact. Abrasion, maceration, and ultraviolet radiation may compromise the skin as a natural barrier to infection. In addition, vigorous exercise may modify exposure to airborne pathogens by increasing frequency of mouth breathing, thus bypassing the nasal filter.

Multiple alterations in specific aspects of immune system function have been described as a result of exercise training. However, it has been very difficult to determine the relationship between these changes and the clinical risk of infection. There is a general perception among elite athletes and coaches that moderate exercise may confer some enhanced protection against upper respiratory infection, which is the most common infectious complaint among athletes. At the same time, there is a general consensus that prolonged intense exertion or "overtraining" may result in decreased resistance to similar infections (1). Scientific data to support these conclusions are limited at this time.

In studies of overweight women randomized to near-daily exercise (brisk walking) for 12 to 15 weeks, test subjects reported 40%-50% fewer days with upper respiratory infection symptoms as compared to those who continued their sedentary lifestyle. Overtraining by exceeding individually defined thresholds has been shown to be associated with a higher percentage of illness (1). However, given that overtraining appears to be an individual-specific phenomenon, it is very difficult to develop general guidelines to minimize risk of infection as a result of such overtraining.

Heavy exertion has been associated with specific changes in immune system variables, including the following traits:

1. Plasma catecholamines, growth hormone, and cortisol levels, all leading to neutrophilia with relative lymphopenia, are increased.
2. Phagocytic function of granulocytes and monocytes is increased.
3. Natural killer cell cytotoxic activity is decreased.
4. Mitogen-induced T cell proliferation is decreased.
5. Delayed-type hypersensitivity response is decreased.
6. Plasma concentrations of cytokines-TNFα, IL-1β, IL-6, IL-10, and IL-1 receptor antagonist are increased.
7. Nasal and salivary IgA production are decreased.

These changes are not usually seen with "moderate" exercise. Thus, whereas changes in immune function clearly occur as a result of strenuous exercise, their clinical significance remains unclear. Multiple studies have been performed to assess the risk of upper respiratory infections related to physical exertion in rowers, swimmers, and marathon runners. These studies rely on subjective reporting of symptoms rather than actual isolation of a pathogen and have yielded data consistent with increased, decreased, and unaltered risk for infection (2). There is a clear need for further research in this area. Understanding will increase as approaches (molecular methods and systems analyses) to the elucidation of immune function become increasingly sophisticated.

Skin and Soft Tissue Infections

Dermatophytes

Risk for infection due to superficial fungi (dermatophytes) is increased in sports as indicated by the synonyms "athlete's foot" for tinea pedis and "jock itch" for tinea cruris. The dermatophytes are separated into three genera: *Microsporum* and *Trichophyton,* both of which have several species, and *Epidermophyton,* of which there is a single species. These fungi only infect the dead keratin layer of the skin (hair and nails).

Toe web infection, usually between the fourth and fifth toes, may cause the skin to seem white, soggy, and macerated or dry, scaly, and fissured (3). A chronic form of tinea pedis may lead to hyperkeratosis at the plantar surface, causing the sole to be covered with fine white scale. This form may be more resistant to therapy. Individuals with tinea pedis should be treated with antifungal agents and wear protective footwear while using shared facilities such as showers and locker rooms (4). Outbreaks of tinea corporis (ringworm)—characterized by well-circumscribed scaling and erythematous annular plaques—have been described related to direct contact from wrestling (5).

Treatment may be topical with allylamines, such as terbinafine, or with imidazoles, such as clotrimazole, miconazole, and econazole (6). Systemic therapy is reasonable for more severe or refractory cases, usually with oral terbinafine 250 mg each day for 2 weeks, itraconazole 200 mg twice a day for 1 week, or fluconazole 150 mg each week for 2-4 weeks. These medications are not approved by the Food and Drug Administration (FDA) for tinea pedis without onychomycosis, and caution is necessary given potential side effects and drug interactions.

Athletes who will be involved in significant direct contact with others, especially wrestlers, should be examined before any such activity. *Athletes with a tinea infection should be excluded from competition if the involved areas cannot be adequately covered.*

Cutaneous Viral Infections

Herpes simplex virus (HSV) infection may be the most common contagion transmitted through direct contact in sports activities. The risk for wrestlers and rugby players, in particular, is well-known and has led to the terms "herpes gladiatorum" and "scrumpox" respectively. Infection occurs by direct inoculation of the virus from a vesicle on the skin of one competitor onto the often abraded skin of another. This method of transmission was the cause of a large outbreak in high school wrestlers attending a training camp in 1989. Many of the wrestlers continued to wrestle after the onset of the vesicular rash. Of the 175 wrestlers, 60 became infected with lesions on the head (73%), extremities (42%), and trunk (28%). Conjunctivitis or blepharitis was also diagnosed in 5 wrestlers (7). Constitutional symptoms were common, indicating probable primary infection. These symptoms may include fever, chills, sore throat, headache, malaise, and regional adenopathy. Given the significant risk for transmission, individuals should not be allowed to compete until vesicles are dry and scabbed. Primary or recurrent HSV infection may be treated with acyclovir, valacyclovir, or famciclovir to decrease the time of viral shedding and time to scabbing of vesicles.

Other viral infections of the skin that may be spread by direct contact include *varicella zoster* virus (VZV), molluscum contagiosum, and verruca caused by human papillomavirus. Individuals with primary VZV infection (chickenpox) may spread disease both through direct contact and through airborne droplet nuclei and should be quarantined until the lesions are crusted. Evidence of protective immunity through natural infection or immunization should likely be a prerequisite for competition, at least in older children and adults, given the increased severity of primary infection as one grows older, including an increased risk for pneumonitis and hepatitis. Localized recurrence of disease (shingles) also should preclude one from skin-to-skin contact in competition and should prompt the practitioner to administer an HIV antibody test.

Cutaneous Bacterial Infections

Person-to-person contact in sports may also readily spread skin and soft tissue infection due to bacteria. *Staphylococcus aureus* and *Streptococcus pyogenes* (Group A *Streptococcus*) are the most commonly implicated and may cause impetigo, folliculitis, furunculosis, and carbunculosis. Impetigo is a highly contagious superficial skin infection causing a vesicular rash which may form bulla (bullous impetigo) or honey-colored crusting (non-bullous) with minimal surrounding erythema (6). In a setting of abrasions and prolonged skin-to-skin contact, such as in wrestling, rugby, and jujitsu, transmission may lead to colonization and then to infection (5).

One well-described outbreak of *Streptococcus pyogenes*-related disease in rugby players led to the development of acute glomerulonephritis ("scrum kidney") in a player and acute salpingitis in a player's girlfriend (8). The index case was a 20-year-old student nurse with a 4-day history of facial impetigo. She was treated with tetracycline but developed fever, abdominal pain, and leukocytosis 3 days later. She was diagnosed with acute salpingitis. Her boyfriend was on the rugby team; he had had facial impetigo for the previous 3 weeks. On investigation, it was determined that another player on the team had been hospitalized 3 days before the student nurse. He had a wound infection and developed facial swelling and decreased urinary output consistent with acute glomerulonephritis. Four more cases of streptococcal pyoderma were diagnosed on the rugby team (all scrum players). These particularly severe complications of skin infection illustrate the need for proper infection control measures for athletic competition, including proper cleansing of wounds or abrasions with an antiseptic soap (such as chlorhexidine) and precluding from competition any individual with wounds that cannot be adequately dressed. Community outbreaks of methicillin-resistant *Staphylococcus aureus* (MRSA) involving athletes have also been described (9).

Given the potential for significant illness related to these infections, individuals with active (especially draining) bacterial skin infections should be discouraged from participation in close contact sports. Also, abrasions or lacerations sustained during competition should be properly cleansed with an antiseptic, such as chlorhexidine, to decrease the risk of local infection. Clinical disease should be treated with proper antimicrobial therapy. In many areas, the first-generation cephalosporins, such as cephalexin, and penicillinase-resistant penicillins, such as dicloxacillin, are effective. Unfortunately, the increasing prevalence of MRSA in certain areas may lead to clinical failure of these medications and may necessitate culture of the lesion for identification and susceptibility-testing versus empiric therapy with agents effective against MRSA, such as trimethoprim-sulfamethoxazole or minocycline.

Contagious Viral Infections

Many outbreaks of specific viral infections have been described in relation to team sports. The genus *Enterovirus* (of the Picornaviridae family) includes the echoviruses, coxsackieviruses A and B, polioviruses, rhinoviruses, and the enteroviruses. Each of these, in turn, is separated into multiple serotypes. These enteroviruses may be responsible for many clinical syndromes, including upper respiratory tract infections, aseptic meningitis, encephalitis, undifferentiated febrile illness, pleurodynia, and myopericarditis (10). Outbreaks of aseptic meningitis and other illness related to echoviruses, as well as coxsackieviruses, have been described among members of high school football teams (11,12). These reports show that, in the setting of an outbreak, attack rates among members of an athletic team may be significantly elevated as compared with others in the community. Transmission may occur by person-to-person contact, as well as by common source exposure. Poor hygienic practices, such as sharing squeeze bottles, dunking cups directly into a water source, or drinking directly from a water cooler spout, should therefore be strongly discouraged (12).

Person-to-person transmission during a football game has also been implicated in an outbreak of a Norwalk-like virus related to gastroenteritis. A game between North Carolina and Florida football teams resulted in illness in 47 players and 18 staff. Primary cases in the outbreak were traced back to a box lunch (turkey sandwich) that was served in North Carolina on the day before the game. Many of these individuals developed nausea, vomiting, and diarrhea before or during the game. As such, skin and uniforms were soiled with feces and vomitus, facilitating spread by person-to-person contact. Interestingly, all of the affected players on the Florida team played on the offense. Given the very similar timing of the illness, this was most likely due to the severity of illness in certain North Carolina defenders who made most of the tackles in the game. This report clearly illustrates the importance of isolating individuals with acute gastroenteritis and excluding them from such competition (13).

Epstein-Barr virus (EBV) infection is highly prevalent and infects most people by age 30. Infection in children is often asymptomatic, whereas college and military age populations experience significant illness. Infectious mononucleosis is the most common presentation, with sore throat, fever, and cervical lymphadenopathy. Splenomegaly occurs in about half of the cases. A peripheral blood count may show more than 50% mononuclear cells with more than 10% atypical lymphocytes. A heterophile antibody is present in about 90% of cases but may appear late in the course of illness. The differential diagnosis for heterophile-negative infectious mononucleosis includes cytomegalovirus infection, acute retroviral syndrome due to primary HIV infection, toxoplasmosis, and viral hepatitis. EBV treatment is supportive. Acetaminophen or nonsteroidal anti-inflammatory drugs (NSAIDs) may be used for symptomatic relief, though NSAIDs should be avoided in the presence of thrombocytopenia or hemolysis. Treatment with corticosteroids is indicated for infection complicated by impending airway compromise, severe thrombocytopenia, or hemolytic anemia. Use of corticosteroids in uncomplicated cases is controversial. Risk of splenic rupture is present, and contact sports and heavy lifting should be avoided for the first 2-3 weeks of illness and until splenomegaly is resolved. Training may be resumed 3 weeks after onset of illness if the spleen is not markedly enlarged or painful, the patient is afebrile, LFTs are normal, and pharyngitis is resolved. Strenuous exercise and contact sports can be resumed 1 month after the onset of illness if there is no splenomegaly and the above conditions are met. One may consider the use of ultrasound for more specific splenic measurements (3,10).

Case Study 7-1

An 18-year-old male football player presents to the training room with a five-day history of an extremely sore throat. The athletic trainer evaluating the patient refers him to your office on the same day.

On exam, the patient appears ill. He has a temperature of 100.8°F; a moderately erythematous pharynx and marked anterior cervical adenopathy are appreciated. The abdominal examination is unremarkable. There is no left upper quadrant tenderness or palpable splenomegaly. Rapid strep test on the patient is negative; however, the mono spot test is positive. The patient is diagnosed with infectious mononucleosis and advised to discontinue his involvement in football or any sort of training activity until a follow-up visit in three weeks. Laboratory tests for liver functions are ordered but prove unremarkable.

Three weeks later, the patient claims that he has had complete resolution of symptoms. The physical exam shows resolution of the adenopathy and no evidence of splenomegaly. The patient is advised that he may resume non-contact training immediately and full-contact training in one week. These recommendations are communicated to the athletic trainer after receiving consent from the patient.

Severe acute respiratory syndrome (SARS) is an illness caused by a coronavirus. The communicability of this illness has been well documented (14). As a result of this syndrome, the 2003 Women's World Cup Soccer tournament was moved from China to the United States. Outbreaks in Canada caused concern among sports organizations that competed there, including the National Basketball Association, Major League Baseball, and the National Hockey League. These cases highlight the fact that physicians who provide care to teams that travel should be aware of local and regional health issues.

Blood-Borne Pathogens

The risk for transmission of blood-borne pathogens (HIV, hepatitis B, hepatitis C) during sports activities is quite low. Given the extreme consequences of such an infection, however, it is imperative to follow guidelines to reduce such risk even further. Hepatitis B appears to be the most transmissible of these agents due to high levels of circulating virus in the blood and increased ability to survive in the environment. Risk for acquisition of HIV seems to be the lowest, with risk for hepatitis C infection somewhere in-between.

Several clusters of hepatitis B infection related to sports activities have been described. Among members of a sumo-wrestling club and among members of an American football team, both in Japan, transmission occurred most likely through percutaneous exposure to bleeding wounds (15,16). Another cluster occurred among a group of Swedish athletes participating in track finding (orienteering). In this case, the most likely source appeared to be contaminated water used to clean wounds sustained during the activity (17). An effective recombinant vaccine is available, and the American Academy of Pediatrics recommends that all children and adolescents be immunized against hepatitis B (17). For this reason, vaccination should be a requirement to participate in team sports.

HIV and hepatitis C virus infections have not been described as resulting from participation in sports activities. Guidelines to prevent such an occurrence have been published (18,19). Return-to-play guidelines for athletes with hepatitis are given in Chapter 8, Table 8-8.

To prevent infection with blood-borne pathogens, "universal precautions" should be followed, These including proper adhesive dressings for any wounds before competition and prompt management of any wounds sustained in competition. If active bleeding occurs, participants should be removed from play as soon as possible for management, and any clothing that is saturated with blood should be changed. Small amounts of dried blood on clothing do not pose a significant infection risk. Health care personnel should follow guidelines set forth by the Occupational Safety and Health Administration (OSHA), including the use of disposable gloves when treating the athlete and the use of disposable towels and proper disinfecting agents for decontamination of environmental surfaces.

Infections Related to Water

Many infections, including some of those mentioned above, are caused or facilitated by exposure to water during sports activities. Acute diffuse otitis externa ("swimmer's ear") is most common in hot, humid environments. Water may become trapped in the ear, leading to irritation. Scratching the area with a finger or foreign object may then lead to skin abrasion, allowing for a mixed infection caused by skin flora. Gram negatives, including *Pseudomonas aeruginosa,* may play a significant role. Fungi also may be encountered, though pathogenicity is unclear; a hypersensitivity reaction may be present. The ear canal may become red and edematous and movement of the pinna may elicit pain. Cleansing of the area with hypertonic saline (3%) and application of Burow's solution (aluminum acetate in water; available over the counter) may be helpful in severe cases. Treatment is usually with neomycin, polymyxin, and hydrocortisone in an otic solution. Oral fluoroquinolones also may be used in severe cases; however, one must use these drugs with caution in athletes due to the potential development of tendonopathies associated with their use. This condition should be differentiated from acute localized otitis externa arising from a furuncle due to *Staphylococcus aureus* or group A *Streptococcus*, for which the treatment would be systemic antibiotics with drainage of a lesion, if appropriate (3,10,20).

Exposure to contaminated fresh water in kayaking, orienteering, or swimming in lakes or rivers may lead to gastrointestinal infection with *Giardia, Cryptosporidium, Salmonella, Shigella*, or *Aeromonas*. After a 10-14 day incubation period, *Giardia* may cause multiple symptoms, including anorexia, bloating, and flatulence, or belching with or without vomiting or diarrhea. For diagnosis, antigen detection assays are superior to direct stool for ova and parasites. Treatment is usually with metronidazole 250 mg three times a day for 5-7 days (3,10,20).

Surface water (lakes, rivers, ponds) may also become contaminated with *Cryptosporidium* from infected humans, wildlife, and livestock (10). Outbreaks related to swimming pool water have also been described, as this agent is relatively resistant to chlorination. Affected individuals develop watery diarrhea, usually with a self-limited course, over 2-4 weeks.

Treatment is primarily symptomatic, as no reliable treatment is available. The diarrhea may be chronic in the immunocompromised (20).

Aeromonas may cause gastroenteritis or may contaminate open wounds, occasionally leading to a severe, rapidly progressive cellulitis. *Salmonella* and *Shigella* may lead to dysentery (bloody diarrhea) (20).

Leptospirosis outbreaks have been associated with participation in certain triathlons and other races involving fresh water exposure. These have occurred both in the US (Lake Springfield, Illinois) and abroad (Segama River, Malaysian Borneo) (21,22). Water is contaminated by wild and domestic animals, which serve as reservoirs for leptospires and shed the organisms in their urine. Infection may occur from direct contact with contaminated water (10). Conjunctival exposure and gastrointestinal exposure through swallowing water likely play a role. The incubation period is usually 5-14 days. The disease generally is biphasic with an acute septicemic phase that may be characterized by fever, headache, myalgias, conjunctival suffusion, abdominal pain, nausea, vomiting, diarrhea, and skin rashes. Muscle tenderness, particularly in the lumbar spine and the calves, may be a prominent clinical finding. The immune phase of illness is marked by defervescence. It may last 4-30 days, and aseptic meningitis is a common finding (10). Weil's disease is a severe form of the infection, noted by impaired renal and hepatic function (22). Fortunately, in the described outbreaks, no athletes developed the most severe complications of the infection. Treatment is usually with doxycycline 100 mg twice a day for outpatients and with intravenous penicillin for hospitalized patients. Chemoprophylaxis may be achieved with doxycycline 200 mg orally each week and has been highly efficacious in protection of military personnel (23). Some participants in the "Eco-Challenge" in Malaysian Borneo took prophylactic doxycycline 100 mg each day with some protective effect, but this was not statistically significant (22).

Vaccine-Preventable Illness

Numerous outbreaks of vaccine-preventable infections have been described on sports teams. Measles, in particular, is highly contagious, as it may be spread by direct contact with droplets or by airborne nuclei. Vaccination with MMR (live-attenuated measles, mumps, and rubella) is recommended (24). Hepatitis B vaccination is also recommended (24). Hepatitis A vaccination, while not formally recommended under NCAA and other guidelines, is quite reasonable, as outbreaks have occurred among sports teams. This vaccine is recommended for individuals living in or traveling to areas with high rates of infection. A combined hepatitis A and B vaccine is now available. Tetanus and diphtheria toxoid (Td) vaccination should be kept up-to-date as well (24).

Varicella vaccination or evidence of immunity would also be a reasonable recommendation. Yearly immunization against influenza should also be considered.

It is difficult to develop specific guidelines with respect to sports participation with fever. It is known that fever negatively affects performance by decreasing strength, endurance, and concentration. It is often recommended that "strenuous" conditioning and competition be avoided in the febrile state ($\geq 38°C$). One should also avoid such exertion in the presence of malaise, myalgias, shortness of breath, vomiting, or diarrhea. Given the frequency of upper respiratory infections, it may be reasonable to continue to exercise in the absence of systemic involvement (fever, lymphadenopathy, myalgias, malaise).

REFERENCES

1. **Nieman DC.** Is infection risk linked to exercise workload? Med Sci Sports Exerc. 2000;32(7):S406-11.
2. **Brenner IKM, Pang NS, Shephard RJ.** Infections in athletes. Sports Med. 1994; 17(2):86-107.
3. **Beck CK.** Infectious diseases in sports. Med Sci Sports Exerc. 2000;32(7):S431-8.
4. **Adams BB.** Which skin infections are transmitted between athletes? Br J Sports Med. 2000;34:413-4.
5. **Goodman RA, Thacker SB, Solomon SL, et al.** Infectious diseases in competitive sports. JAMA. 1994;271:862-7.
6. **Habif TP, Campbell JL, Quitadamo MJ, Zug KA.** Skin Disease: Diagnosis and Treatment. St. Louis: Mosby; 2001:196-205.
7. **Belongia EA, Goodman JL, Holland EJ, et al.** An outbreak of herpes gladiatorum at a high school wrestling camp. N Engl J Med. 1991;325:906-10.
8. **Ludlam H, Cookson B.** Scrum kidney: epidemic pyoderma caused by a nephritogenic *Streptococcus pyogenes* in a rugby team. Lancet. 1986;331-3.
9. **Lindenmayer JM, Schoenfeld S, O'Grady R, Carney JK.** Methicillin-resistant *Staphylococcus aureus* in a high school wrestling team and the surrounding community. Arch Intern Med. 1998;158:895-9.
10. **Mandell GL, Bennett JE, Dolin R.** Principles and Practice of Infectious Diseases. Philadelphia: Churchill Livingstone; 2000:1888-919.
11. **Baron RC, Hatch MH, Kleeman K, MacCormack JN.** Aseptic meningitis among members of a high school football team: an outbreak associated with echovirus 16 infection. JAMA. 1982;248:1724-7.
12. **Alexander JP, Chapman LE, Pallansch TJ, et al.** Coxsackievirus B_2 infection and aseptic meningitis: a focal outbreak among members of a high school football team. J Infect Dis. 1993;167:1201-5.
13. **Becker KM, Moe CL, Southwick KL, MacCormack JN.** Transmission of Norwalk virus during a football game. N Engl J Med. 2000;343:1223-7.
14. **Wenzel RP, Edmond MB.** Managing SARS amid uncertainty. N Engl J Med. 2003;348:1947-8.

15. **Kashiwagi S, Hayashi J, Ikematsu H, et al.** An outbreak of hepatitis B in members of a high school sumo wrestling club. JAMA. 1982;248:213-4.

16. **Tobe K, Matsuura K, Ogura T, et al.** Horizontal transmission of hepatitis B virus among players of an American football team. Arch Intern Med. 2000;160:2541-5.

17. **American Academy of Pediatrics.** Human immunodeficiency virus and other blood-borne pathogens in the athletic setting. Pediatrics. 1999;104:1400-3.

18. **Mast EE, Goodman RA, Bond WW, et al.** Transmission of blood-borne pathogens during sports: risk and prevention. Ann Intern Med. 1995;122:283-5.

19. **National Collegiate Athletic Association.** Bloodborne Pathogens and Intercollegiate Athletics. NCAA Guideline 2II. Overland Park, KS; August 2000.

20. **Buescher ES.** Infections associated with pediatric sport participation. Pediatri Clin North Am. 2002;49(4):743-51.

21. **Centers for Disease Control and Prevention.** Update: leptospirosis and unexplained acute febrile illness among athletes participating in triathlons-Illinois and Wisconsin, 1998. MMWR Morb Mortal Wkly Rep. 1998;47:673-6.

22. **Selvar J, Bancroft E, Winthrop K, et al.** Leptospirosis in "Eco-Challenge" athletes, Malaysian Borneo, 2000. Emerg Infect Dis. 2003;9(6):702-7.

23. **Takafuji ET, Kirkpatrick JW, Miller RN, et al.** An efficacy trial of doxycycline chemoprophylaxis against leptospirosis. N Engl J Med. 1984;310:497-500.

24. **National Collegiate Athletic Association.** Medical Evaluations, Immunizations and Records. NCAA Guideline 1b. Overland Park, KS; June 2000.

8

■ ■ ■

Gastrointestinal Issues
in Sports Medicine

Balakrishnan (Balu) Natarajan, MD

In a large number of studies over the past 20 years, athletes in many sports have reported gastrointestinal symptoms. Large numbers of marathon runners have reported such symptoms (1). One questionnaire, sent to more than 600 endurance athletes in the Netherlands, found a 79% prevalence of lower gastrointestinal symptoms among triathletes while running. The effect of symptoms on activity, however, appeared to be minimal; nearly all of these athletes continued activity despite their symptoms, and less than 6% of them used medication for relief (2). Gastrointestinal symptoms in athletes may be caused by problems resulting from the specific physiologic effects of physical activity, such as lower abdominal cramping and frequent bowel movements among runners, or they may be the manifestations of illnesses that occur in athletic and nonathletic populations alike. The clinician must therefore consider not only a wide differential diagnosis when caring for the athlete with gastrointestinal symptoms but also the special needs and risks of this patient group, for whom management of the GI problem must also account for a safe return-to-sport plan.

Physiologic Effects of Exercise

Splanchnic Blood Flow

During exercise, the body undergoes significant physiologic changes, leading to a hypoperfusion of the gastrointestinal tract (3). In the first few minutes of activity, 15% of central blood volume is shunted to working skeletal muscle. As a person continues that activity, the body's core temperature elevates, leading to a shunting of 20% blood volume to the skin for cooling. In order to maintain central blood volume, flow is directed away from other organs, including the gastrointestinal tract. In the process, the athlete can experience up to 80% reduction of normal intestinal blood flow. Hypoperfusion of the gastrointestinal tract can be exacerbated by volume depletion, a hot environment, and poor acclimation to the heat.

Neuroendocrine Changes

Many neuroendocrine and humeral changes are associated with intense activity (4). Levels of vasoactive intestinal peptide, secretin, pancreatic polypeptide, somatostatin, peptide histidine isoleucine, gastrin, glucagon, motilin, catecholamines, endorphins, and prostaglandins all change during exercise. In addition, cortisol, norepinephrine, and epinephrine levels have been found to be elevated after long-distance running. With so many variables and their complex interactions, the root causes and clinical significance of these exercise-related changes are hard to determine (4).

Effects on Immune Function

The protective effect of the gastrointestinal mucosa may be diminished under high mechanical and biochemical stresses, such as those experienced by the endurance athlete. This can lead to an increased uptake of toxins and immunogens in the gastrointestinal tract, leading to a reduction of physical performance and increased propensity for infection (5). Elevated plasma endotoxin levels have been found among triathletes and ultramarathoners. In one study, nausea, vomiting, and diarrhea correlated significantly with endotoxin levels (4). Some authors have proposed that the athlete's diet may have a significant effect on gastrointestinal immunity (5).

Potential Protective Effects

In contrast to these potentially deleterious effects, physical activity may also have a positive effect on the gastrointestinal system. Exercise may reduce the risks of colon cancer, cholelithiasis, and constipation (6). The underlying mechanisms for these observations are poorly understood.

Common Gastrointestinal Problems

There are many gastrointestinal injuries and illnesses (Table 8-1). Common causes of gastrointestinal symptoms in athletes include too much anxiety and stress, upper gastrointestinal motility problems, lower gastrointestinal motility problems, gastrointestinal bleeding, blunt abdominal trauma, and infectious and viral illnesses that are likewise common in the general population.

Anxiety and Stress Reaction

Precompetitive anxiety can have both facilitative and debilitative effects among athletes (7). Gastrointestinal manifestations can include dyspepsia, heartburn, abdominal cramping, diarrhea, and vomiting (8). In one study, 24% of athletes with lower gastrointestinal symptoms attributed them to stress (4). There may be a physiologic explanation for this observation; stress has been associated with alterations in gastric acid secretion, gastric and colonic blood flow, and intestinal motility. The widespread use of ergogenic aids warrants direct questions about their use, because they can be associated with both neuropsychologic and gastrointestinal effects.

Treatment of stress typically does not require medication and may be aided by a sports psychologist, who may use a combination of reassurance, education, behavioral modification, and relaxation exercises (8).

Upper Gastrointestinal Motility Problems

Upper gastrointestinal symptoms, such as dyspepsia, heartburn, anorexia, nausea, and vomiting, have been described in athletes in numerous studies (9-11). Most surveys have analyzed the experience of runners, but symptoms have been described among swimmers and cyclists as well. Few studies have analyzed gastrointestinal symptoms in the traditional team setting.

Table 8-1	Common Causes of Abdominal Symptoms
Infectious	• Gastroenteritis • Hepatitis • Appendicitis/diverticulitis/cholecystitis • Urinary tract infection • Pelvic inflammatory disease
Neoplastic	• Gastrointestinal tract solid tumor • Lymphoma
Endocrine	• Thyroid disease • Pancreatic and biliary disease
Medication	• Prescription, over-the-counter, or illicit drugs • Supplements
Autoimmune	• Inflammatory bowel disease
Trauma	• Gastrointestinal organs, genitourinary organs
Vascular	• Cardiac ischemia • Mesenteric ischemia • Dehydration/hypovolemia
Other	• Peptic ulcer disease • Irritable bowel syndrome • Constipation • Specific foods or beverages • Ruptured ovarian cyst • Ectopic pregnancy • Nephrolithiasis • Hyperthermia

The cause of these symptoms may be multifold; research has attempted to define the contributory effects of many factors, as listed in Table 8-2.

The frequency, amplitude, and duration of esophageal contractions decline with increasing exercise intensity (3). In one study involving an intraesophageal pH probe, running produced significantly more minutes of gastroesophageal reflux (GER) than rest (12). GER was associated with symptoms of belching in that series. In another study involving a pH probe, volunteers were analyzed for GER during rest and during running, lifting, and biking. Running was associated with the most symptoms (13).

Research has been helpful in identifying the potential interaction between exercise and gastric emptying time. At lower levels of exertion, gastric emptying increases, possibly as a consequence of the mechanical effect of abdominal contractions. As intensity increases, however, higher levels of catecholamines and humeral factors, along with hypoperfusion of the gastrointestinal tract, may lead to decreased gastric emptying times (9). This may explain why surveys have found that runners complain more during hard runs than easy runs. There also may be a physiologic gastrointestinal adaptation over time; novice runners are typically more symptomatic than experienced runners (10).

Gastric juice content and acidity have not been found to be a major contributor to upper gastrointestinal symptoms (9). Exertion does not seem to alter gastric acidity. Some studies have attempted to reduce effects of exercise with the use of medication. While a few studies have found symptomatic relief among runners using ranitidine and cimetidine, study numbers were small, and long-term effects of the use of such medications in athletes are unknown (9,12,14,15). More recently, a study analyzed the effects of omeprazole on GER. While an ambulant pH system demonstrated reduced GER, runners did not report symptomatic relief. Thus, gastric acidity is likely not the sole explanation for gastrointestinal symptoms among runners (16).

Despite numerous studies, no single cause has been determined for upper gastrointestinal symptoms in athletes. A diagnostic approach to these symptoms is detailed later in this chapter.

Table 8-2   Potential Etiologies of Upper Gastrointestinal Symptoms in Athletes

- Esophageal contractions and their changes with exercise intensity
- Reduced esophageal motility due to hypoperfusion
- Changes in lower esophageal sphincter tone and associated gastroesophageal reflux
- Changes in gastric emptying time
- Contents of gastric juice

Lower Gastrointestinal Motility Problems

Most surveys have found lower gastrointestinal symptoms to be even more prevalent among athletes than upper gastrointestinal symptoms. Major side effects of activity, particularly running, include lower abdominal cramping, bowel movement urge, increased frequency of bowel movements, and diarrhea (9). These effects, commonly referred to as "runner's trots, " increase in direct relation to the level of physical exertion (8). As with upper gastrointestinal symptoms, the cause is unknown and may be multifactorial. Research has focused on the variables listed in Table 8-3.

Case Study 8-1

A 22-year-old cyclist presented with 2 weeks of abdominal cramps and loose stools associated with activity. He reported increased intensity of training due to an upcoming competition, and he related the use of a new sports drink and supplements to enhance his performance.

The physical examination was normal.

Analysis of the nutritional content of the sports drink revealed a 12% carbohydrate concentration. The cyclist replaced his sports drink with one that had a 6% carbohydrate concentration, and his symptoms resolved over the next week.

Few studies have analyzed the biomechanical effects of exercise. One group measured vibration of the abdominal region during running and bicycling and found significantly greater results among subjects while running. Study numbers, however, were small, and further research is necessary to determine if biomechanical effects explain the generally higher percentage of symptoms among runners than cyclists (17).

One study has looked at the effects of reduced gastrointestinal blood flow among marathoners. Correlating gastrointestinal symptoms with volume status, the authors found that body weight loss was a significant predictor (9). Among those long-distance runners who lost more than 4% of their body weight, 80% had gastrointestinal symptoms. This at least indirectly supports the theory of splanchnic hypoperfusion.

Table 8-3   Potential Etiologies of Lower Gastrointestinal Symptoms in Athletes

- Mechanical effects of activity
- Hypoperfusion of the splanchnic circulation
- Reduced absorption of water from stool
- Alterations in colonic motility
- Diet
- Changes in neuroendocrine modulation

Some investigators have attempted to define the role of orocecal transit time in athletes' symptoms. Analyses of both orocaecal and whole-gut transit time have shown equivocal results (18). Unfortunately, it is difficult to control for diet, underlying processes such as irritable bowel syndrome, and timing of oral intake in relation to physical activity.

To further elucidate the question of colonic motility, one group followed a number of subjects, observed diet and bowel habits, and studied transit times. Results were likewise equivocal, and the authors concluded that colonic function is not significantly affected by exercise (9). They proposed that changes in diet, which may be associated with increasing activity, could lead to changes in orocecal transit times.

A telephone survey of triathlon participants attempted to answer the question of dietary influence. These athletes reported that large amounts of fat, fiber, and protein were associated with gastrointestinal symptoms (4). Other studies have not confirmed these results. While some investigators have tried to determine the optimal level of carbohydrate in fluid supplements, they have not drawn consistent conclusions with regard to prevention of gastrointestinal complaints.

As with the proximal gastrointestinal tract, no clear cause has been identified with regard to lower gastrointestinal symptoms in athletes.

Gastrointestinal Bleeding

Gastrointestinal bleeding among athletes can range from occult blood loss to frank hematochezia. Some extreme cases have been described in which subtotal colectomy was required after long distance events (19). Studies of ultramarathoners have found that 85% have heme-positive post-race stools (8). The percentages are much lower among marathoners and cyclists, but may be as high as 22% (9).

Case Study 8-2

A 62-year-old male ran his fourteenth marathon. He presented after the event to the medical tent with lower abdominal cramping and bloody diarrhea. He reported occasional cramps and loose stools while running but no previous hematochezia. Prior to the marathon, he had been asymptomatic and had trained for this marathon appropriately. He denied the use of medications. Physical examination was unrevealing.

Because his abdominal pain progressed, the patient was sent to the hospital and underwent CT scan of the abdomen, which revealed focal thickening of the sigmoid colon.

The patient was taken to the operating room to restore blood flow to the ischemic sigmoid colon. He tolerated the procedure well but retired from marathon running.

Post-event endoscopic studies have demonstrated gastric antral erosions, patchy areas of hyperemia, eroded gastrointestinal mucosa, and ischemic colitis (9); most of these findings have been observed within 48 hours of endurance events. When athletes have undergone endoscopy 4 or more days after activity, examinations have been normal. Most investigators believe that these observations support the concept of hypoperfusion of the splanchnic circulation during exercise. Other causes of bleeding may include the use of NSAIDs and, in theory, repetitive microtrauma to the abdominal viscera, but these theories have not been fully supported by investigation.

In the case of gross bleeding, a root cause must be determined. Gross gastrointestinal bleeding in an athlete may require aggressive evaluation and therapy.

Blunt Abdominal Trauma

Blunt abdominal trauma is rare in the endurance events described earlier, but is more common in contact sports. Important traumatic injuries are listed in Table 8-4.

The most common of these entities is epigastric contusion. An unguarded blow to the epigastric region can affect the neural solar plexus, leading to temporary spasm of the diaphragm with consequent respiratory paralysis. Athletes describe this phenomenon as "getting the wind knocked out" (20,21). Knee and abdominal flexion typically resolve symptoms.

A rectus sheath hematoma occurs after direct trauma to the abdomen, leading to muscular hemorrhage. Athletes report sudden, severe abdominal pain, and rapid swelling can occur (20). It is important to watch for this entity, since significant bleeding can occur and can occasionally require surgical repair of a ruptured vessel.

Diaphragmatic rupture is caused by blunt chest or abdominal trauma, and leads to a herniation of abdominal contents into the chest. Symptoms include dyspnea and chest pain, as well as the symptoms of bowel obstruction. This injury is associated with other major organ ruptures or fractures in a large percentage of cases. Patients will occasionally present with symptoms hours after the initial injury (20).

Table 8-4   Important Injuries Sustained after Blunt Trauma to the Abdomen

• Epigastric contusion	• Rupture of the spleen
• Rectus sheath hematoma	• Laceration of the liver
• Rupture of the diaphragm	• Rupture of the stomach and intestines

Splenic rupture, while rare, is the most frequent cause of death due to abdominal injury in sport (20). The overall incidence in sport is unknown. Due to the capsular structure of the spleen, bleeding can be asymptomatic until many days after the initial trauma. Symptoms may include sharp abdominal pain on the left side, followed by constant, dull discomfort in the abdomen or left flank. Diaphragmatic irritation can lead to referred shoulder discomfort.

Liver lacerations are not very common in most contact sports (20). They are usually associated with high-speed accidents and a blow to the right upper quadrant of the abdomen. Patients will present with right upper abdominal pain, and treatment is guided by the severity of the laceration.

Gastric and intestinal rupture are rare (20). Patients will present with signs and symptoms of an acute abdomen, and they require urgent abdominal exploration and repair.

All of these entities can be distinguished diagnostically with the assistance of computed tomography, diagnostic peritoneal lavage, and ultrasound. Diagnostic testing and treatment for blunt trauma involving the abdomen are detailed later in this chapter.

Medical Illness

Athletes are prone to medical illnesses like the rest of the population. Inflammatory bowel disease, peptic ulcer disease, GER, and pancreatitis should be considered. In some situations, athletes may be especially vulnerable to infections, due to travel and the sharing of quarters with other team members. These infections include gastroenteritis, "traveler's diarrhea," hepatitis, and infectious mononucleosis.

Typically viral, acute gastroenteritis peaks in the winter among city dwellers and in the summer among those who participate in rural or outdoor sports (8). Symptoms are usually self-limited and include fevers, myalgias, nausea, emesis, abdominal cramping, and loose stools or diarrhea. Rare cases of *Giardia* have been described among athletes (19). "Traveler's diarrhea," which affects the international athlete in particular, should be ruled out, since treatment requires the use of antibiotics.

Hepatitis A, which is an acute process, causes 25% of viral liver infections in the United States and spreads by fecal-oral transmission (21). It is not associated with long-term complications. Conversely, hepatitis B and C pose challenges to the physician due to their chronicity and the potential disability involved. In fact, 10% of hepatitis B patients and 70% of hepatitis C patients will progress to chronic hepatitis (22). Hepatitis patients present with headache, fatigue, fevers, nausea, emesis, abdominal pain, decreased appetite, light-colored stools, and dark-colored urine. Jaundice develops 7-14 days after constitutional symptoms. Hepatitis B symptoms tend to be the most severe (21). Among athletes, hepatitis B may be transmitted through contaminated water used to clean wounds sustained during the sports event and through percutaneous exposure to bleeding wounds. Liver function tests will be markedly elevated, and viral serologies can be used to distinguish among the different entities. Hepatitis C infections have not been reported to be transmitted through sports activity.

Infectious mononucleosis may be a gastrointestinal concern in patients with splenomegally.

Diagnostic Approach to Abdominal Pain

Because of the breadth of diagnoses that may present with abdominal symptoms, a systematic approach is necessary (Figure 8-1). First, the chronicity of symptoms should be considered. If symptoms are acute, then the patient should be assessed to rule out a surgical abdomen. The history should include questions about blunt trauma.

Blunt Abdominal Trauma

Sideline physical examination may not be reliable in the event of blunt trauma (21). Evaluation of vital signs and of the abdomen often yields nonspecific findings. Focal tenderness, rebound tenderness, hypoactive bowel sounds, radiation of pain to the back or shoulder, and signs of intravascular volume depletion warrant close observation and further evaluation. Because the spleen is most likely to be injured and the liver is second, CT may be employed in ruling out organ rupture or laceration. Occasionally, a person may be too unstable to evaluate by CT; in such patients, diagnostic peritoneal lavage or ultrasound may be used as alternatives. Unfortunately, diagnostic peritoneal lavage cannot detect subcapsular or retroperitoneal bleeding (23).

Acute Symptoms (No Blunt Abdominal Trauma)

If blunt trauma is not involved but symptoms are acute, specific elements of the history can help to identify a surgical abdomen (24). Symptoms that favor a surgical abdomen are listed in Table 8-5; symptoms that favor a nonsurgical abdomen are listed in Table 8-6.

As with blunt abdominal trauma, focal tenderness, rebound tenderness, hypoactive bowel sounds, radiation of pain to the back or shoulder, and signs of intravascular volume depletion warrant close observation and further evaluation. A rectal examination and pelvic examination are important components of the evaluation.

Once a surgical abdomen is ruled out in a person with acute symptoms, the clinician should look for clues that suggest an acute medical process. Cardiac ischemia should be considered and ruled out as needed with cardiac enzymes and electrocardiogram. Mesenteric ischemia should be considered when abdominal discomfort is out of proportion to physical

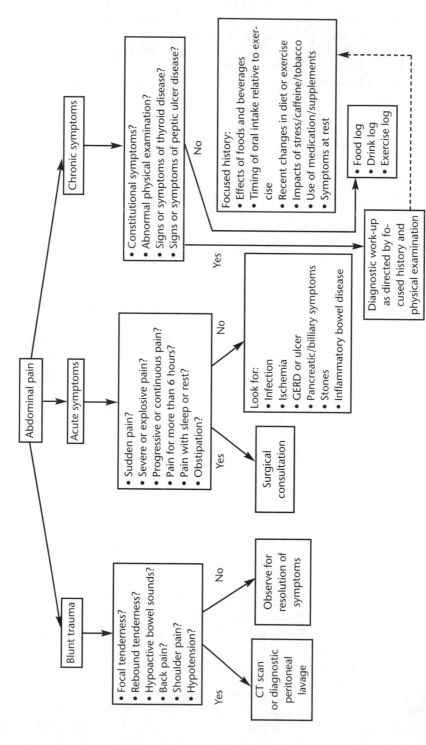

Figure 8-1 Diagnostic approach to abdominal pain.

Table 8-5   Symptoms that Suggest a Surgical Abdomen

- Sudden pain
- Severe or explosive pain
- Progressive and continuous pain
- Pain lasting more than 6 hours
- Pain associated with sleep or relative inactivity
- Obstipation

Table 8-6   Symptoms that Suggest a Nonsurgical Abdomen

- Gradual, mild, or moderate pain
- Intermittent or recurrent pain
- Pain that resolves in less than 6 hours
- Fever and chills
- Diarrhea

examination findings. While mesenteric angiography is the diagnostic gold standard, CT can often be helpful in confirming the diagnosis.

Classic signs and symptoms of gastroenteritis and hepatitis have been described earlier in this chapter. These and other infections, such as diverticulitis, urinary tract infection, and pelvic inflammatory disease, should be considered, particularly in the febrile patient.

Remaining causes of acute abdominal pain in the athlete include GERD, peptic ulcer disease, pancreatic and biliary disease, nephrolithiasis, inflammatory bowel disease, and hyperthermia. History and physical examination, along with judicious use of laboratory testing and endoscopy, can distinguish among these. Patients at risk for inflammatory bowel disease should be assessed for oral ulcers and dermatologic manifestations. Athletes who present after an endurance event should be checked for hyperthermia, which can be a cause of abdominal discomfort. In these individuals, a rectal temperature is the only reliable indicator of core temperature.

Chronic Symptoms

Chronic symptoms may be due to neoplasm, thyroid disease, cholclithiasis, peptic ulcer disease, GERD, irritable bowel syndrome, or diet. Patients should be assessed for constitutional symptoms, night sweats, weight changes, temporal wasting, lymphadenopathy, and enlargement of the liver or spleen (3). A thorough thyroid examination should be performed, and attention should be given to associated reflexes, ocular findings, and dermatologic signs. For those patients who have chronic symptoms suggestive of esophageal or gastroduodenal pathology, upper endoscopy may be helpful.

Table 8-7   Focused History for Athletes with Gastrointestinal Symptoms

- Effects of various foods and beverages
- Timing of oral intake in relation to exercise
- Recent changes in training or diet
- Impact of stress, caffeine, tobacco, and alcohol on symptoms
- Use of medications or supplements
- Symptoms that occur during periods of rest or relative inactivity

---

Athletes who do not have an acute abdomen and who do not exhibit characteristics of the previously mentioned medical illnesses are likely to have either irritable bowel syndrome or a gastrointestinal motility problem secondary to the combination of oral intake and exercise. In these individuals, history should focus on the issues listed in Table 8-7.

A detailed history, which may include a food, drink, and exercise log maintained over a period of days or weeks, may be helpful in determining a treatment plan to reduce symptoms.

With the above approach, the clinician should be able to determine which gastrointestinal symptoms among athletes require emergent treatment, and which can be seen over a period of time.

Treatment and Return to Sport

Blunt Abdominal Trauma

Treatment of the athlete after blunt trauma to the abdomen is based on the severity of the injury sustained. In the case of liver laceration or splenic rupture, the patient may need surgical intervention. Even if the injury does not require laparotomy, the athlete will need close observation to ensure stability. Thus, return to play should not be considered until abdominal contents are thought to be fully healed. When this determination has been made, a period of noncontact activity is indicated, followed by a gradual return to contact sports. While specific guidelines for return to play do not exist, most authors suggest a minimum of 4 months of rest before returning athletes to collision sports after serious visceral injury.

Post-Operation

Athletes should be managed carefully after abdominal surgery. Two months postoperatively, skin wounds have achieved only half of their tensile strength (9). For most abdominal wounds, guidelines suggest supervised exercise at 4 weeks after surgery, noncontact athletics at 8 weeks, and unrestricted return to sports at 12 weeks. For appendectomies and hernia operations, the guidelines reduce these waiting periods by 50% (9).

Table 8-8   Return-to-Play Guidelines for Athletes with Hepatitis

- Persons with acute viral hepatitis may continue physical activity and mild-to-moderate training as tolerated by overall well-being and clinical condition but should not participate in strenuous activity or competitive sports until liver function tests have returned to normal.
- Persons with chronic persistent hepatitis should be allowed to participate in moderate physical activity. Routine medical follow-up is advised.
- Persons with chronic active hepatitis or cirrhosis should not participate in strenuous competitive sports but should be encouraged to partake in a low-level and graduated training program under the supervision of an experienced physician.

Infections

Infections should be treated based on the microbial source. Athletes with infectious processes are vulnerable to further illness or injury because of dehydration and febrile state. They also place teammates and opponents at risk through close contact.

Athletes with gastroenteritis should be held out of competition until they are no longer febrile and no longer experience myalgias or diarrhea. They should also be euvolemic. When they do return, participants should attempt at least a few days of light activity before engagement at the usual level of intensity. Athletes should be made aware that gastrointestinal infections are preventable, and they should be encouraged to wash hands after contact with others. Additionally, they should eat adequately cooked food, wash all raw fruits and vegetables, and avoid sharing of beverage cans and water bottles.

Hepatitis treatment is based on the specific viral cause and chronicity. For athletes with hepatitis, consult Table 8-8 for proposed return-to-play guidelines (22).

Treatment for infectious mononucleosis is generally supportive. Analgesics may be needed for oropharyngeal symptoms.

Other Medical Illnesses

Treatment of the remaining medical illnesses should be based on the individual disease process. When these illnesses have been treated and have resolved, gradual return to full activity is advisable.

In the athlete suspected of having exercise-associated motility symptoms, a log of food intake, exercise, and symptoms should be documented over a period of 1 week. By doing so, the athlete may be able to identify triggers of symptoms and modify foods or timing of oral intake accordingly.

If these efforts are not helpful, the approaches listed in Table 8-9 may help reduce symptoms (3).

Table 8-9   Reducing Gastrointestinal Symptoms During Exercise

- Suggest a light meal several hours prior to competition, followed by jogging to stimulate gastrocolic reflex.
- If the athlete is not used to drinking a lot of fluids, encourage more fluid intake to improve hydration and reduce relative gastrointestinal ischemia.
- Adjust fiber in the athlete's diet, then follow symptoms.
- In endurance athletes, reduce mileage and intensity 20-40%, then increase slowly to previous levels to encourage gradual physiologic adjustments.
- Medications are typically not recommended due to lack of evidence about long-term side effects in the athlete.

Treatment of gastrointestinal bleeding requires identification and management of the underlying source. In the case of bleeding due to relative gastrointestinal ischemia, treatment should be aimed at improved splanchnic flow. Appropriate hydration is important in this endeavor (8).

Conclusion

Although gastrointestinal symptoms are frequently seen in the athlete, serious illness is rare. A detailed history and physical examination should aid the clinician in ruling out surgical processes and serious medical illnesses. For the majority of patients with mild, chronic symptoms, modification of diet and activity can be helpful in improving quality of exercise.

REFERENCES

1. **Riddoch C, Trinick T.** Gastrointestinal disturbances in marathon runners. Br J Sports Med. 1988;22(2):71-4.
2. **Peters HP, Bos M, Seebregts L, et al.** Gastrointestinal symptoms in long-distance runners, cyclists, and triathletes: prevalence, medication, and etiology. Am J Gastroenterol. 1999;94(6):1570-81.
3. **Natarajan B, Torres JL, Mellion MB.** Gastrointestinal problems. In: Mellion MB, et al., eds. Team Physician's Handbook, 3rd ed. Philadelphia: Hanley & Belfus; 2002:244-8.
4. **Peters HP, Akkermans LM, Bol E, Mosterd WL.** Gastrointestinal symptoms during exercise. Sports Med. 1995;20(2):65-76.
5. **Berg A, Muller HM, Rathmann S, Deibert P.** The gastrointestinal system-an essential target organ of the athlete's health and physical performance. Exerc Immunol Rev. 1999;5:78-95.
6. **Peters HP, DeWries WR, Vanberge-Henegouwen GP, Akkermans LM.** Potential benefits and hazards of physical activity and exercise on the gastrointestinal tract. Gut. 2001;48(3):435-9.
7. **Jones G, Hanton S.** Pre-competitive feeling states and directional anxiety interpretations. J Sports Sci. 2001;19(6):385-95.

8. **Bray JE.** Gastrointestinal problems in athletes. In: Mellion MB, et al., eds. Sports Medicine Secrets, 3rd ed. Philadelphia: Hanley & Belfus; 2003:250-4.

9. **Green GA.** Gastrointestinal disorders in the athlete. Clin Sports Med. 1992;11(2):453-70.

10. **Keeffe EB, Lowe DK, Goss JR, Wayne R.** Gastrointestinal symptoms of marathon runners. West J Med. 1984;141:481-4.

11. **Worme JD, Doubt TJ, Singh A, et al.** Dietary patterns, gastrointestinal complaints, and nutrition knowledge of recreational triathletes. Am J Clin Nutr. 1990; 51:690-7.

12. **Krauss BB, Sinclair JW, Castell DO.** Gastroesophageal reflux in runners. Ann Intern Med. 1990;112:429-33.

13. **Clark SC, Krauss BB, Sinclair J, Castell.** Gastroesophageal reflux induced by exercise in healthy volunteers. JAMA. 1989;261(24):3599-601.

14. **Moses FM, Baska RS, Peura DA, Deuster PA.** Effect of cimetidine on marathon-associated gastrointestinal symptoms and bleeding. Dig Dis Sci. 1991;36(10):1390-4.

15. **Baska RS, Moses FM, Deuster PA.** Cimetidine reduces running-associated gastrointestinal bleeding. Dig Dis Sci. 1990;35:956-60.

16. **Peters HP, DeKort AF, Van Krevelen H, et al.** The effect of omeprazole on gastro-oesophageal reflux and symptoms during strenuous exercise. Aliment Pharmacol Ther. 1999;13(8):1015-22.

17. **Rehrer NJ, Meijer GA.** Biomechanical vibration of the abdominal region during running and bicycling. J Sports Med Phys Fitness. 1991;31(2):231-4.

18. **Gil SM, Yazaki E, Evans DF.** Aetiology of running-related gastrointestinal dysfunction. How far is the finishing line? Sports Med. 1998;26(6):365-78.

19. **Eichner ER, Scott WA.** Exercise as disease detector. Phys Sportsmed. 1998; 26(3):41-52.

20. **Chang CJ, Graves DW.** Athletic injuries of the thorax and abdomen. In: Mellion MB, et al., eds. Team Physician's Handbook, 3rd ed. Philadelphia: Hanley & Belfus; 2002:441-59.

21. **Sevier TL, Roush MB.** Infections in athletes. In: Safran MR, et al., eds. Manual of Sports Medicine. Philadelphia: Lippincott-Raven; 1998:201-15.

22. **Harrington DW.** Viral hepatitis and exercise. Med Sci Sports Exerc. 2000;32(7):S422-30.

23. **Patton RM.** Thoracic and abdominal problems (including genitourinary injuries). In: Mellion MB, et al., eds. Sports Medicine Secrets, 3rd ed. Philadelphia: Hanley & Belfus; 2003:336-43.

24. **Bergman RT.** Assessing acute abdominal pain: a team physician's challenge. Phys Sportsmed. 1996;24(4):72-82.

9

Anemia, Blood Doping, and Other Hematologic Considerations in Athletes

Donald M. Christie Jr, MD

Blood lets the resting body "come alive." It delivers oxygen and energy substrates to active muscles and, at the same time, carries away metabolic wastes. Blood plays an essential role in water and mineral homeostasis, and it helps dissipate the heat produced by exercise. The right quantity and quality of red cell mass and plasma are crucial to optimal athletic performance.

Athletes may become anemic for the same reasons as nonathletes. Yet, by virtue of the body's responses to the stresses of training and competition and the often-extraordinary needs for "raw materials" that may put them at greater risk for deficiency states, athletes deserve special consideration whenever hematological evaluation appears necessary.

This chapter focuses on topics associated with blood that are especially pertinent to the care of athletes: pseudoanemia; iron-deficiency states (occult blood loss, dietary insufficiency, heavy training); exercise-associated hemolytic anemia ("footstrike" hemolysis); hemoglobinopathies and sports participation; unethical performance enhancement through blood doping; and athletes as blood donors.

Clinical Presentation

In many people, anemia is often discovered quite by happenstance when a complete blood count is performed in the course of a "routine" or other screening examination. On the other hand, unless an athlete has a pertinent personal or family history, a physician need not *routinely* assess hematological parameters in the course of a preparticipation screening examination (1). However, when this same "healthy" patient complains of undue fatigue or unexplained deterioration in performance, the sports physician must understand the likely effects of exercise on blood and blood production in order to evaluate the problem fairly.

A rapidly developing anemia-from hemorrhage or major hemolysis-produces immediate symptoms from sudden loss of blood volume and oxygen-carrying capacity, whereas a slowly developing anemia (often days to weeks in the making) may cause, especially in trained athletes accustomed both to the fatigue and the exhilaration of hard training and competition, only vague symptoms of fatigue, somewhat more than customary dyspnea on exertion, and a decrement in endurance performance. (The very different clinical presentations are in large part understood when considering the cardiovascular responses to different rates of blood loss, as shown in Table 9-1.) Significant deterioration in performance may appear only in very hard-training elite athletes and may be too mild to be noted otherwise in good, but not superb, performers. Enter the special perspective of sports medicine!

Case Study 9-1

A high school track coach advised his 17-year-old star sprinter to consult his physician for an unexplained deterioration in racing times. The young man at first denied any problem but, after further interviewing, he reported melena, which he had not wanted to mention to either his mother or his coach. He claimed no use of NSAIDs, other drugs, or alcohol.

Normal resting supine and sitting vital signs were taken. Aside from pallor of mucus membranes and nail beds, there were no abnormal physical findings. The dark stool was found to be strongly guaiac positive. The hematocrit value was 0.17 (17%). Upper gastrointestinal barium contrast fluoroscopy showed an active duodenal ulcer.

Treatment of ulcer disease in athletes should include rest from the stresses of training and competition, along with ferrous sulfate supplementation of an iron-rich diet. If no further GI blood loss is observed and normal red cell indices and serum iron studies are restored, this athlete may return to his training program next season.

Pseudoanemia of Athletes

A hematological variant seen in healthy, endurance-trained athletes, pseudoanemia does not represent a pathological process at all but a laboratory deception brought about by the body's early-phase adaptation to training.

Blood volume represents the sum of plasma volume and red cell volume (with a negligible contribution from leukocytes and platelets—the

Table 9-1   Cardiovascular Responses to Anemia

Cardiovascular Responses to Rapidly Developing Anemia
(from Sudden Blood Loss)

- Decreased plasma volume
- Decreased cardiac output
- Orthostatic hypotension
- Increased peripheral resistance as blood is shunted to central organs (viscera)

Cardiovascular Responses to Slowly Developing Anemia
(from "Slow Leak," Minor Hemolysis, Deficiency States)

- Increased plasma volume
- Increased peripheral vascular dilatation, producing decreased peripheral resistance (decreased blood pressure)
- Increased cardiac output from increased stroke volume
- Increased 2,3-diphosphoglycerate (DPG) binding in RBCs, causing a rightward shift in the oxyhemoglobin dissociation curve and enhancing the unbinding of O_2 at any given blood O_2 tension

"buffy coat"). Changes in these two major components generally are independent of the other and occur at very different rates. Red cell volume typically expands and contracts over weeks and months, as synthesis of erythropoietin (EPO), the principal regulating hormone, is modulated by renal oxygen tension that, barring cardiovascular or lung disease, reflects the oxygen tension of inspired air. The hypoxemia produced by intense exercise, as well as the associated secretion of adrenergic amines, androgens, and growth hormone, play a role in stimulating marrow red cell production. Plasma volume, on the other hand, expands and contracts over the course of minutes to days as a function of changes in extracellular fluid volume, plasma proteins, and pre- and post-capillary hydrostatic pressure—the balance of water and electrolytes modulated in large measure by the effects of secreted renin, aldosterone, antidiuretic hormone, and catecholamines (2).

Commencing endurance training increases an athlete's blood volume about 10% within a few days due to the plasma expansion of compensatory retention of salt and water and synthesis of albumin (3). Over 3 to 4 weeks, however, red cell mass increases and relative plasma volume decreases to result in the same red cell-to-plasma volume ratio as before training. Thus, if one happens to determine the hematocrit within the first 2 weeks of an athlete's training, one finds a decreased red cell-to-plasma volume ratio (a false or "pseudo" anemia) which, within another week or two, fades into normalcy as a new steady-state of the now-increased blood volume is achieved.

The increase in aerobic capacity noted several weeks after embarking on an endurance training program can be attributed, in part, to this augmentation in both red cell mass and plasma volume, obeying the mandates of Fick's Law governing maximal oxygen uptake by facilitating both oxygen carrying capacity and cardiac output, as well as to cardiovascular, pulmonary, and local muscle training adaptations. Alas, some overly ambitious and win-at-any-cost athletes have attempted to capitalize on unnatural expansion of each of these components (red cell mass and plasma volume) in order to surreptitiously and unethically boost endurance performance (see the section on Blood Doping later in this chapter).

Sophisticated methods assessing actual red cell volume (e.g., radioactive isotope labeling, carbon monoxide rebreathing, dye dilution) are impracticable in clinical circumstances. The hematocrit test, interpreted in the context of the duration of an athlete's training program, state of hydration, and the exclusion of blood loss or of decreased erythropoiesis from dietary deficiencies (see the section on Iron Deficiency and Depletion below), guides the astute clinician in distinguishing pseudoanemia—the dilutional "false" anemia of athletes, an acute response to endurance training—from a true decrease in red cell quantity and quality.

Iron Deficiency and Depletion

Athletes develop classical iron *deficiency* anemia for the same reasons as anyone else: major red cell loss (whether obvious or occult), insufficient intake of dietary iron, or impaired absorption and incorporation of iron. They may also become iron *depleted* without developing frank anemia, a condition possibly detrimental to performance. Such depletion or latent deficiency may occur despite usually adequate dietary intake and in the absence of blood loss, possibly reflecting impaired iron absorption and an increased elimination in sweat and shed epithelium (4).

Blood Loss

Among the well-known causes of blood loss are "classic" gastrointestinal ulcers and erosions (including those associated with the use of aspirin and aspirin-like medicines, drugs frequently used by athletes as well as by nonathletes), gastrointestinal and genitourinary tract tumors, and menorrhagia. In athletes, additional causes of blood loss include intense aerobic exercise and long, hard runs in hot weather, both of which may result in gastrointestinal and genitourinary bleeding. This is presumably caused by a combination of "shaking trauma" and ischemic visceral mucosal changes produced by dehydration and shunting of blood to skin and exercising muscle, resulting in transient ischemic injury (5-9) (see Chapter 8). Such blood loss is more prevalent in runners than in cyclists, lending some credence to the "shaking trauma" hypothesis, as well as to that of dehydration and visceral ischemia. While some patients may report abdominal cramping and even hematochezia or gross hematuria, many will have no specific complaint associated with such blood loss.

The alert clinician keeps these exercise-related sources of blood loss in mind, but given that such lesions have been shown to heal within a few days with rest and replenishment of fluid and electrolytes, the sports physician may have to do serial testing for stool occult blood, before and after intense exercise, to verify suspected exercise-induced gastrointestinal bleeding or a provocative field test, such as an interval workout on a suitably hot and dehydrating day, to confirm or refute a suspicion of exercise-induced hematuria.

One shouldn't be surprised to find a high incidence of this phenomenon, as mirrored in a study of interval workouts in middle-distance runners, 90% of whom showed at least one episode of post-workout microscopic hematuria over 4 weeks of biweekly workouts (8). (Blood loss from exercise-related hemolysis is discussed later in this chapter.) Gastrointestinal and genitourinary tumors are rare in young athletes, although they must be kept in mind (9,10), especially when additional risk factors prompt a more extensive evaluation.

Insufficient Dietary Intake

One might assume that athletes, with their greatly increased fuel needs and voracious appetites, would consume more than adequate amounts of iron. However, this may not be the case, especially in rapidly growing teenagers; athletes who, for whatever reason, tend to eat little or no meat; those who, in fact, eat grossly inadequate amounts of food, especially inadequate amounts of iron-rich foods; and women with heavy menstrual bleeding. *Strict vegetarians, while usually consuming adequate folate, may ingest inadequate amounts of iron and vitamin B_{12}.*

An athlete's eating habits often reflect concerns about weight, body image, and perceived cultural norms for size and shape more than sound nutrition principles. The problem of insufficient dietary iron intake plagues young women (because of their menses) more than young men (11-13). Amenorrheic women athletes, although not losing iron through menses, may nevertheless consume inadequate amounts of iron, folate, vitamin B_{12}, and protein, and are at greater risk for deficiency anemias. Kopp-Woodroffe and colleagues recorded the interesting and revealing stories of four young women athletes with this problem and their rewarding responses to a concerted treatment program that modified dietary and exercise regimens (13).

Iron Deficiency (Depletion) Without Anemia

In the earliest stage of iron deficiency—namely, iron depletion—the depletion of iron stores begins before total iron binding capacity (transferrin) increases and before serum iron and percent transferrin saturation decrease. Some have speculated that iron depletion alone leads to reduced physical capacity and produces nonspecific symptoms, such as fatigue, headache, and muscle cramping, presumably secondary to iron deficiency in myoglobin and metabolic enzymes. Thus, when athletes report undue fatigue or poor performance not easily explained by lack of sleep, poor training, or overtraining, iron depletion may be suspected, even when hemoglobin concentrations are not yet below the normal range. Low or borderline-low serum ferritin levels or a high soluble transferrin receptor (sTfR) level may provide a clue to this condition.

Repletion of iron stores might be expected to help lagging performance in these patients (14,15), but a closer look at the evidence shows that this is not certain (16).

Diagnosis

Finding a low hemoglobin concentration or hematocrit—that is, detecting "anemia"—should prompt the clinician to look for the classic changes of iron-deficiency anemia (Table 9-2): low hemoglobin concentration (or hematocrit); reduced red cell number; low serum iron and ferritin; high iron binding capacity (transferrin); diminished transferrin saturation, microcytosis (low mean cell volume, or MCV); elevated or normal reticulocyte count in the early stages of anemia (or in later stages "normal" or even low, when the marrow is unable to respond appropriately to erythropoietin stimulus for want of sufficient iron stores); and reduced mean corpuscular hemoglobin concentration (MCHC). These values are often reflected in microcytosis and hypochromia, an abnormal red cell morphology characterized by the appearance of small, pale cells seen during careful examination of a well-prepared Wright's-stained smear of peripheral blood. Measurement of the soluble transferrin receptor may improve sensitivity in assessing iron deficiency states in athletes.

Assessment of Iron Status

When one suspects iron depletion or "subclinical" (latent) iron deficiency (an intermediate category between "depletion" and overt anemia), assessment of

Table 9-2   Qualitative Test Results in Iron Deficiency States and Anemia

Stage	Hb	Fe	Ferritin	TIBC	%Sat	sTfR
Iron depletion	N	N	Low or low-N	N	N	High
Latent deficiency	N	Low	Low	High	Low	High
Overt anemia	Low	Low	Low	High	Low	High
Chronic disease	Low	Low	N to high-N	Low to low-N	Low	N

Hb = hemoglobin concentration; Fe = serum iron; Ferritin = serum ferritin; TIBC = total iron binding capacity; %Sat = percent transferrin saturation; sTfR = soluble transferrin receptor; N = within normal reference limits; Low = below normal limits; High = above normal limits body iron stores is necessary. ("Subclinical" is a misnomer if one truly suspects iron deficiency of any degree; the causes of undue fatigue or worsening performance are important "clinical" clues in their own right.)

In a "healthy" sedentary adult, serum ferritin is a valid surrogate measure of marrow iron stores. Heavy physical exercise, on the other hand, produces changes in blood constituents that, in many respects, mimic those noted in acute and chronic inflammatory states, including changes in ferritin levels and other markers of iron metabolism (16-18).

In the "anemia of chronic disease," inflammatory cytokines interfere with absorption and utilization of iron, as well as with the production and action of EPO (18). Markers of inflammation, such as increases in C-reactive protein, fibrinogen, and leukocytes, are seen with acute, intense activity, as well as with chronic overtraining (16,17,19). Serum ferritin may also increase such that, in heavy training in athletes with true iron deficiency or depletion, ferritin levels may not be low but, misleadingly, "low-normal."

A better marker is soluble transferrin receptor (sTfR) (20). Transferrin-bound iron attaches to targeted cells, such as erythroblasts, by interacting with a specific membrane receptor-transferrin receptor, a soluble form of which can be measured in serum. Soluble TfR reflects marrow erythropoiesis and is a better indicator than serum ferritin of true iron deficiency in athletes, as well as in the elderly and those with chronic disease, in whom serum ferritin levels may not reliably reflect body iron stores (21,22). The transferrin receptor-ferritin index (the ratio of sTfR level to log ferritin level) may improve the sensitivity of the diagnosis of iron deficiency in athletes, as well as in those with chronic disease states and acute and chronic inflammation (see Table 9-2) (21,23). Soluble TfR appears unaffected by intravascular hemolysis (24). Physicians should make sure their clinical reference laboratories perform accurate and reliable sTfR assays.

Rarely, direct assessment of marrow iron stores may be needed to confidently distinguish iron deficiency anemia from the anemia of chronic disease or overtraining. Alternatively, one could look at response to iron supplementation—the "relative" change in hemoglobin and ferritin, as well as sTfR levels, for example—while holding constant variables such as training volume.

"Relative anemia" is a useful concept to keep in mind when evaluating an athlete in whom one suspects anemia or subclinical iron deficiency but whose initial hemoglobin or iron parameter values may be in the "low-normal" range. By looking at the changes, in laboratory values over time, the physician may observe what effect an intervention—be it rest, change in training, improved diet, or use of iron supplements—may have had on the athlete's blood and thus more confidently affirm or refute the working diagnosis. Thus serial study of an athlete's laboratory values may help solve a diagnostic conundrum.

Treatment

Once a source of blood loss leading to iron deficiency is recognized and treated, or when it seems apparent from the patient's evaluation that the "cause" of iron deficiency or depletion is insufficient dietary iron, the physician can then counsel appropriate changes in diet. Whipple and colleagues demonstrated 80 years ago that no food beats liver and lean beef in speeding recovery from anemia due to blood loss (25). Note that the heme-iron of meat is better absorbed than the nonheme-iron in plants. For athletes unwilling or unable to consume larger amounts of iron-rich foods, such as meat, beans, nuts, whole-grain cereal products, and dark-green leafy vegetables, prescribe twice daily intake of ferrous iron, the only form absorbed by the gut.

The traditional dose of ferrous sulfate, 325 mg, in conventional tablet or liquid form, is more than can possibly be absorbed at one time, and one should prescribe a lesser dose, in a range of 32 to 65 mg, taken once or twice daily on an empty stomach, with the caution that the patient might experience abdominal cramping and constipation and observe dark, almost black, stools (11). Smaller initial doses may also minimize gastrointestinal distress. Supplementing iron intake with extra helpings of lean red meat is a "nicer" way of augmenting one's usual iron intake, to say nothing of the extra zinc, magnesium, vitamin B_{12}, and high-quality protein they also provide.

While few athletes fail to respond to adequate dietary or oral iron supplementation and require parenteral iron therapy, the clinician must never assume that therapy is complete until a few key tests—hemoglobin or hematocrit, ferritin, and soluble transferrin receptor (or, if sTfR is not available, serum iron, iron binding capacity, and percent transferrin saturation)—repeated every 4 weeks over a 3-month period verify marrow response, restoration of iron stores, and achievement of a normal quantity and quality of red cells as evidenced by normal red cell indices and morphology. Symptoms attributed to iron depletion and deficiency or to overt anemia should likewise resolve.

The goals of therapy for patients in iron-deficiency states can be summarized as

- Discovery and resolution of cause of iron depletion or deficiency
- Restoration of depleted iron reserves
- Restoration of red cell quantity and quality
- Resolution of symptoms
- Prevention of further deficiency

Screening

While routine screening of blood and iron values is not recommended for all athletes (1), physicians are justified in screening athletes at "high risk" for iron depletion or iron deficiency: menstruating women, especially those in endurance sports in which a low body weight seems important (for example, distance running, Nordic skiing, gymnastics); vegetarians; and very hard training athletes, especially those also trying to lose fat weight. At the same time as the clinician oversees treatment of patients with iron deficiency or iron depletion, he or she counsels others not to routinely consume iron supplements. Too much of this good thing is not better!

Footstrike Hemolysis

A form of accelerated red cell destruction, also known as "march hemoglobinuria," footstrike hemolysis has long been noted in soldiers and others whom march or run particularly long and hard on firm surfaces and on hot, dehydrating days (26). The hemoglobulinuria seen with footstrike hemolysis occurs 1 to 3 hours after the exercise bout. Local trauma to red cells coursing through this pedal gauntlet is an appealing hypothesis to explain the phenomenon, yet it is not the whole story (4,27-29). The "trauma" of repetitive, forceful muscle contraction may contribute to this hemolysis as well. Laboratory findings may include hemoglobinuria and decreased haptoglobin levels, which are sometimes difficult to assess in the presence of contracted plasma volume (dehydration). A mild reticulocytosis appears if the hemolytic stress is sufficient. However, Fallon and Bishop (30) found no consistent or convincing reticulocyte response to ultralong distance running, and some view chronic decrease in haptoglobin as yet another marker of trained athletes (31), implying that a low-grade, accelerated red cell destruction may accompany ongoing heavy training.

A few athletes will report seeing "bloody" urine (red-brown or coffee-colored) after a heavy workout or race. For many clinicians, this phenomenon is detected only if one checks the urine for free hemoglobin (as opposed to the hematuria composed of intact red cells from genitourinary tract bleeding, or myoglobin from rhabdomyolysis). On the other hand, increased numbers of red cells noted upon microscopic urine analysis, not just a positive test for hemoglobin, indicate actual genitourinary tract bleeding.

Hemoglobinopathies

The pathophysiology and resulting precarious circulatory and metabolic compensations in people with thalassemia major and sickle cell disease preclude their participation in vigorous physical activity and limit them to low-intensity exercise, such as walking, golf, and bowling. Athletes with the heterozygous form of sickle cell disease (HbSC) have impaired oxygen transport and lower exercise tolerance (32). Tissue hypoxia, such as that induced by intense exercise and compounded by dehydration, may trigger red cell sickling. Athletes with sickle trait also must be cautioned to avoid intense or prolonged exercise, with its attendant stresses of hypoxemia, heat, and dehydration, as well as exercise at high altitude, for such factors may provoke sickling, rhabdomyolysis, and "sickling-collapse," if not sudden death (33-35). Those with thalassemia minor (ß-thalassemia trait)— not an uncommon finding in an era of automated hematological screening that detects a very low MCV—can train and compete as well as anyone else. In all cases, performing accurate, reliable hemoglobin electrophoresis is essential to precisely identifying and distinguishing these conditions.

The informed physician should reassure and counsel affected athletes (and their trainers, coaches, and families) about the usually benign nature of these traits and what kinds of high-stress training and competition to avoid.

Blood Doping

A Brief (Shameful) History

While this chapter has focused on aspects of anemia and hematological conditions pertinent to athletes and other active people, attention must also be given to another problem: attempts to enhance performance by artificially and unethically increasing red cell mass or plasma volume.

Acute infusion of red cells into a conditioned athlete or, to a lesser extent, sudden plasma volume expansion results in a significant increase in aerobic capacity (36-39). In the 1970s, rumors circulated about unusual performance improvements in major competitions, including some distance races in the 1976 Olympic Games, as a result of blood transfusion. Indeed, rumor was laid to rest with the revelation of the shameful use of transfusions by some members of the United States cycling team at the 1984 Los Angeles Games (40,41).

Recombinant erythropoietin (rEPO) became commercially available in the late 1980s, and thereafter followed an epidemic of sudden death in otherwise superbly fit European cyclists, raising suspicions that surreptitious use of rEPO had backfired, presumably from a fatal arrhythmogenic complication of blood hyperviscosity produced by a combination of elevated red cell mass and dehydration, perhaps compounded by use of ergogenic adrenergic compounds. In testimony before a French investigative judge in October 2000, French cycling star Richard Virenque finally admitted to "doping" and alluded to the widespread use of rEPO and other drugs in European professional cycling (42). Alas, that did not cure him and others of further obfuscation and self-serving excuses (43). Just two years earlier, the fabled Tour de France had nearly collapsed in the wake of scandal after discoveries by French police of illegal drugs, including rEPO, in the possession of some riders and support personnel.

The most recent chapters in this saga of "blood, pure and corrupted" began with the disqualification of six members of the host country team at the 2001 Nordic Skiing World Championships in Lahti, Finland. These dishonored "heroes" in their own land had traces of a metabolite of hydroxyethyl starch (HES, an emergency plasma expander) detected on doping control. One speculates that these skiers had used acute plasma expansion for its immediate boost to aerobic capacity or for "hemodilution" purposes to mask a red cell mass increased by earlier, difficult-to-detect, use of rEPO.

Further variations on this theme of physiological deceit were seen just a year later at the 2002 Olympic Winter Games in Utah, when three medallists in Nordic events were disqualified after testing positive for darbepoetin alfa, a newer, longer-acting version of rEPO. Further, after the Olympics a trash bag filled with used blood collection paraphernalia was found in the Utah house just vacated by the Austrian national team (44,45). In the 2003 Nordic Skiing World Championships in Val di Fiemme, Italy, a Finnish skier was disqualified after darbepoetin detection (46).

A postscript to the saga of the infamous "Lahti Six" suggests that what has been detected and officially disciplined up until now is only the figurative tip of the iceberg of a pervasive problem among elite Nordic skiers (at least among European racers; no North American Nordic skier was implicated in these World Championship and Olympic scandals). Reporting the results of prerace hemoglobin and reticulocyte testing at the 2001 Lahti World Championships, Stray-Gundersen and colleagues (47) noted that, in samples obtained from 82 of 90 top-10 finishers in all 9 races, 34 (43%) were "highly abnormal" (> 3 SD above the mean based on data from the 1989 World Championships and the International Olympic Committee Erythropoietin 2000 project), and 9 (11%) were "abnormal" (> 2 SD but < 3 SD above the mean). Based on an expected prevalence of less than 0.3% and less than 2.5% for the "highly abnormal" and "abnormal" groups, respectively, the authors concluded that the findings were highly suspicious for pervasive blood doping practices at this elite level, where the 10% improvement in performance that a combination of increased red cell mass and plasma volume may afford can make the difference between last place and a gold medal.

Blood Doping in the "Treatment" of Thalassemia Minor

One might conclude that increasing red cell mass would be of interest only to endurance sport athletes, yet the use of rEPO to "treat" a Division I football player with ß-thalassemia trait provoked considerable discussion and debate (48-51). The team physician reasoned that the "anemia" [hematocrit 0.37 (37%), Hb 118 g/L (11.8 g/dL)], not unexpected given the microcytosis associated with thalassemia trait, was detrimental to the player's performance, which was being monitored by professional teams. He frequently needed intravenous rehydration during halftime, and his undue fatigue after a series of plays, especially in the second half of a game, required respites from regular play. The pretreatment EPO level was reported as low, yet this could have simply reflected inadequate tissue oxygenation, not failure of renal EPO synthesis.

A total of eleven injections of rEPO, delivered over four weeks, produced "dramatic" results: Hct 0.499 (49.9%), Hb 162 g/L (16.2 g/dL), with the athlete reporting "more energy" and observed to have improved "stamina" (49). For this strength-agility sport athlete, whose primary energy sources are immediately available ATP and creatine phosphate, as well as anaerobic glycolysis (not oxidative phosphorylation of fatty acids and glycogen), no report of baseline and post-treatment aerobic capacity and anaerobic threshold was given. Other than noting the apparent failure to maintain fluid and electrolyte balance (witness the halftime intravenous fluid "rescues") in this athlete, whose frequent dehydration could be attributed to the nature of his sport, the physician did not comment on the patient's nutrition, hydration, and training practices. A further problem with this "therapy" was the potential for adverse consequences of the increase in blood viscosity when hematocrit was artificially boosted by one-third.

Athletes as Blood Donors: Why Not?

Athletes (and their coaches) may inquire about the wisdom of *donating* blood. They want to fulfill their civic duty, yet wonder if will it hurt their performance or interfere with their training. Our knowledge of hematology and exercise physiology implies that the modest, temporary decrease in red cell mass caused by venesection of 1 unit-about 100 g/L (1 g/dl) of Hb or 0.03 points (3%) of the Hct, replaced over the following 3 or 4 weeks-plus the short-lived drop in plasma volume (about 10%, restored within a day or so), would produce a temporary decrement in aerobic capacity (52). It might also interfere with very heavy workouts, just as athletes at high altitudes discover they cannot exercise as intensely for as long a time as they can at sea level.

These temporary disadvantages, although significant to an elite-level endurance athlete during the competition season, or at a crucial time of training immediately preceding that season, should be seen as moot during the off-season. Physicians can, in good conscience, encourage athletes to join their friends in line at the bloodmobile, to view the day of donation as a "rest" day in their training schedules, and to drink lots of fluids and tread cautiously through the following day, when plasma volume will be fully restored (53).

Conclusion

Physicians caring for athletes and other active people must appreciate the physiological and pathological effects of exercise on the blood, as well as the manner in which an athlete's nutrition may play upon the sufficiency, or inadequacy, of normal blood production. Physicians may be called on to evaluate cases unique to hard-training athletes (perhaps those exhibiting subtle deficiency states) or make recommendations about suitability and safety of sports for people with hemoglobinopathies. When it is a question of performance-enhancing corruption of blood, physicians must keep ethics, safety, and valid medical indications in mind. The sports physician has a responsibility to help athletes define success in terms other than simply winning a race or game.

REFERENCES

1. Preparticipation Physical Evaluation, 3rd ed. American Academy of Family Physicians, American Academy of Pediatrics, American Medical Society for Sports Medicine, American Orthopedic Society for Sports Medicine, and American Osteopathic Academy of Sports Medicine. The Physician and Sports Medicine, McGraw-Hill Healthcare, Minneapolis, MN; 2005.

2. **Convertino VA.** Blood volume: its adaptation to endurance training. Med Sci Sports Exerc. 1991;23(12):1338-48.

3. **Sawka MN, Convertino VA, Eichner ER, et al.** Blood volume: importance and adaptations to exercise training, environmental stresses, and trauma/sickness. Med Sci Sports Exerc. 2000;32(2):332-48.

4. **Ehn L, Carlmark B, Hoglund S.** Iron status in athletes involved in intense physical activity. Med Sci Sports Exerc. 1980;12:61-4.

5. **Siegel AJ, Hennekens CH, Solomon HS, Van Boeckel B.** Exercise-related hematuria: findings in a group of marathon runners. JAMA. 1979;241(4):391-2.

6. **Moses FM, Brewer TG, Peura DA.** Running-associated proximal hemorrhagic colitis. Ann Intern Med. 1988;108(3):385-6.

7. **Schwartz AE, Vanagunas A, Kamel PL.** Endoscopy to evaluate gastrointestinal bleeding in marathon runners. Ann Intern Med. 1990;113:632-3.

8. **Jones GR, Newhouse IJ, Jakobi JM, et al.** The incidence of hematuria in middle distance track running. Can J Appl Physiol. 2001;26(4):336-49.

9. **Cohen RA, Brown RS.** Microscopic hematuria. N Engl J Med. 2003;348:2330-8.

10. **Elliot DL, Goldberg L, Eichner ER.** Hematuria in a young recreational runner. Med Sci Sports Exerc. 1991;23(8):892-4.

11. **Clement DB, Sawchuck LL.** Iron status and sports performance. Sports Med. 1984;1:65-74.

12. **Haymes EM.** Nutritional concerns: need for iron. Med Sci Sports Exerc. 1987;19(5 Suppl 1):S197-200.

13. **Kopp-Woodroffe SA, Manore MM, Dueck CA, et al.** Energy and nutrient status of amenorrheic athletes participating in a diet and exercise training intervention program. Int J Sport Nutr. 1999;9:70-88.

14. **Hinton PS, Giordano C, Brownlie T, Haas JD.** Iron supplementation improves endurance after training in iron-depleted, nonanemic women. J Appl Physiol. 2000;88:1103-11.

15. **Friedmann B, Weller E, Mairbaurl H, Bartsch P.** Effects of iron repletion on blood volume and performance capacity in young athletes. Med Sci Sports Exerc. 2001;33(5):741-6.

16. **Garza D, Shrier I, Kohl HW, et al.** The clinical value of serum ferritin tests in endurance athletes. Clin J Sport Med. 1997;7(1):46-53.

17. **Fallon KE.** The acute phase response and exercise: the ultramarathon as prototype exercise. Clin J Sport Med. 2001;11:38-43.

18. **Krantz SB.** Pathogenesis and treatment of the anemia of chronic disease. Am J Med Sci. 1994;307:353-9.

19. **King DE, Carek P, Mainous AG III, Pearson WS.** Inflammatory markers and exercise: differences related to exercise type. Med Sci Sports Exerc. 2003;35(4):575-81.

20. **Cook JD.** The nutritional assessment of iron status. Arch Latinoam Nutr. 1999;49(3 Suppl 2):11-4.

21. **Rimon E, Levy S, Sapir A, et al.** Diagnosis of iron deficiency anemia in the elderly by transferrin receptor-ferritin index. Arch Intern Med. 2002;162:445-9.

22. **Joosten E, Van Loon R, Billen J, et al.** Serum transferrin receptor in the evaluation of the iron status in elderly hospitalized patients with anemia. Am J Hematol. 2002;69(1):1-6.

23. **Beguin Y.** Soluble transferrin receptor for the evaluation of erythropoiesis and iron status. Clin Chim Acta. 2003;329(1-2):9-22.

24. **Malczewska J, Blach W, Stupnicki R.** The effects of physical exercise on the concentrations of ferritin and transferrin receptor in plasma of female judoists. Int J Sports Med. 2000;21(3):175-9.

25. **Whipple GH, Robscheit-Robbins FS.** Blood regeneration in severe anemia. II. Favorable influence of liver, heart and skeletal muscle in diet. Am J Physiol. 1925;72:408-18.

26. **Stahl WC.** March hemoglobinuria. JAMA. 1957;164:1458-60.

27. **Dufaux B, Hoederoth A, Streitberger I, et al.** Serum ferritin, transferrin, haptoglobin, and iron in middle- and long-distance runners, elite rowers, and professional racing cyclists. Int J Sports Med. 1981;2:43-6.

28. **Algazy KM.** Spinner's hematuria [letter]. N Engl J Med. 2002;346(21):1676.

29. **Selby GB, Eichner ER.** Endurance swimming, intravascular hemolysis, anemia and iron depletion: new perspective on athlete's anemia. Am J Med. 1986;81(5):791-4.

30. **Fallon KE, Bishop G.** Changes in erythropoiesis assessed by reticulocyte parameters during ultralong distance running. Clin J Sport Med. 2002;12(3):172-8.

31. **Spitler DL, Alexander WC, Hoffler GW, et al.** Haptoglobin and serum enzymatic response to maximal exercise in relation to physical fitness. Med Sci Sports Exerc. 1984;16(4):366-70.

32. **Oyono-Enguelle S, Le Gallais D, Lonsdorfer A, et al.** Cardiorespiratory and metabolic responses to exercise in HbSC sickle cell patients. Med Sci Sports Exerc. 2000;32(4):725-31.

33. **Helzlsouer KJ, Hayden FG, Rogol AD.** Severe metabolic complications in a cross-country runner with sickle cell trait. JAMA. 1983;249(6):777-9.

34. **Koppes GM, Daly JJ, Coltman CA Jr, Butkus DE.** Exertion-induced rhabdomyolysis with acute renal failure and disseminated intravascular coagulation in sickle cell trait. Am J Med. 1977;63:313-7.

35. **Eichner ER.** Deadly collapse in sickle-trait athletes: sickling on the run. Sports Med Digest. 2002;24(11):121, 123.

36. **Ekblom B, Goldbarg AN, Gullbring B.** Response to exercise after blood loss and reinfusion. J Appl Physiol. 1972;330:175-80.

37. **Williams MH, Wesseldine S, Somma T, Schuster R.** The effect of induced erythrocythemia upon 5-mile treadmill run time. Med Sci Sports Exerc. 1981;13:169-75.

38. **Brien AJ, Simon TL.** The effects of red blood cell reinfusion on 10-km race time. JAMA. 1987;257:2761-5.

39. **Sawka MN, Young AJ, Muza SR, et al.** Erythrocyte reinfusion and maximal aerobic power. JAMA. 1987;257(11):1496-9.

40. **Cramer RB.** Olympic cheating: the inside story of illicit doping and the US cycling team. Rolling Stone. 1985 Feb 14:25-30.

41. **Rostaing B, Sullivan R.** Triumphs tainted with blood. Sports Illustrated. 1985 Jan 22.12-7.

42. **Associated Press.** Tour de France drug scandal: Virenque admits to doping. 2000 Oct 24.

43. **Art S.** Top cyclist again embroiled in doping controversy. The New York Times. 1999 May 12.

44. **Christie D.** Soldier Hollow redux: reflections on blood, pure and corrupted. http://www.SkiFaster.net. 2002 1 Mar. Available from URL: http://www.skifaster.net

45. **Christie D.** The doping scandals of Salt Lake. http://www.SkiFaster.net. 2002 May 12. Available from URL: http://www.skifaster.net

46. B-sample of Kaisa Varis proves use of doping. Helsingin Sanomat. 2003 Mar 14. Available from URL: http://www.helsinginsanomat.fi.english/

47. **Stray-Gundersen J, Videman T, Penttila I, Lereim I.** Abnormal hematologic profiles in elite cross-country skiers: blood doping or? Clin J Sport Med. 2003;13:132-7.

48. **Eichner ER.** Finding a way: rationalizing erythropoietin in sports. Sports Med Digest. 2002;24(6):61-3.

49. **Smith KB.** EPO for the treatment of thalassemia minor: is it doping? [Letter]. Sports Med Digest. 2002;24(9):102.

50. **Spivak JL.** EPO in thalassemia minor: is it doping? [Invited Commentary]. Sports Med Digest. 2002;24(9):103.

51. **Green G, Smith B.** Using recombinant human erythropoietin in a football player with thalassemia minor: the wrong medicine [Invited Commentary]. Sports Med Digest. 2002;24(9):102, 104.

52. **Panebianco RA, Stachenfeld N, Coplan NL, Gleim GW.** Effects of blood donation on exercise performance in competitive cyclists. Am Heart J. 1995;130(4):838-40.

53. **Schnirring L.** Donating blood: what active people need to know. Phys Sportsmed. 2001;29(6):11, 15.

10

■ ■ ■

Genitourinary Problems
in Athletes

Philip H. Cohen, MD

Athletes may be afflicted by a wide variety of genitourinary problems. Some of these conditions are relatively sport-specific, whereas others are common to many different athletic endeavors. Some genitourinary problems may result from trauma related to sports activity, though such injuries generally are uncommon. Major trauma may, of course, result in genitourinary injury, but less obvious forms of trauma, such as the "repetitive" or chronic trauma seen with sports like long distance running and cycling, may also incur injuries. Although not always sustained during sports activities, atraumatic conditions, including hernia, hematuria, and proteinuria, have special considerations in athletes.

Anatomy

The upper genitourinary tract consists of the kidneys, the renal vasculature, and the ureters. The kidneys are bean-shaped organs, approximately 10-12 cm in length, that lie in the paravertebral gutters on either side of the spine at the T12-L3 vertebral levels. Here, in their retroperitoneal position, the kidneys are well-protected by a fibrous capsule and surrounding mass of perirenal fat, as well as the local musculature and the lower ribs. On each side, a renal artery runs from the abdominal aorta to enter the kidney at the hilum. The renal vein exits each kidney at the hilum and drains into the inferior vena cava. The renal pelvis conducts urine from the major calyces into the ureter, which, in turn, courses inferiorly along the psoas, crossing anterior to the common iliac artery, and then entering the bladder at the trigone (1,2).

The lower genitourinary tract includes the urinary bladder and the posterior urethra. The bladder is a strong, muscular sac that lies (in its empty state) in the pelvis, inferior to the peritoneum and posterior to the symphysis pubis. In the male, the neck of the bladder is firmly attached to the pelvis by the puboprostatic ligaments. In females, the inferior portion of the bladder is loosely attached to the urogenital diaphragm by the pubovesical ligaments (1,2). Thus, males are more susceptible to shearing injury at this location than females (3).

In the female, the urethra is a short, muscular tube running from the neck of the bladder, through the urogenital diaphragm, to the external urethral orifice. Due to its short length (4 cm) and great distensability, the female urethra is rarely injured (1,4). In males, the urethra is about 20 cm long and is divided into anterior and posterior portions by the urogenital diaphragm. The posterior portion comprises the prostatic urethra (3 cm long and very distensable) and membranous urethra (2.5 cm long at the least distensable and narrowest part of the urethra, firmly fixed). The junction of these two segments is a common location for shearing injuries (2,5). The prostate gland completely encircles the prostatic urethra; palpation of a high-riding prostate during digital rectal exam in a patient who has sustained pelvic trauma may signify a rupture of the membranous urethra (6). The anterior urethra, the longest portion, passes from the bulb of the penis, through the corpus spongiosum, to the external urethral orifice (1,2).

The female external genitalia include the labia majora and minora, clitoris, urethral orifice, and vaginal vestibule. The internal female genitalia consist of the vagina, uterus, ovaries, and Fallopian tubes. The male external genitalia consist of the anterior urethra, penis, scrotum, and testicles. Although the male external genitalia protrude further from the body and are thus more susceptible to injury, the female external genitalia may also be injured by direct trauma. The perineum is the diamond-shaped region extending from the tip of the coccyx to the symphysis pubis, overlying the pelvic outlet. The urogenital diaphragm closes the anterior part of the pelvic outlet and the posterior part is closed by the levator ani muscles (1,2). A detailed discussion of the perineum is beyond the scope of this chapter, but it is important to note that clinical syndromes, including neuropathies and incontinence, may arise from injury to the structures in this area.

Traumatic Conditions

Renal Injuries

Renal injuries are relatively uncommon, occurring in less than 2% of trauma cases in one large study (7). Yet, the kidney is the most commonly injured organ in the urinary tract, and renal injuries complicate 8%-10% of all cases of major abdominal trauma (8,9). Blunt trauma accounts for 90% or more of renal injuries, whereas penetrating wounds are much less common (7-9). Isolated renal injury is rare in adults; 80%-95% of these injuries are associated with injury to other organs (7,8). The incidence of renal injury in sporting event participants is less well-studied, especially in adults. One retrospective review (10) found that, among trauma patients at a children's hospital, more than 40% of the renal injuries occurred during some form of sporting activity, which is similar to estimates by other authors (11) (although less than 3% of renal injuries in this study occurred during team sports participation). A high degree of vigilance must be maintained when evaluating a child with abdominal trauma; symptoms of intra-abdominal injury may not become apparent for up to 24 hours after a bicycle accident, for example (12). In another study, among 18 skiers who had sustained splenic injury, 10 were found to have concomitant renal injury (13).

Kidney injuries can be classified according to their severity and the structures involved. Grade I injuries are minor and usually consist of contusions, or small lacerations which do not require surgical intervention. Grade II injuries are represented by deep lacerations with involvement of the collecting system. Grade III injuries involve major lacerations, fracture of the kidney, or renal pedicle injury. Grade IV injuries occur when the kidney is avulsed from the ureteropelvic junction and vascular pedicle. The majority of Grade I and II injuries can be treated conservatively, whereas catastrophic injuries (Grade III and IV) often necessitate surgical intervention and may require nephrectomy (8).

A patient who sustains renal trauma may report flank, back, or abdominal pain; hematuria is also very common. However, the absence of these signs does not rule out renal injury (11,14). Localized tenderness to palpation is common but nonspecific. Exam findings indicative of vertebral or rib fracture, or injury to other inra-abdominal organs, should raise suspicion of a possible associated renal injury. More severe injuries may present with more pain and significant hematuria, although the degree of hematuria does not correlate well with injury severity (9). The presence of an enlarging flank mass indicates a torn renal capsule with a secondary retroperitoneal hematoma. Catastrophic renal injuries usually present with signs and symptoms of hypovolemic shock, although this may not be immediately obvious. In fact, renal vascular injuries may not cause any hematuria (15). Thus, it is crucial to closely monitor any athlete with suspected renal trauma, even if initial evaluation suggests a minor injury (16).

Urinalysis, CBC, and blood chemistries, including blood urea nitrogen (BUN) and creatinine, should be obtained. CT is the imaging test of choice, as it has excellent capacity for detecting renal contusions and lacerations, urine extravasation, and retroperitoneal bleeding (11). CT has been shown to have a sensitivity of 90%-100% for renal injuries (8,17,18), although its specificity is significantly lower (8,19). Helical CT may be especially useful, as its decreased acquisition time minimizes artifact in acutely injured patients who may have difficulty remaining still (20,21). IVP, formerly the preferred imaging test in renal trauma evaluation, can still be very useful if the patient is too unstable for CT, as IVP can be performed intraoperatively (17,22,23). However, IVP is less accurate in detecting smaller renal contusions and lacerations (8) and, unlike CT, does not allow evaluation of concomitant abdominal or pelvic injuries. In selected patients, such as those with serious renal injury or inconclusive CT imaging, MRI may offer better injury delineation, although it is more costly and time-consuming (24,25). Ultrasound has been studied in the evaluation of renal trauma, but, to date, sensitivity has been poor (8). Arteriography can be extremely valuable in the evaluation of renal vascular injuries and can also be used for therapeutic applications such as embolization to control bleeding (17).

Initial management of the patient with suspected renal trauma should focus on rapid but thorough clinical evaluation with close supervision, even if only a minor injury is suspected. Grade I and II injuries may be treated with careful monitoring and strict rest. Most of these injuries heal within 6-8 weeks (11,14). Return-to-activity decisions are based on injury severity and the type of activities in which the patient participates. Microscopic hematuria must be fully resolved, and, for more significant injuries, repeat CT should demonstrate complete healing and show no sign of complication, such as urinoma (11,15). Consider having the contact athlete wear a flak jacket or similar protective equipment. All patients with renal trauma should be followed up for at least one year to watch for the development of post-traumatic complications, such as hypertension, hydronephrosis, and impaired renal function. Patients with Grade III injuries typically have been managed surgically, but recent evidence suggests that some of these patients may be followed conservatively. Grade IV injuries need urgent surgical treatment and often require nephrectomy (8,17,26). For athletes who have sustained catastrophic renal injuries, return to contact sports is not advocated for at least 6-12 months, if return is feasible at all (15). Patients who have undergone nephrectomy or who have sustained post-traumatic complications need to be counseled about the potentially devastating consequences of returning to contact sports and given precautions about the use of medications such as NSAIDs.

Bladder Injuries

Acute bladder injuries are uncommon in sports but may complicate pelvic fracture or may occur with a direct blow to the distended bladder. More than 98% of patients with bladder rupture will have gross hematuria (8). The diagnosis of a bladder injury can be made with CT, CT cystography, or conventional cystography (27,28); care must be taken to rule out a urethral injury before inserting the catheter to perform cystography. Treatment of intraperitoneal bladder ruptures requires direct repair; extraperitoneal ruptures may, depending on the exact nature of the injury, be treated operatively or treated nonoperatively with catheter drainage. Contusions and minor lacerations are treated conservatively (8,28).

Repetitive bladder trauma commonly occurs in sports such as long distance running and may cause gross hematuria ("runner's bladder"). Microscopic hematuria has been reported to occur in up to 20% of marathon runners, more than 50% of ultramarathon runners, and more than 55% of football, track, and lacrosse athletes (15). This may be due to repeated impact of the posterior bladder wall against the bladder base, causing a contusion. Hypoxia-mediated increases in glomerular permeability and increased glomerular filtration pressure may also allow increased passage of red blood cells into the urine (8,29). This condition resolves spontaneously with rest, and urinalysis should show resolution of the hematuria within several days to a week (8,11,15). Persistent hematuria necessitates further evaluation (see below). Recurrences can be minimized by not fully evacuating the bladder before strenuous activity, thereby "cushioning" the bladder against the repeated microtrauma.

Urethral Injuries

Urethral injuries are rare in sports. They typically result from a straddle injury, in which the athlete falls astride a solid object, or from major trauma, often involving pelvic fracture (9,30,31). Straddle injuries may damage the anterior urethra, causing immediate pain, edema, and ecchymosis. Blood may be present at the meatus, and the patient may be unable to void (30). A retrograde urethrogram should be obtained before attempting to pass a Foley catheter. For partial tears, treatment may include long-term catheterization to allow urethral healing, whereas complete tears often require surgical intervention. Improper or late treatment of these injuries may result in a high rate of complications, such as strictures or erectile dysfunction (8,32). Urethral injuries in females are especially uncommon and are almost always associated with pelvic fractures (8). A notable exception is the "forced water douche," which can occur when a female water skier falls and water is forcefully injected into the genitourinary tract; this may not only injure the urethra but also the vulva and vagina and may result in salpingitis (30).

Genital Injuries

Acute penile injuries are uncommon in sports, as athletic supporters and cups afford reasonable protection to the flaccid penis. Most injuries are lacerations or contusions due to direct trauma; vascular injury may occur and should not be overlooked. The erect penis may sustain "fracture," that is, traumatic rupture of the tunica albuginea and corpus cavernosum. The patient may recall a sudden "cracking" sound, and will present with severe pain, swelling, and ecchymosis. The penis may be bent to the affected side (8,9,30). This injury is a urologic emergency, requiring immediate surgical repair. Some patients may be too embarrassed to admit that the injury occurred during sexual activity and instead may claim that it was "sports-related."

Scrotal injuries are often the result of direct, blunt trauma. Scrotal contusions can be treated with support, ice, and analgesics. Often, in cases of blunt trauma, the testicles are injured also; therefore one must fully evaluate for signs of testicular injury. Mild testicular contusions are common and present with pain and nausea. Conservative treatment is recommended, but a thorough exam and close observation are warranted to rule out more serious injury. Hydroceles may arise after trauma, due to impaired reabsorption of tunica vaginalis secretions. These lesions transilluminate, and can be treated conservatively, but close follow-up is recommended to rule out an underlying tumor.

Traumatic hematoceles do not transilluminate and may be difficult to distinguish from a testicular rupture. If there is an expanding mass that does not transilluminate, difficulty in palpating the epididymis, or pain out of proportion to the injury, one must suspect a testicular or epididymal fracture (8,9,11,30). This requires emergent evaluation by a urologist. Surgical exploration is recommended if a major testicular injury is deemed likely. Ultrasound can be very helpful in evaluating the injured testicle, but surgery should not be delayed if the ultrasound can not be performed right away. Immediate surgical intervention has been shown to save the injured testicle in approximately 90% of cases, as opposed to a 33%-50% save rate with conservative management or delayed surgery (33,34).

Chronic trauma to the dorsal branch of the pudendal nerve, cavernous nerve, and genital branch of the genitofemoral nerve may result in penile and scrotal sensory changes, and erectile dysfunction (9,30,35). This has been reported in up to 8% of long-distance cyclists, in whom the nerves may be compressed between the bike seat and the symphysis pubis, resulting in an ischemic or traumatic neuropathy. These symptoms tend to resolve with rest, and may be ameliorated by appropriate adjustment of the seat, proper riding form, use of padded cycling shorts, intermittent standing on the pedals during long rides, and use of a seat with a channel cut out to decrease pressure on the nerves (36-38). Urethritis, prostatitis, and urinary tract infections have also been associated with long-distance cycling and seem to respond to similar measures as above, which decrease perineal pressure. Care must be taken to exclude the more common causes of these conditions, and standard treatment with antibiotics should be undertaken as appropriate (38). Recent evidence has shown that up to 90% of mountain bikers who bike more than 3,000 miles per year have lower sperm counts, decreased sperm motility, and more scrotal abnormalities than noncyclists. Due to the potential fertility implications, it has been suggested that mountain bikers need to use appropriate suspension and shock absorption systems in addition to adhering to the above recommendations for long-distance cyclists in general (39,40).

Injuries to the female external genitalia in sports mainly consist of vulvar hematomas and contusions. These can usually be treated with rest, ice packs, and analgesics. However, thorough gynecologic and urologic evaluation is warranted in cases of significant trauma or penetrating injury. In addition, in these cases, a high index of suspicion should be maintained for the possibility that the injury was caused by sexual assault (8,30).

Atraumatic Conditions

The Acute Scrotum

Atraumatic cases of an acute scrotum typically are caused by testicular torsion, appendiceal torsion, or epididymo-orchitis (41). Although these conditions are not commonly considered as sports-related, they can occur in athletes and should not be misdiagnosed as contusions or other injuries incurred during sports activities. Testicular torsion occurs most commonly in neonates and adolescents and presents with sudden, severe testicular pain, often associated with nausea and vomiting. Physical examination usually reveals a high-riding, tender, swollen testis with a transverse lie. The overlying scrotum may be inflamed and swollen, and the cremasteric reflex is usually absent. Elevating the testicle usually does not relieve the pain (9,41,42).

Testicular torsion is a urologic emergency. An attempt may be made at manual detorsion, by rotating the testis away from the midline; an immediate and marked reduction in pain implies success, but retorsion may occur. Color Doppler ultrasound or nuclear scintigraphy will reveal diminished or absent testicular blood flow in cases where the diagnosis is unclear but should not delay immediate surgical exploration if suspicion of torsion is high (41,42). If detorsion is accomplished within 6 hours of symptom onset, testicular salvage rates are around 100%, but decrease significantly thereafter (43,44).

Appendiceal torsion is more common in prepubertal boys and usually presents with slowly increasing scrotal pain. The exam may reveal tenderness isolated to the superior testicular pole; the "blue dot sign," a small, bluish discoloration at the superior pole, may also be present. This condition can be treated with rest, scrotal elevation, and analgesics (41,42).

Epididymitis is more common in adolescents and older individuals. It presents with insidiously increasing scrotal pain, over hours to days, and may be associated with fever, dysuria, and abnormal discharge. The epididymis itself is extremely tender to the touch, but the testis is not tender unless an associated orchitis is present. Scrotal erythema and edema may be present, but, unlike in cases of testicular torsion, the cremasteric reflex is present, and elevating the affected testicle usually decreases the pain. In sexually active men younger than age 35, *Chlamydia trachomatis* and *Neisseria gonorrhoeae* are the most common pathogens. In older men, enteric species cause the majority of cases. Urinalysis should be obtained to evaluate for pyuria, with bacterial culture and appropriate amplification techniques for detecting *C. trachomatis* and *N. gonorrhoeae*. Treatment involves rest, elevation of the affected hemiscrotum, analgesics, and appropriate antibiotic coverage for the patient and his sexual partner(s) (41,42).

Scrotal Masses

Testicular cancer is the most common malignancy in males aged 15-34 years, with an incidence of approximately 3 per 1,000 men (43); a second peak of incidence is found among middle-aged males (44). A history of cryptorchidism is the major risk factor, increasing the risk of subsequent malignancy by up to a factor of 40 (45). Other risk factors include gonadal dysgenesis, Klinefelter's syndrome, DES exposure, immunocompromised states, and a close relative with testicular cancer (44,46). Although no clear associations have been found between these malignancies and athletics, the use of anabolic steroids has been reported to be involved in the pathogenesis of certain testicular and prostate tumors (47). Testicular cancers are often picked up during a preparticipation screening exam (PPSE) or during testicular self-exam (TSE) performed by the patient. The usual presentation is a painless, firm mass that disrupts the integrity of the testicle and is separate from the epididymis and spermatic cord. These lesions do not transilluminate. As the vast majority of testicular cancers can be cured if detected and treated early, urgent ultrasonography and urologic referral are needed for the patient with a suspicious mass (43). The PPSE is an excellent time to teach TSE to young athletes.

Hydroceles, spermatoceles, and other cystic lesions of the testicle and epididymis are benign lesions, which generally transilluminate. However, a hydrocele may be a manifestation of an underlying malignancy and therefore requires careful evaluation. Ultrasonography is an excellent technique for better delineating these lesions (48). Varicoceles, which are varicosities of the internal spermatic veins, usually manifest as a "bag of worms" next to the testicle. Typically, they do not require treatment other than reassurance and use of proper support (9,30). However, larger varicoceles have been associated with impaired testicular function, including subnormal fertility (49). Previously, it has been thought that varicocelectomy was the treatment of choice in these cases; however, recent data indicate that the benefits of surgical therapy may not be as great as previously thought (50). Urologic consultation and full discussion with the patient (and partner or family members, as appropriate) are recommended for larger lesions.

Hernias

Inguinal hernias are abnormal protrusions of peritoneal-lined sacks through a weakness in the abdominal wall (51). Indirect hernias are the most common type in both males and females, although they are five to ten times more common in males (52). Indirect hernias exit the internal inguinal ring lateral to the inferior epigastric vessels and pass into the inguinal canal; in some cases, they extend into the scrotum. Direct hernias protrude directly from the abdomen into the floor of the inguinal canal, posterior to the spermatic cord, and medial to the inferior epigastric vessels. Indirect inguinal hernias are due to a congenital weakness caused by a patent processus vaginalis, whereas direct inguinal hernias are more often related to increasing age and strenuous physical activity such as weightlifting (52,53).

In either case, symptomatic patients typically complain of a bulge in the groin, which may be noted to worsen with standing or Valsalva and resolve with recumbency. Mild discomfort is common, but severe pain is indicative of hernia strangulation. Inguinal hernias are often asymptomatic and may only be serendipitously detected during a PPSE. Evaluation with the patient standing may reveal a visible mass in the groin that often reduces with recumbency. With the examiner's finger palpating the external ring, a mass may be felt that may "tap" the examiner's finger when the patient performs the Valsalva maneuver. The hernia may be reducible with gentle pressure (52,53). Hernias that can not be reduced are said to be incarcerated and should be referred for surgical repair. Incarcerated hernias are not necessarily symptomatic; however, if the hernia is not reducible and is tender and tense, one should suspect a strangulated hernia. This is a surgical emergency in which the hernia contents become ischemic and nonviable. A patient with a strangulated hernia typically shows signs of intestinal obstruction and may become septic rapidly.

Femoral hernias occur when intra-abdominal contents protrude into the femoral sheath in the femoral canal. These lesions are prone to incarceration and occur much more commonly in females than in males. They tend to be related to exertion and pregnancy (52).

In some cases, history and physical may not provide a clear diagnosis in the athlete with groin pain. In these situations, imaging modalities should be considered to better delineate the pathology. For example, herniography has recently been shown to demonstrate inguinal hernia in approximately 25% of patients with groin pain of unclear etiology (54). An athlete with an inguinal hernia should be referred to a surgeon for consideration of repair. The best type of repair for that athlete may depend on many factors, including the particular stresses the athlete experiences in his or her sport. Therefore, consultation with a surgeon well-versed in treating athletes is recommended. Return-to-play depends on many factors, including the patient's general health, type and intensity of sport, and type of surgical procedure. In recent years, laparoscopic hernia repairs have gained favor due to their shorter recovery times and lower incidence of persistent pain and numbness compared with open techniques. One study utilizing laparoscopic repair with an anatomically contoured mesh has reported a

97% rate of return to unrestricted sports by 6 weeks (55). However, surgical complications, although uncommon, may be slightly more frequent with laparoscopic techniques (56).

Chronic Groin Pain

Chronic groin pain in athletes represents a diagnostic and therapeutic challenge. A broad differential diagnosis must be considered, including local musculoskeletal etiologies (Table 10-1).

Athletic Pubalgia (Sportsman's Hernia)

Athletic pubalgia refers to chronic inguinal or pubic pain in athletes, which only occurs with certain movements and is not attributable to a true hernia or other diagnosis (57). Athletic pubalgia, often called "sportsman's hernia" (or "Gilmore's groin"), is a recently recognized syndrome characterized by a wide spectrum of pathology. Data on prevalence are incomplete, but the condition appears to be much more common in males than in females

---

Table 10-1   Differential Diagnosis of Chronic Groin Pain

Local musculoskeletal etiologies
      Adductor strain
      Athletic pubalgia
      Osteitis pubis
      Iliopsoas bursitis
      Avulsion fracture
Referred pain
      Lumbosacral radiculopathy
      Femoral neck stress fracture
      Avascular necrosis of femoral head
      Acetabular labral tear
      DJD of femoral head
Nerve compression (ilioinguinal, obturator, iliohypogastric)
Infections
      Genitourinary tract infection
      Abscess
      Osteomyelitis
Inflammatory conditions
      Inflammatory bowel disease
      Vasculitis
Abdominal pathology
      Abdominal aortic aneurysm
      Neoplasm
      Ovarian cyst
      Endometriosis
      Appendicitis

(58,59). Most patients with sportsman's hernia present with unilateral groin pain and/or proximal adductor pain that worsens with sudden movements, especially acceleration, twisting or cutting moves, and kicking. Valsalva maneuvers reproduce the pain in less than 10% of patients (58). The pain may be sharp and is often centered at the inguinal canal, near the insertion of the rectus abdominus. Pain may radiate to the adductor region or the testicles (58,59). A common feature in sportsman's hernia is that the symptoms abate with rest but recur when the athlete attempts to return to sporting activities. The patient may have been previously diagnosed with a "groin strain" and typically has attempted treatment with NSAIDs, physical therapy, and rest, to no avail. The pain is usually bad enough that it prevents the athlete from participating fully in his or her sport (58,59). In many cases, especially in runners, the onset of pain is insidious. In other cases, especially in soccer and hockey players, the athlete may remember a specific move that correlated with the onset of pain (58,59).

In most cases, the cause seems to be a disruption of part of the posterior inguinal wall. Multiple authors (58-63) have reported finding various injuries, including tears of the conjoined tendon (the common tendon of internal oblique and transversus abdominus), abnormalities of the rectus abdominus insertion, tearing away of the transversalis fascia from the conjoined tendon, and defects in the external oblique aponeurosis. It is thought these injuries are caused by excessive shear forces across the pelvis during sporting activities, resulting in weakening or tearing of the these structures. Entrapment of terminal branches of the iliohypogastric nerve by defects in the external oblique aponeurosis also has been reported (64).

Physical exam often reveals pain with resisted hip adduction; pain with resisted sit-ups is less common. Tenderness may be noted near the pubic origin of adductor longus or over the inguinal canal and conjoined tendon but is much less common at the pubic symphysis (58,59). No inguinal hernia is appreciable, but the external inguinal ring may feel dilated. On physical exam, it is often difficult to differentiate between sportsman's hernia, osteitis pubis, rectus abdominus strains, and adductor tendonosis. Diagnostic imaging may be useful for excluding other causes of pain, but it has a very low sensitivity for detecting the pathology associated with sportsman's hernia. As mentioned, a wide differential must be considered (58,59,65).

Treatment often consists of an initial attempt at conservative therapy. A 2- to 3-month physical therapy program focusing on dynamic pelvic stabilization may be effective for some patients (66). If conservative therapy fails, surgical referral is warranted. If the patient is a high-level athlete in whom the diagnosis appears clear and other pathology has been ruled out, initial surgical referral is appropriate. It is extremely important that referral be made to a surgeon with specific expertise and experience in treating sportsman's hernia. Multiple surgical techniques have been described (59), but all attempt to repair the soft tissue defects in the posterior abdominal wall and pelvic floor. In addition, adductor release has been advocated as an important component of surgical therapy in selected patients (58). Despite the wide spectrum of pathology and different surgical approaches, most authors report excellent success rates after surgery (58,61,67-70).

Hematuria and Proteinuria

As previously mentioned, microscopic hematuria associated with exercise is relatively common and usually benign (29). In these cases, resolution of the hematuria should occur within 24 to 72 hours after cessation of exercise (15). If hematuria persists or the history and physical suggest a pathologic process, further evaluation is indicated. It is important to realize that a dipstick test for blood in the urine may test positive for not only red blood cells but also for free hemoglobin (e.g, from hemolysis) or myoglobin (e.g, in rhabdomyolysis). Therefore, a microscopic urinalysis must always be performed if the dipstick test is positive. Also, reddish urine may not necessarily indicate hematuria; various drugs and chemicals, such as phenazopyridine, rifampin, nitrofurantoin, and food dyes, can impart a reddish hue to the urine (9,15).

Obtaining a thorough history is crucial in investigating persistent hematuria. Various entities need to be considered (71), including glomerular and nonglomerular renal disease, as well as extra-renal disorders. Extra-renal causes of microscopic hematuria can be classified as upper tract, lower tract, or systemic disorders (Table 10-2). In athletes whose sports involve repeated footstrikes, "march hemoglobinuria" (also known as "footstrike hemolysis") must be considered. This entity may present with hemoglobinuria one to three hours after the exercise bout and is thought to be caused by hemolysis of RBCs as they are traumatized during passage through the foot. It may be characterized by hemoglobinuria and evidence of mild hemolysis such as decreased serum haptoglobin. A similar syndrome has been noted after repetitive hand trauma in martial artists and conga drum players (9,15,72).

Complete microscopic urinalysis is the most important initial test in the laboratory evaluation of hematuria. The presence of RBC casts, acanthocytes, or a predominance of dysmorphic RBCs, suggests glomerular disease. If accompanied by significant proteinuria, renal insufficiency, or other worrisome clinical findings, this should trigger a complete nephrology workup (71,73). If the patient has isolated glomerular microscopic hematuria with normal renal function and no proteinuria, he or she may be followed with repeat clinical evaluation, urinalysis, and measurement of renal function every 6-12 months (71). In the appropriate clinical settings, coagulopathy testing, sickle cell prep, urine culture, and evaluation for sexually transmitted diseases should be undertaken.

If nonglomerular disease is suspected and the above investigations are unrevealing, imaging of the upper urinary tract should be performed. Helical CT is an excellent imaging choice, as it has exquisite sensitivity

Table 10-2   Differential Diagnosis of Persistent Isolated Hematuria in Athletes

Glomerular causes	IgA nephropathy
	Post-streptococcal glomerulonephritis
	Hereditary nephritis (Alport's syndrome)
	Other forms of glomerulonephritis
	Thin basement membrane disease
Nonglomerular causes	
Upper tract	Nephrolithiasis
	Pyelonephritis
	Renal trauma
	Polycystic kidney disease
	Medullary sponge kidney
	Renal cell carcinoma
	Papillary necrosis
	Wilms' tumor
	Hemoglobinopathy (sickle cell anemia)
	Renal tuberculosis
	Urethral stricture
	Renal infarct/Arteriovenous malformation
Lower tract	Cystitis, urethritis, prostatitis
	Prostate and bladder neoplasms
	"Runner's bladder"
	Trauma
	Schistosomiasis
	Urethral stricture
Systemic/Other causes	Coagulopathy (iatrogenic or other)
	Vasculitis
	Urine contamination with menstrual effluent
	Exercise hematuria
	Psychiatric (self-mutilation)
Causes of red/dark urine without actual hematuria	March hemoglobinuria
	Rhabdomyolysis/myoglobinuria
	Intravascular hemolysis
	Medications (phenazopyridine, rifampin)
	Food colorings

for detecting nephrolithiasis and allows for clear evaluation of renal morphology. It is also superior to IVP and ultrasound for detecting renal masses, especially those less than 3 cm in size (74,75). IVP can still be very useful as an initial test for evaluating the upper genitourinary tract if CT is unavailable, but it may not be able to differentiate between cystic and solid masses. Renal ultrasound is a safe and relatively inexpensive modality and can be used during pregnancy and in patients with renal failure or contrast agent hypersensitivity. However, due to its lower sensitivity for detecting small masses, further imaging may be required (71,76). If an upper tract origin is not identified, voided urine cytology and cystoscopy are recommended to evaluate for urothelial malignancies in patients over age 40 or with risk factors for transitional cell carcinoma (71,73).

With appropriate evaluation, athletes with benign, sports-associated hematuria may continue to exercise. It is clear that renal blood flow (RBF) and glomerular filtration rate (GFR) decrease in proportion to intensity of exercise (15). Recent animal data (77) suggest that moderate exercise may be safe in polycystic kidney disease, but human data are lacking. Therefore, athletes who are found to have significant renal abnormalities need appropriate consultation before returning to high-intensity sports.

Proteinuria is very common in athletes, occurring in up to 70%-80% of athletes after exercise (78). A higher incidence of proteinuria is seen with more intense exertion; it is thought that this is due to an increased filtration fraction and enhanced glomerular membrane permeability, resulting in increased flow of protein into the lumen (15). This proteinuria usually resolves within 24-48 hours after exercise (79). Other causes of transient proteinuria include fever, stress, and exposure to cold (15). As with hematuria, a thorough history and physical exam must be performed. If the proteinuria resolves with rest, no further testing is recommended; if it persists, further evaluation is warranted, especially for common causes, such as hypertension and diabetes mellitus. Initial testing should include full microscopic urinalysis, CBC, chemistry panel, blood glucose, and 24-hour urine for protein and creatinine. As with hematuria, dipstick testing may give false-positive readings; very concentrated specimens, gross hematuria, dehydration, alkaline urine, and certain medications may trigger a mildly positive result, as may the presence of mucus, semen, or pus in the urine (15,80,81). Serum and urine protein electrophoresis may be warranted to evaluate for multiple myeloma (15,80). Heavy proteinuria (> 2 g per day) or other concerning findings should prompt a full renal workup and appropriate consultation.

Lower levels of proteinuria in the otherwise healthy patient may indicate orthostatic proteinuria, a benign condition (80,82,83) afflicting 3%-5% of adolescents and young adults, in which proteinuria occurs when the person is upright but resolves when supine. Testing involves collecting a 16-hour daytime urine sample, with the last void being just before bedtime. The next morning, another sample is obtained, reflecting the 8 hours of recumbency overnight. The daytime sample will show increased protein excretion, whereas the overnight sample will be normal (less than 50 mg). Orthostatic proteinuria requires no treatment, although monitoring with annual urinalysis and routine blood pressure checks seems prudent (80).

Patients with moderate nonorthostatic proteinuria but no sign of specific renal or systemic pathology may be classified as having isolated proteinuria. These patients have a 20% risk of developing worsening renal function over a ten-year period (80,84). Further evaluation such as renal biopsy may be appropriate (85).

Because benign, sports-associated hematuria and proteinuria are so common, and due to the potential harm that can be caused by false-positives and extensive workups, screening for these entities in athletes generally is not recommended (15,71,86).

Urinary Tract Infections

Although no studies definitively confirm causality, urethritis (87), cystitis (38), and prostatitis (88,89) have been linked to long-distance cycling. It is thought that urethral inflammation from constant bike seat irritation may predispose to bacterial urethritis (90); this may also result in conditions favoring the development of cystitis, although no conclusive evidence is available.

Due to increasing antibiotic resistance among common urinary tract pathogens, clinicians must consider the use of various antibiotics for treating these infections. It is particularly important that clinicians caring for athletes realize that fluoroquinolones have been associated with multiple cases of degeneration and rupture of weight-bearing tendons, especially the Achilles tendon. In addition, quinolones have been associated with chondropathic changes in animal models (91-95). Therefore, it is recommended that quinolones be used with caution in athletes and that athletes be instructed to report signs of tendinitis immediately, as these signs may presage impending rupture. Quinolones should not be used in children or pregnant women. If possible, other antibiotic choices should be used for athletes involved in running and jumping sports, especially if a long duration of therapy is contemplated.

Sexually Transmitted Infections

As a group, young athletes may exhibit a higher rate of risk-taking behaviors (including unsafe sexual practices) and have been shown to have a higher rate of sexually transmitted infections than their nonathlete peers (96,97). In particular, male athletes have a higher prevalence of unsafe sex behaviors than do female athletes (98,99). Given the overall high rate of risk-taking behaviors among adolescents and young adults, it is recommended that risk-factor screening be performed as part of the athletic PPSE and that appropriate counseling be given.

Stress Urinary Incontinence

The involuntary loss of urine during exercise is common among female athletes. The mechanism is multifactorial and involves a weakening of the pelvic floor support structures. Neuromuscular dysfunction and collagen abnormalities may also play a role. These factors prevent proper compression of the urethra, creating a lack of resistance with respect to the pressure in the bladder and thus allowing urine to leak out when intra-abdominal pressure increases, as with cough, sneeze, or strenuous exertion (100). Stress urinary incontinence (SUI) is most likely to occur in sports that involve repetitive jumping and running motions or high-impact landings (101). Overall prevalence rates among 20-year-old nulliparous female athletes may be as high as 28%-50% (100-102), with rates as high as 67% reported in gymnasts and basketball players (102). Risk factors include increased age and parity, obesity, hypoestrogenemia, and involvement in high-impact sports (101). Decreased foot flexibility (i.e., rigid, high-arched foot) has been correlated with an increased risk for SUI, presumably due to decreased absorption of shock (103). SUI has also been found to be more prevalent among women with eating disorders than among athletes without eating disorders (104). A careful history and physical exam, including pelvic and rectal exam, are warranted.

Many athletes note improvement with moderate reduction of fluid intake before exertion; avoidance of alcohol, caffeine, and other diuretic agents; regular voiding; and performance of Kegel exercises to strengthen the pelvic floor (100,105,106). Use of sanitary napkins and barrier devices can be useful to decrease leakage. Other treatment strategies include biofeedback, vaginal cones, tampons, pessaries, bladder neck support devices, and electrical stimulation (100,105,106). Tampons and pessaries have each been shown to be more effective for athletes than not using a mechanical device (107). Women who are hypoestrogenemic may benefit from a topical vaginal estrogen cream (101). Certain medications, such as imipramine and α-adrenergic agonists, have been shown to increase bladder outlet resistance and to ameliorate SUI symptoms (108). Phenylpropanolamine had shown promising results but has been removed from the market due to its association with hemorrhagic strokes.

For women who do not obtain satisfactory results with the above conservative measures, surgery may be an option. Urethral sling procedures seem to have better effectiveness and durability than needle suspension procedures and lower rate of illness than retropubic suspensions (110). Although cure rates are in the 80%-90% range (110), patients who undergo a surgical procedure for SUI should still be encouraged to follow the behavioral recommendations noted above.

The Athlete with a Single Kidney or Testicle

This is a controversial area in sports medicine. Although contact sports present an inherent threat, the evidence shows that risk of damaging the remaining organ in organized sports activities is extremely low (10,11). A survey of members of the American Medical Society for Sports Medicine (AMSSM) found that 54% would allow participation in contact and collision sports for an athlete with a single kidney, after full discussion of the potential risks (111). In patients who have an ectopic kidney, hoseshoe kidney, or other anatomic variation predisposing them to greater risk of injury, most experts would agree that participation in contact sports should not be allowed (9,112). The American Academy of Pediatrics does not recommend banning athletes with a single testicle from contact sports but considers use of a protective cup mandatory (113). It is recommended that the athlete (and their family members, as appropriate) be fully counseled about the potential risks and benefits of participating in contact sports.

Renal Complications of Exercise and Associated Behaviors

Acute renal failure (ARF) in athletes is uncommon but potentially devastating. Mechanisms of ARF in exercise are multiple. As previously noted, strenuous exercise decreases RBF and GFR, which can result in renal ischemia (15). Prolonged ischemia may subsequently cause acute tubular necrosis (ATN) (114).

Rhabdomyolysis from excessive exertion can cause myoglobinuria with subsequent ATN and ARF. Volume depletion and heat stress can increase an athlete's risk (15), as can obesity and poor conditioning. The level of activity reported by the patient may not seem excessive at the time but may still lead to significant tissue breakdown. Other potential factors, including sickle cell trait or disease, endocrinopathies, myopathies, and the use of medications such as "statins" and drugs such as alcohol, amphetamines, cocaine, creatine, Ecstasy, ephedrine, and PCP, should aggressively be sought after. Athletes may present complaining of fatigue, malaise, back pain, nausea, and myalgias. Dark or "tea-colored" urine may be noted, and the patient may seem dehydrated. Muscle tenderness and swelling may be present. Exertional rhabdomyolysis may also occur in the setting of heat stroke, which can be rapidly fatal; thus, it is imperative that heat illness be immediately identified and treated.

Prompt evaluation and treatment are essential in preventing ARF, which may complicate 15% of cases of rhabdomyolysis. However, research indicates that isolated exertional rhabdomyolysis may have a better prognosis than if there are other inciting causes. Myoglobinuria is often first noted by a positive dipstick test for blood, with no RBCs seen on microscopic analysis. Creatine kinase levels and hepatic enzymes are often markedly elevated. Hyperkalemia, hyperuricemia, hyperphosphatemia, and hypocalcemia may be seen; these may predispose to arrhythmias, so cardiac monitoring is recommended.

Rehydration with intravenous fluids and close monitoring of clinical status are essential. Alkalinization of the urine is recommended by some, but no controlled studies have shown it to be effective. Diuretics, including mannitol, should generally be avoided, as they do not improve, and may actually worsen, outcomes. N-acetylcysteine and other agents may have renal protective effects, but data are limited at present. Serial measurements of renal function, electrolyte and metabolic status, and the ruling out of associated complications (such as DIC and compartment syndromes) are required. In severe cases, hemodialysis may be necessary (115-117).

Athletes who use NSAIDs, analgesics, and other medications are at higher risk for renal complications of exercise. NSAIDs decrease renal prostaglandin synthesis, further decreasing renal blood flow and predisposing to ischemia and ATN (15,118). Over time, NSAIDs may cause or worsen hypertension through multiple renally mediated mechanisms (119). COX-2 selective NSAIDs seem to have the same potential for renal complications as do traditional NSAIDs (119,120). Therefore, NSAIDs should not be used during strenuous activities, and long-term use needs to be closely monitored by the clinician. Proper fluid intake is necessary to decrease the risk of volume contraction and development of prerenal azotemia.

Analgesic nephropathy due to chronic consumption of acetaminophen, phenacetin, NSAIDs, or similar medications is a well-known entity. This typically results in papillary necrosis and can result in chronic interstitial nephritis ands eventually end-stage renal disease (121,122).

The high-protein diets favored by many athletes have been shown to deliver a large acid load to the kidneys, resulting in increased risk for stone formation and increased calcium loss with potential risk for decreased bone mineral density (123,124). These diets may also speed the rate of decline in patients with chronic renal insufficiency (124). It is recommended that athletes who regularly participate in moderate to intense aerobic exercise consume 1.2 to 1.8 g of protein/kg/day, with up to 2 g/kg/day for high-intensity strength athletes. No benefit has been found at levels above 2 g/kg/day (125).

Genitourinary Effects of Ergogenic Aids

The use of creatine supplements by athletes has spurred concern over its potential nephrotoxic effects. Animal data have shown that creatine supplementation can worsen cystic kidney disease (126). There are no data at present to show that long-term creatine supplementation has an adverse effect on renal function in healthy athletes (127,128). There are sporadic case reports of elevated serum creatinine levels resolving after cessation of creatine use. However, for those athletes who use creatine, regular monitoring of renal function is recommended (129).

Anabolic steroids can cause testicular atrophy, prostate enlargement, erectile dysfunction, and libido changes in men, and potentially irreversible virilization in women (130,131). These agents have also been linked to an increased risk for Wilms' tumor, as well as prostate and testicular cancers (132). Anabolic steroids are controlled substances, and, due to their potential dangers and classification as doping agents, the IOC, the NCAA, and most professional sports organizations have banned them.

REFERENCES

1. **Moore KL.** Clinically Oriented Anatomy, 2nd ed. Baltimore: Williams & Wilkins; 1985.

2. **Hall-Craggs ECB.** Anatomy as a Basis for Clinical Medicine, 2nd ed. Baltimore: Urban & Scwarzenberg; 1990.

3. **Taffet R.** Management of pelvic fractures with concomitant urologic injuries. Orthopedic Clin N Am. 1997;28:389-95.

4. **Watnik NF, Coburn M, Goldberger M.** Urologic injuries in pelvic ring disruptions. Clin Orthopaedics Related Res. 1996;329:37-45.

5. **Webster GD, Guralnick ML.** Reconstruction of posterior urethral disruption. Urologic Clin N Am. 2002;29:429-41.

6. **Coppola PT, Coppola M.** Emergency department evaluation and treatment of pelvic fractures. Emerg Med Clin N Am. 2000;18:1-27.

7. **Baverstock R, Simons R, McLoughlin M.** Severe blunt renal trauma: a 7 year retrospective review from a provincial trauma centre. Can J Urol. 2001;8:1372-6.

8. **Dreitlein DA, Suner S, Basler J.** Genitourinary trauma. Emerg Med Clin N Am. 2001;19:569 90.

9. **Dombrowski RT.** Genitourinary problems of athletes. In: Baker CL, ed. The Hughston Clinic Sports Medicine Book. Baltimore: Williams & Wilkins; 1995:129-34.

10. **McAleer IM, Kaplan GW, LoSasso BE.** Renal and testis injuries in team sports. J Urol. 2002;168:1805-7.

11. **Amaral JF.** Thoracoabdominal injuries in the athlete. Clin Sports Med. 1997; 16:739-53.

12. **Cantor RM, Leaming JM.** Evaluation and management of pediatric major trauma. Emerg Med Clin N Am. 1998;16:229-56.

13. **Sartorelli KH, Pilcher DB, Rogers FB.** Patterns of splenic injury seen in skiers. Injury. 1995;26:43-6.

14. **Peterson NE.** Genitourinary trauma. In: Feliciano DV, Moore EE, Mattox KL, eds. Trauma, 3rd ed. Stamford, CT: Appleton & Lange; 1996:661-93.

15. **Cianflocco AJ.** Renal complications of exercise. Clin Sports Med. 1992;11:437-51.

16. **Wexler RK, Parmar A.** Renal laceration in a high school football player. Phys Sportsmed. 2003;31:43.

17. **Tillou A, Romero J, Asensio JA, et al.** Renal vascular injuries. Surg Clin N Am. 2001;81:1417-30.

18. **Harris AC, Zwirewich CV, Lyburn ID, et al.** CT findings in blunt renal trauma. Radiographics. 2001;21:S201-14.

19. **Porter JM, Singh Y.** Value of computed tomography in the evaluation of retroperitoneal organ injury in blunt abdominal trauma. Am J Emerg Med. 1998;16:225-7.

20. **Novelline RA, Rhea JT, Bell T.** Helical CT of abdominal trauma. Radiol Clin N. Am. 1999;37:591-612.

21. **Schreyer HH, Uggowitzer MM, Ruppert-Kohlmayr A.** Helical CT of the urinary organs. Eur Radiol. 2002;12:575-91.

22. **Morey AF, McAninch JW, Tiller BK, et al.** Single shot intraoperative excretory urography for the immediate evaluation of renal trauma. J Urol. 1999;161:1088-92.

23. **Carpio F, Morey AF.** Radiographic staging of renal injuries. World J Urol. 1999;17:66-70.

24. **Ku JH.** Is there a role for magnetic resonance imaging in renal trauma? Int J Urol. 2001;8:261-7.

25. **Kawashima A, Sandler CM, Corl FM, et al.** Imaging of renal trauma: a comprehensive review. Radiographics. 2001;21:557-74.

26. **Knudson MM, Maull KI.** Non-operative management of solid organ injuries: past, present, and future. Surg Clin N Am. 1999;79:1357-71.

27. **Vaccaro JP, Brody JM.** CT cystography in the evaluation of major bladder trauma. Radiographics. 2000;20:1373-81.

28. **Hsieh CH, Chen RJ, Fang JF, et al.** Diagnosis and management of bladder injury by trauma surgeons. Am J Surg. 2002;184:143-7.

29. **Abarbanel J, Benet AE, Lask D, Kimche D.** Sports hematuria. J Urol. 1990;143:887-90.

30. **McKeag DB, Hough DO.** Common sports-related injuries and illnesses—thorax and abdomen. In: McKeag DB, Hough DO. Primary Care Sports Medicine. Dubuque, IA: Brown & Benchmark; 1993:343-94.

31. **Lofthouse GA.** Traumatic injuries to the extremities and thorax. Clin Sports Med. 1994;13:113-35.

32. **Jezior JR, Schlossberg SM.** Excision and primary anastomosis for anterior urethral stricture. Urol Clinic N Am. 2002;29:373-80.

33. **Noujaim SE, Nagle CE.** Acute scrotal injuries in athletes: evaluation by diagnostic imaging. Phys Sportsmed. 1989;17:125.

34. **Munter DW, Faleski EJ.** Blunt scrotal trauma: Emergency department evaluation and management. Am J Emerg Med. 1989;7:227-33.

35. **Silbert PL, Dunne JW, Edis RH, Stewart-Wynne EG.** Bicycling induced pudendal nerve pressure neuropathy. Clin Exp Neurol. 1991;28:191-6.

36. **Andersen KV, Bovim G.** Impotence and nerve entrapment in long distance amateur cyclists. Acta Neurol Scand. 1997;95:233-40.

37. **Thompson MJ, Rivara FP.** Bicycle-related injuries. Am Fam Physician. 2001;63:2007-14.

38. **Weiss BD.** Clinical syndromes associated with bicycle seats. Clin Sports Med. 1994;13:175-86.

39. **Frauscher F.** Paper presented to 2003 Annual Meeting of the Radiological Society of North America. Chicago, IL; 2003.

40. **Frauscher F, Klauser A, Stenzl A, et al.** US findings in the scrotum of extreme mountain bikers. Radiology. 2001;219:427-31.

41. **Galejs LE, Kass EJ.** Diagnosis and treatment of the acute scrotum. Am Fam Physician. 1999;59:817-24.

42. **Marcozzi D, Suner S.** The nontraumatic, acute scrotum. Emerg Med Clin N Am. 2001;19:547-68.

43. **Epperly TD, Moore KE.** Health issues in men. Part 1: Common genitourinary disorders. Am Fam Physician. 2001;63:2331-2.

44. **Savory LM.** Preventive services for the middle-aged adult (41-64 years). Clin Fam Practice. 2000;2.

45. **Docimo SG, Silver RI, Cromie W.** The undescended testicle: diagnosis and management. Am Fam Physician. 2000;62:2037-44.

46. **Epperson WJ, Frank WL.** Male genital cancers. Prim Care. 1998;25:459-72.

47. **Froehner M, Fischer R, Leike S, et al.** Intratesticular leiomyosarcoma in a young man after high dose doping with Oral-Turinabol: a case report. Cancer. 1999;86:1571-5.

48. **Coakley FV, Hricak H, Presti JC Jr.** Imaging and management of atypical testicular masses. Urol Clin N Am. 1998;25:375-88.

49. **Fretz PC, Sandlow JI.** Varicocele: current concepts in pathophysiology, diagnosis, and treatment. Urol Clin N Am. 2002;29:921-37.

50. **Evers JLH, Collins JA.** Assessment of efficacy of varicocele repair for male subfertility: a systematic review. Lancet. 2003;361:1849-52.

51. **Townsend CM Jr, Beauchamp RD, Evers BM, Mattox KL, eds.** Sabiston Textbook of Surgery, 16th ed. Philadelphia: WB Saunders; 2001:783-800.

52. **Carabasi RA, Cohn IIE, Jarrell DE, et al.** Surgical principles. In: Jarrell BE, Carabasi RA, eds. Surgery. Media, PA: Harwal; 1986-48-52.

53. **Lacroix VJ.** A complete approach to groin pain. Phys Sportsmed. 2000;28:66-86.

54. **Kesek P, Ekberg O, Westlin N.** Herniographic findings in athletes with unclear groin pain. Acta Radiol. 2002;43:603-8.

55. **Bell RC, Price JG.** Laparoscopic inguinal hernia repair using an anatomically contoured three-dimensional mesh. Surg Endosc. Published online: 10 September 2003; Springer-Verlag.

56. **McCormack K, Scott NW, Go PM, et al.** EU Hernia Trialists Collaboration. Cochrane Database Syst Rev. 2003;(1):CD001785.

57. **Taylor DC, Meyers WC, Moylan JA, et al.** Abdominal musculature abnormalities as a cause of groin pain in athletes. Inguinal hernias and pubalgia. Am J Sports Med. 1991;19:239-42.

58. **Meyers WC, Foley DP, Garrett WE, et al.** Management of severe lower abdominal or inguinal pain in high-performance athletes. Am J Sports Med. 2000;28:2-8.

59. **Kemp SR, Batt ME.** The "sports hernia": a common cause of groin pain. Phys Sportsmed. 1998;26-36.

60. **Gilmore OJ.** Gilmore's groin. Sportsmed Soft Tissue Trauma. 1992;3:12-4.

61. **Hackney RG.** The sports hernia: a cause of groin pain. Br J Sportsmed. 1993;27:58-62.

62. **Simonet WT, Saylor HI. III, Sim L.** Abdominal wall muscle tears in hockey players. Int J Sports Med. 1995;16:126-8.

63. **Williams P, Foster ME.** "Gilmore's groin"—or is it? Br J Sports Med. 1995;29:206-8.

64. **Ziprin P.** External oblique aponeurosis nerve entrapment as a cause of groin pain in the athlete. Br J Surg. 1999;86:566-8.

65. **Morelli V, Smith V.** Groin injuries in athletes. Am Fam Phys. 2001;64:1405-14.

66. **Hölmich P, Uhrskou P, Ulnits L, et al.** Effectiveness of active physical training as treatment for long-standing adductor-related groin pain in athletes: randomized trial. Lancet. 1999;353:439-43.

67. **Poglase AL, Frydman GM, Farmer KC.** Inguinal surgery for debilitating chronic groin pain in athletes. Med J Austr. 1991;155:674-7.

68. **Malycha P, Lovell G.** Inguinal surgery in athletes with chronic groin pain: the "sportsman's" hernia. Austr N Z J Surg. 1992;62:123-5.

69. **Urquhart DS, Packer GJ, McLatchie GR.** Return to sport and patient satisfaction after surgical treatment for groin disruption. Sports Exerc Injury. 1996;1:37-42.

70. **Brannigan AE, Kerin MJ, McEntee GP.** Gilmore's groin repair in athletes. J Orthop Sports Phys Ther. 2000;30:329-32.

71. **Cohen RA, Brown RS.** Microscopic hematuria. N Engl J Med. 2003;348:2330-8.

72. **Cecil RL, Goldman L, Bennett JC.** Cecil Textbook of Medicine, 21st ed. Philadelphia: WB Saunders; 2000:884.

73. **Grossfeld GD, Wolf JS Jr, Litwan MS, et al.** Asymptomatic microscopic hematuria in adults: summary of the AUA best practice policy recommendations. Am Fam Phys. 2001;63:1145-54.

74. **Jamis-Dow CA, Choyke PL, Jennings SB, et al.** Small (< or = 3 cm) renal masses: detection with CT vs US and pathologic correlation. Radiology. 1996;198:785-8.

75. **Warshauer DM, McCarthy SM, Street L, et al.** Detection of renal masses: sensitivities and specificities of excretory urography/linear tomography, US, and CT. Radiology. 1988;169:363-5.

76. **Grossfeld GD, Carroll PR.** Evaluation of asymptomatic microscopic hematuria. Urol Clin N Am. 1998;25:661-76.

77. **Darnley MJ, DiMarco NM, Aukema HM.** Safety of chronic exercise in a rat model of kidney disease. Med Sci Sports Exerc. 2000;32:576-80.

78. **Alyea EP, Parish HH, Durham NC.** Renal response to exercise-urinary findings. JAMA. 1958;167:807-13.

79. **Neviackas JA, Bauer JM.** Renal function abnormalities induced by marathon running. South Med J. 1981;74:1457-60.

80. **Carroll MF, Temte JL.** Proteinuria in adults: a diagnostic approach. Am Fam Physician. 2000;62:1333-40.

81. **Kashif W, Siddiqi N, Dincer HE, et al.** Proteinuria: how to evaluate an important finding. Clev Clin J Med. 2003;70:535-47.

82. **Springberg PD, Garrett LE Jr, Thompson AL Jr, et al.** Fixed and reproducible orthostatic proteinuria: results of a 20 year follow-up study. Ann Intern Med. 1982;97:516-9.

83. **Rytand DA, Spreiter S.** Prognosis in postural (orthostatic) proteinuria: forty to fifty year follow-up of six patients after diagnosis by Thomas Addis. N Engl J Med. 1981;305:618-21.

84. **Abuelo JG.** Proteinuria: diagnostic principles and procedures. Ann Intern Med. 1983;98:186-91.

85. **Trachtman H, Bergwerk A, Gauthier B.** Isolated proteinuria in children: natural history and indications for renal biopsy. Clin Pediatr. 1994;33:468-72.

86. **Kurowski K, Chandran S.** The preparticipation athletic evaluation. Am Fam Physician. 2000;61:2683-90, 2696-8.

87. **Hershfeld NB.** Pedaller's penis. Can Med Assoc J. 1983;128:366-7.

88. **O'Brien KP.** Sports urology: the vicious cycle. N Engl J Med. 1981;304:1367-8.

89. **Dickson TB.** Preventing overuse cycling injuries. Phys Sportsmed. 1985;13:116-23.

90. **Mellion MB.** Common cycling injuries: Management and prevention. Sports Med. 1991;11:52-70.

91. **Cunha BA.** Antibiotic side effects. Med Clin North Am. 2001;85:149-85.

92. **Bass PF, Jarvis JW, Mitchell CK.** Urinary tract infections. Prim Care: Clin Office Pract. 2003;30.

93. **Oliphant CM, Green GM.** Quinolones: a comprehensive review. Am Fam Physician. 2002;65:455-64.

94. **O'Donnell JA, Gelone SP.** Fluoroquinolones. Infect Dis Clin North Am. 2000;14:489-513.

95. **Casparian JM, Luchi M, Moffat RE, Hinthorn D.** Quinolones and tendon ruptures. South Med J. 2000;93:488-91.

96. **Nattiv A, Puffer JC, Green GA.** Lifestyles and health risks of collegiate athletes: a multi-center study. Clin J Sport Med. 1997;7:262-72.

97. **Nattiv A, Puffer JC.** Lifestyles and health risks of collegiate athletes. J Fam Pract. 1991;33:585-90.

98. **Kokotailo PK, Henry BC, Koscik RE, et al.** Substance use and other health risk behaviors in collegiate athletes. Clin J Sport Med. 1996;6:183-9.

99. **Kokotailo PK, Koscik RE, Henry BC, et al.** Health risk taking and human immunodeficiency virus risk in collegiate female athletes. J Am Coll Health. 1998;46:263-8.

100. **Elia G.** Stress urinary incontinence in women. Phys Sportsmed. 1999;27:39.

101. **Greydanus DE, Patel DR.** The female athlete: before and beyond puberty. Pediatr Clin North Am. 2002;49:553-80.

102. **Nygaard IE, Thompson FL, Svengalis SL, Albright JP.** Urinary incontinence in elite nulliparous athletes. Obstet Gynecol. 1994;84:183-7.

103. **Nygaard IE, Glowacki C, Saltzman CL.** Relationship between foot flexibility and urinary incontinence in nulliparous varsity athletes. Obstet Gynecol. 1996;87:1049-51.

104. **Bø K, Borgen JS.** Prevalence of stress and urge urinary incontinence in elite athletes and controls. Med Sci Sports Exerc. 2001;33:1797-802.

105. **Nygaard IE, Kreder KJ, Lepic MM, et al.** Efficacy of pelvic floor muscle exercises in women with stress, urge, and mixed urinary incontinence. Am J Obstet Gynecol. 1996;74:120-5.

106. **Visco AG, Figuers C.** Nonsurgical management of pelvic floor dysfunction. Obstet Gynecol Clin North Am. 1998;25:849-65.

107. **Nygaard I.** Prevention of exercise incontinence with mechanical devices. J Reprod Med. 1995;40:89-94.

108. **Wein AJ, Rovner ES.** Pharmacologic management of urinary incontinence in women. Urol Clin North Am. 2002;29:537-50.

109. Reference deleted in proof.

110. **Niknejad K, Plzak LS III, Staskin DR, Loughlin KR.** Autologous and synthetic urethral slings for female incontinence. Urol Clin North Am. 2002;29:597-611.

111. **Anderson CR.** Solitary kidney and sports participation. Arch Fam Med. 1995;4:885-8.

112. **Terrell T, Woods M, Hough DO.** Blunt trauma reveals a single kidney: A disqualification dilemma. Phys Sportsmed. 1997;25.

113. **Grafe MW, Paul GR, Foster TE.** The preparticipation sports examination for high school and college athletes. Clin Sportsmed. 1997;16:569-91.

113. **Sinert R, Kohl L, Rainone T, Scalea T.** Exercise-induced rhabdomyolysis. Ann Emerg Med. 1994;23:1301-6.

114. **Agrawal M, Swartz R.** Acute renal failure. Am Fam Physician. 2000;61:2077-88.

116. **Sauret JM, Marinides G, Wang GK.** Rhabdomyolysis. Am Fam Physician. 2002;65:907-12.

117. **Abernethy VE, Lieberthal W.** Acute renal failure in the critically ill patient. Crit Care Clin. 2002;18:203-22.

118. **Sanders LR.** Exercise-induced acute renal failure associated with ibuprofen, hydrochlorothiazide, and triamterene. J Am Soc Nephrol. 1995;5:2020-3.

119. **Frishman WH.** Effects of nonsteroidal anti-inflammatory drug therapy on blood pressure and peripheral edema. Am J Cardiol. 2002;89:18-25D.

120. **Wright JM.** The double-edged sword of COX-2 selective NSAIDs. Can Med Assoc J. 2002;167:1131-7.

121. **Dubach UC, Rosner B, Pfister E.** Epidemiologic study of abuse of analgesics containing phenacetin: renal morbidity and mortality (1968-1979). N Engl J Med. 1983;308:357-62.

122. **Michielsen P, de Schepper P.** Trends of analgesic nephropathy in two high-endemic regions with different legislation. J Am Soc Nephrol. 2001;12:550-6.

123. **Reddy ST, Wang CY, Sakhaee K, et al.** Effect of low-carbohydrate high-protein diets on acid-base balance, stone-forming propensity, and calcium metabolism. Am J Kidney Dis. 2002;40:265-74.

124. **Denke MA.** Metabolic effects of high-protein, low-carbohydrate diets. Am J Cardiol. 2001;88:59-61.

125. **Rankin JW.** Role of protein in exercise. Clin Sports Med. 1999;18:499-511.

126. **Edmunds JW, Jayapalan S, DiMarco NM, et al.** Creatine supplementation increases renal disease progression in Han: SPRD-cy rats. Am J Kidney Dis. 2001;37:73-8.

127. **Mayhew DL, Mayhew JL, Ware JS.** Effects of long-term creatine supplementation on liver and kidney functions in American college football players. Int J Sport Nutr Exerc Metab. 2002;12:453-60.

128. **Poortmans JR, Francaux M.** Long-term oral creatine supplementation does not impair renal function in healthy athletes. Med Sci Sports Exerc. 1999;31:1108-10.

129. **Poortmans JR, Francaux M.** Adverse effects of creatine supplementation: fact or fiction? Sports Med. 2000;30:155-70.

130. **Congeni J, Miller S.** Supplements and drugs used to enhance athletic performance. Pediatr Clin North Am. 2002;49:435-61.

131. **Greydanus DE, Patel DR.** Sports doping in the adolescent athlete: the hope, hype, and hyperbole. Pediatr Clin North Am. 2002;49:829-55.

132. **Joyce JA.** Anesthesia for athletes using performance-enhancing drugs. AANA J. 1991;59:139-44.

11

■ ■ ■

Dermatologic Problems in Athletes

George C. Baker, MD, MBA

S kin problems are extremely common in persons participating in sports. As might be imagined, skin injuries account for a major proportion of sports-related injuries. Such injuries are prone to infection due to close physical contact with other persons and with environmental pathogens. These injuries can result in significant lost time in training and also can lead to disqualification from sports events.

This chapter is meant to serve as a basic, practical, and straightforward guide to relatively common dermatologic problems in athletes, as well as in any person who participates in sports (for example, for recreation). It is important to remember, however, that athletes can exhibit any skin disorder, not just those particularly associated with sports. As in any other area of clinical medicine, dermatologic problems that are common in the general population will be common in athletes as well, and the physician examining the athlete's skin disorder should consider not just the sports-related diagnoses in the differential. Further, underlying chronic skin disorders (for example, psoriasis and chronic dermatitis) can predispose the athlete to infection and injury obtained during the sports activity (for example, through person-to-person contact).

Viral Infections

Warts

Warts (verrucae) are caused by many subtypes of human papilloma virus (HPV), a DNA virus. Warts usually appear as flesh-colored, rough papules on exposed surfaces and can coalesce into small to large plaques, especially on areas such as palms and soles. Certain subtypes of HPV are associated with certain anatomic locations. The virus must penetrate the stratum corneum (outer dead layer of epidermis) to cause infection. This process can occur through cuts, abrasions, or puncture wounds. Compromised epidermis from chronic friction or maceration (for example, sweating) can predispose the patient to infection. Swimming pool decks and communal showers are typical locations for the spread of plantar warts. Palmar warts are frequently seen in athletes who share weight-lifting equipment. Skin-to-skin contact can spread the wart virus during contact sports.

Treatment for warts often involves the use of destructive modalities, including wart paring, liquid nitrogen cryotherapy, salicylic acid applications (liquid and patches), and blistering agents. Other modalities include curettage (scraping off the wart tissue), laser treatment, topical imiquimod, and duct tape occlusion. Warts can be stubborn and resistant to therapy, particularly when they are located on periungual and plantar surface areas. Sometimes multiple treatments and/or modalities must be used for a successful outcome.

Although many warts may spontaneously resolve, active treatment is recommended to prevent spread of the virus to other body areas or to other persons. If the patient tolerates the treatment, the wart may be frozen and a liquid blistering compound with Band-Aid occlusion can be applied for 8 or more hours. Occasionally, it is suggested that the patient also use over-the-counter salicylic acid preparations. A return visit 2 to 4 weeks later is recommended because retreatment is often necessary, especially if the warts involve the hands and fingers.

Warts are a very annoying yet curable problem. Although the lesions are potentially contagious, prohibiting the athlete with warts from participating in sports, especially if treatment is in progress, is generally not advocated. Such a policy of prohibition could possibly eliminate many otherwise healthy participants from their desired sports activities.

Herpes Gladiatorum

Herpes infections and transmission are common among wrestlers. Again, direct skin-to-skin contact is the mode of transmission. Herpes simplex virus type 1 is the causal agent. As with tinea corporis gladiatorum, most of the lesions occur on the head, neck, and upper extremities. Lesions are usually preceded by several hours of a burning or tingling sensation. They appear as multiple small, clustered, clear vesicles, arising on normal or slightly erythematous skin. The vesicles become purulent and eventually dry and crust over before healing. This process usually takes from 7-10 days. Fever, malaise, and regional lymphadenopathy, often tender, may be common accompanying signs and symptoms. Healing may be complicated by secondary bacterial infection (impetigo). Ocular involvement may be a serious complication.

Case Study 11-1

A 20-year-old college wrestler presented with a burning, itching eruption on the right lateral deltoid area. The lesions began one day earlier, with small red bumps that progressed overnight into clear, grouped vesicles on slightly erythematous skin covering an area approximately 3 by 2 cm. The patient had a similar eruption 8 months ago, but he sought no medical attention at that time; the eruption spontaneously healed within 2 weeks. He had no other known health problems.

The patient was diagnosed with herpes gladiatorum. Treatment consisted of applications of penciclovir cream every 2 hours while awake, along with acyclovir 400 mg orally three times a day for five days. The patient was given clearance for return to play in 10 days.

Treatment of herpes simplex virus (HSV) infections includes topicals (acyclovir ointment, penciclovir cream) and systemic agents (acyclovir, famciclovir, valacyclovir). Recent guidelines for treatment of HSV type 1 fever blisters include valacyclovir 2 grams orally twice a day for one day. To this, the physician can add penciclovir cream q 2 hours to the lesion(s) while awake. Another (more common) option for HSV type 1 lesions on the face or body is prescription of acyclovir 400 mg orally three times a day for 3-5 days, based on the case severity and patient history. Again, the addition of penciclovir cream q 2 hours to the lesions while awake is favored. However, these are only general guidelines; dosage and treatment duration vary depending on severity and other factors.

HSV infections are controllable but, unfortunately, not curable. It is virtually impossible to be 100% confident that there is no viral shedding taking place at the site of an HSV infection at a given moment in time. There may be viral shedding, even in the absence of signs and/or symptoms. Individuals should not be allowed to compete until vesicles are dried and scabbed. It is probably safe to return to play 10 days after initiation of the appropriate antiviral therapy. This time frame presumes a recurrence, rather than a primary HSV infection, which may last longer than just a few days.

Varicella Zoster Virus

Varicella zoster virus (VZV) in its primary form (chicken pox) causes vesicular skin lesions with systemic symptoms of fever and malaise. Patients with this disorder should not be allowed to participate in sports until systemic symptoms have resolved and all skin lesions have crusted. Localized recurrence of VZV (shingles) may be precipitated by severe physical stress. Vesicular lesions should be covered, and athletes should limit contact sports until the lesions have scabbed and crusted.

Molluscum Contagiosum

Molluscum contagiosum may appear as solitary or multiple dome-shaped ways or umbilicated papules. It is caused by two poxviruses and may occur in participants in sports with skin-to-skin contact (1). Lesions may be removed mechanically with curregage or cryotherapy with liquid nitrogen. Topically applied medication, such as 5% podophyllin or 5% imiquimod, may also be used (2). Athletes may resume competition that involves direct contact if the lesion has healed or if it is covered.

Fungal Infections

Tinea

Tinea is a fungal infection caused by dermatophytic fungi. Dermatophytes are a group of fungi (including three genera: *Trichophyton, Microsporum,* and *Epidermophyton*) capable of infecting keratinized epithelium including those of skin, hair and nails.

Tinea Pedis (Athlete's Foot)

Tinea pedis ("athlete's foot") is a common dermatophytic infection that may cause a combination of erythema, scaling, maceration, vesicles/bullae, and often pruritus. Tinea pedis may spread to the groin and buttocks (tinea cruris or "jock itch"), trunk and extremities (tinea corporis), hands (tinea manuum), and nails (onychomycosis). Tinea pedis often results in cracks of the epidermis, providing a portal of entry for pathogenic bacteria. Topical antifungal agents include clotrimazole, econazole, miconazole, ketoconazole, oxiconazole, naftifine, terbinafine, and ciclopirox olamine. Widespread tinea may require oral antifungals (for example, terbinafine or itraconazole). Athletes with tinea pedis should wear protective footwear when using shared facilities (3).

Tinea Corporis (Ringworm)

Trichophyton tonsurans and *Trichophyton rubrum* account for most of the cases of tinea corporis ("ringworm") in wrestlers. As with herpes gladiatorum, the head, neck, and upper extremities are the most commonly affected areas. Direct skin-to-skin contact is the method for transmission; direct skin-to-skin transmission of tinea corporis has been reported in wrestlers (4.) The lesions of tinea corporis usually appear as scaly plaques with a raised erythematous border, often with central clearing. They may be solitary or multiple. The lesions are most often pruritic.

Treatment options for tinea corporis include topical and/or oral antifungal medications. Again, topical agents include clotrimazole, econazole, miconazole, ketoconazole, oxiconazole, naftifine, terbinafine, and ciclopirox olamine. Naftifine, terbinafine , or ciclopirox olamine is recommended twice a day for 4 weeks to minimize recurrences. Although oral antifungals such as terbinafine, ketoconazole, fluconazole, and itraconazole may be used, there are possible systemic side effects and potential drug interactions to consider.

It is difficult to know the exact moment when a tinea infection is no longer contagious. However, after treating the lesions twice a day for one week with terbinafine, naftifine, or ciclopirox olamine, return to play may be considered. At a week's time into such a treatment regimen, the risk of contagion should be minimal.

Bacterial Infections

Impetigo

Staphylococcus aureus and *Streptococcus pyogenes* are the causative organisms of impetigo. Lesions are most commonly located on the head, neck, and upper extremities. A break or cut in the epidermis is needed for these pathogenic bacteria to enter and cause infection. Trauma from sports activities can facilitate such entry. Warm, moist, macerated skin occluded by uniforms and equipment can compromise the skin's ability to resist bacterial entry. Impetigo begins as an erythematous macule that rapidly evolves into a vesiculopustule that breaks, leaving an erythematous erosion covered with honey-colored crust. Satellite lesions may occur around the original lesion(s). Bullous impetigo begins as flaccid bullae become purulent and eventually covered with crust. Local pain, lymphadenopathy, and leukocytosis may accompany cases of impetigo.

Case Study 11-2

An 18-year-old male soccer player presented with a 2-day history of rapidly spreading honey-colored crusted plaques 1-2 cm in size on the face. The lesions began under his right nostril and spread from the upper lip to the cheeks within a couple of days. His past medical history was significant for mild asthma, atopic dermatitis, and allergic rhinitis. A diagnosis of impetigo was made. Because he was at significant risk for spreading the infection to other areas of his skin and to other persons, he was treated with oral anti-*Staph* antibiotics, as well as mupirocin cream or ointment twice a day. In this situation, treatment was therefore continued for a full 10 days, rather than just 7 days. Clearance for return to play was given in 10 days.

Patients with one or more components of the atopic triad (atopic dermatitis, asthma, and allergic rhinitis) are often carriers of *Staphylococcus aureus* in the nose. Those patients with atopic dermatitis often have dry, itchy skin on the face and other areas. Scratching the facial skin disrupts the protective epidermal covering and predisposes the skin to infection from the nasal bacteria.

Antibiotic therapy is indicated for impetigo. Topical mupirocin twice a day for 7-10 days is appropriate for small, localized cases; more extensive cases require 1-2 weeks of systemic antibiotics appropriate for *Staph* and *Strep* bacteria. Local areas of skin infection should be kept covered with a dressing to prevent transmission. First-genertion cepahlosporins are usually adequate for treatment; however, one should be aware of increasing "clusters" of methicillin-resistant *Staphylococcus aureus* (MRSA) skin infections in athletes (5). Clinical failure of first-line medication necessitates culture of the lesion. Antibacterial cleansers, such as Betadine or Hibiclens, may be helpful in wound care.

In general, for mild cases of impetigo, one may give a return-to-play "green light" at one week into therapy. In the team setting, any mild active cases should be treated with both topical mupirocin cream or ointment twice a day for 1 week, along with 1 week of cephalexin 500 mg orally four times a day or (in penicillin allergic patients) azithromycin 500 mg orally for one dose, followed by 250 mg orally qd for the next 4 days. More extensive cases require 10 days of antibiotic therapy. All team members having potential contact with the infected player also should cleanse the skin with an antibacterial cleanser and be monitored closely for the first signs of infection. Handwashing is particularly important. However, wholesale distribution of oral antibiotics to all team members is not always necessary, because most pathogenic bacteria have a difficult time penetrating normal skin.

Furuncles (Boils)

Furuncles are red, hot, tender nodules that evolve from a staphylococcal folliculitis. While simple furunculosis may be treated with nothing more than localized heat application, appropriate anti-*Staph* antibiotics may be necessary when the condition involves athletes who may spread infection.

Pitted Keratolysis

Common in athletes, pitted keratolysis is caused by *Micrococcus sedentarius* and/or *Corynebacterium* species. These organisms invade the stratum corneum, which is compromised by sweating and maceration. The lesions are small pits on the plantar surface, predominantly on weight-bearing surfaces. The affected foot is usually malodorous.

Treatment includes topical and oral erythromycin and topical clindamycin. Helpful preventative measures include using absorbent foot powder, changing socks frequently, and changing out of athletic shoes as soon as the activity is over.

Pseudomonas

Pseudomonas aeruginosa infections are commonly associated with water. *Pseudomonas* folliculitis from hot tubs, whirlpools, and swimming pools presents as pruritic follicular papules and pustules on exposed areas. Most cases resolve spontaneously. Cases requiring antibiotic therapy respond to ciprofloxacin.

Pseudomonas may also cause green nails, otitis externa, and web-space infection, particularly in swimmers. Topical gentamicin may be helpful in treating these conditions.

Phototoxicity

Certain medications (for example, sulfonamides, tetracyclines) and topical contactants (for example, perfumes, limes, and lemons) may induce a phototoxic reaction when the predisposed patient receives ultraviolet radiation from sunlight. These reactions may resemble an exaggerated sunburn with erythema, edema, vesicles or bullae, weeping, associated pain, malaise, and fever. Athletes should be aware of these connections and protect themselves with sunscreens and appropriate protective clothing.

Environmental and Mechanical Dermatoses

Of course, cuts, scrapes, scratches, abrasions, bruising, and so forth are common in athletics, particularly the contact sports. Discussions of most of these common problems are discussed elsewhere. The conditions more specific to dermatology are discussed below.

Callosities

The corn (clavus) is a common thickening of the epidermis (hyperkeratosis) caused by repeated pressure or rubbing of a bony prominence of the foot. Corns most often occur on the top of the fifth toe. Tight-fitting shoes are a predisposing factor. Soft corns, often in the fourth-fifth toe web space, may be painful. The area of hyperkeratosis may become soft and macerated, resembling tinea pedis. Bacterial superinfection may occur in such cases, requiring antibiotics.

A callus also represents epidermal hyperkeratosis, but the lesions are usually larger and less focal than corns. They are also caused by repeated pressure or rubbing. Properly fitting shoes and cushioning socks may help to remedy the problem. Other modalities of callus removal include paring, salicylic acid pads, and 40% urea cream.

Collagenous Athlete's Nodules

A variety of collagenous nodules occur in athletes. These nodules occur at sites of trauma, pressure, and friction and are usually asymptomatic. They are flesh-colored papules or nodules presenting on the feet of surfers ("surfer's nodules"), the knuckles of boxers, and the feet of football and soccer players. In certain symptomatic cases, excision of the lesion may be required for relief.

Piezogenic Pedal Papules

Piezogenic pedal papules are lesions presenting as small skin-colored papules on the lateral heels. They often represent small herniations of the fat caused by vigorous exercise, such as running. Treatment is usually unnecessary, although the lesions may be painful.

Talon Noir (Black Heel) and Tennis Toe (Black Toe, Jogger's Toe)

Talon noir, caused by traumatic force on the calcaneal skin, represents a small hematoma. Its significance lies in the possible confusion with a melanoma. Paring of the lesion will reveal the clotted blood.

Tennis toe represents a subungual hematoma and is most commonly seen on the great toe. It is caused by forcing of the toes into the front of the shoe during quick stops and starts in sports such as tennis, racquetball, squash, jogging, or basketball. The condition may be painful. A subungual melanoma must be considered in the differential diagnosis, particularly if the black color involves the proximal nail fold.

Jogger's Nipples

Jogger's nipples are caused by the constant friction of shirts in runners. The nipples may be painful and eroded. Wearing soft fabric shirts or Band-Aids may prevent the condition.

Friction Blisters

Friction blisters, caused by shearing forces resulting in midepidermal necrosis, are a common problem in athletes. Sweating, heat, and maceration of the epidermis predispose the skin to friction blisters. Properly fitted footwear, cushioning socks, and foot powder can help to prevent blisters on the sole. Golfers and racket sports players can prevent palmar blisters by wearing appropriate gloves.

Urticarial Reactions

A variety of urticarial reactions may occur during athletics, the most common being cholinergic urticaria. During exercise, when the body core is heated, small urticarial papules with surrounding erythematous flares may appear on the skin. Systemic features, including nausea, vomiting, headache, wheezing, dizziness, and dyspnea, may accompany these papules.

Other varieties of urticaria may occur in athletes, including solar urticaria, cold urticaria, aquagenic urticaria, pressure urticaria, and (rarely) exercise-induced anaphylaxis. These varieties are less common than cholinergic urticaria.

Contact Dermatitis

A variety of athletic equipment may cause contact sensitization in athletes. Chemical components of shoes (rubber, glues, leather tanning agents) may cause sensitization. Most commonly, a shoe contact dermatitis will be seen on the dorsal feet and toes, sparing the skin not touched by the shoe. Erythema, scaling, maceration, vesiculation, weeping, and lichenification may all be seen. Secondary bacterial infection may occur, requiring antibiotic therapy.

Swimming goggles, especially of black neoprene rubber, may contain sensitizers. Contact dermatitis in the periorbital area develops in sensitive individuals. Goggles without black neoprene are available. Other swimming equipment, such as masks, fins, snorkels, ear plugs, and nose clips, may also contain sensitizers. Nonsensitizing versions of such swimming equipment are available.

Treatment of contact dermatitis first involves determining the causative agent(s). Patch testing by the dermatologist may determine the cause(s). Once the agent is identified, avoidance is the best medicine. For active dermatitis, treatment may include wet compresses, topical and systemic steroids, antihistamines, and possibly antibiotics for secondary infection.

Acne

Acne mechanica is an exacerbation of acne vulgaris occurring in areas of the skin rubbed by athletic equipment, such as helmets, chin guards, and shoulder straps. Football and hockey players are most commonly affected. Many options for treatment of acne are available, including acne washes and cleansers, topical antibiotics, benzoyl peroxide gels, retinoids, oral antibiotics, and isotretinoin for severe cases.

Anabolic steroid use by athletes may result in severe acne. Steroids have potentially severe and damaging side effects, and physicians should be aware of the possibility of abuse of these drugs by athletes presenting with severe acne.

Aquatic Dermatoses

Swimming pool granuloma, caused by *Mycobacterium marinum*, is characterized by a verrucous plaque, often ulcerated, on the dorsal hand and/or knee. Infection requires traumatically implanting the organism by scraping or cutting the skin on the pool surface. Usually, several weeks are required before the characteristic lesion forms. Treatment options include surgical excision or minocycline 100 mg twice a day for 4-8 weeks.

Swimmers in seawater face a variety of organisms that can inflict painful stings, including jellyfish, Portuguese man-of-war, sea anemones, fire corals, and true corals. All of these organisms belong to the phylum Cnidaria and possess stinging capsules called *nematocysts*. The nematocysts contain toxins, which can be injected into the skin of the unsuspecting human victim. Such stings can range in severity from mild discomfort (for example, true corals), to severe pain, bullae, and tissue necrosis (for example, Portuguese man-of-war), to even a life-threatening systemic reaction or anaphylaxis (for example, box jellyfish). In addition to the immediate reactions, delayed hypersensitivity reactions (allergic contact dermatitis) and permanent deep tissue injuries may ensue. Treatment for these injuries depends on the organism involved but may involve vinegar, baking soda, or meat tenderizer (papain), along with analgesics and, in severe cases, support of vital functions.

Other sea creatures, such as sponges, starfish, sea urchins, and sea cucumbers, may inflict injuries that result in dermatitis and/or systemic symptoms. Certain venomous fish can cause serious and painful injuries to humans. These organisms, including the stingray, catfish, and scorpion fish, have spines with associated venom glands. When the spines penetrate the victim, the toxin is injected into the wound. Secondary bacterial infections may require systemic antibiotic therapy.

Swimmer's itch is an eruption on uncovered parts of the body caused by penetration of schistosome cercariae. Fresh- and salt-water varieties are known. An initial urticarial eruption becomes papular or papulovesicular within a day, accompanied by intense pruritus. There may be pain, edema, and systemic symptoms such as headache and fever. Treatment is symptomatic. The condition is seen in the northern US and Canada.

In contrast to swimmer's itch, seabather's eruption (also known as sea lice or marine dermatitis) occurs on areas of the body covered by the bathing suit. It is caused by stings of marine coelenterate larvae that become trapped under the bathing suit. Macular, papular, or urticarial lesions begin hours after exposure. These may itch or burn and progress to vesiculopapules that heal within a week or so. Treatment is symptomatic. The condition is seen in Florida.

Exacerbation of Chronic Dermatoses

The sweating and friction that accompany athletics often exacerbate chronic dermatologic conditions. Acne mechanica is one such chronic dermatoses (discussed in detail earlier in this chapter). Treatment of severe acne with oral isotretinoin may result in fatigue and musculoskeletal discomfort, which can interfere with athletic training and competition. Other common conditions that may be exacerbated during athletics include atopic dermatitis (eczema), psoriasis, and seborrheic dermatitis. However, it is uncommon to have to cease therapy for these conditions because of patient participation in athletics.

Conclusion

Skin problems in persons participating in athletics are very common, and certain sports may predispose the participant to specific dermatological conditions. It is important for the clinician to recognize signs and symptoms of such conditions. When there are difficult diagnostic or treatment situations, referral to a dermatologist may prove helpful.

REFERENCES

1. **Smith KJ, Skelton H.** Molluscum contagiosum: recent advances in pathogenic mechanisms and new therapies. Am J Clin Deratol. 2002:3(8):535-45.

2. **Stulberg DC, Huthchinson AG.** Molluscum contagiosum and warts. Am Fam Physician 2003;6T(6):1233-40.

3. **Habif TP, Campbell JL, Quitadamo MJ, Zug KA.** Skin Disease: Diagnosis and Treatment. St. Louis: Mosby; 2001:196-205.

4. National Collegiate Athletic Association newsletter. October 27, 2003.

5. **Lindenmayer JM, Schoenfeld S, O'Grady R, Carney JK.** Methicillin-resistant *Staphylococcus aureus* in a high school wrestling team and the surrounding community. Arch Intern Med. 1998;158:895-9.

SELECTED REFERENCES

Textbooks

Arndt KA, Bowers KE, Alam M, et al, eds. Manual of Dermatologic Therapeutics, 6th spiral ed. Philadelphia: Lippincott Williams & Wilkins; 2002.

Freedberg IM, Eisen AZ, Wolff K, et al, eds. Fitzpatrick's Dermatology in General Medicine, 6th ed. New York: McGraw-Hill; 2003.

Lynch PJ, Sams WM Jr, eds. Principles and Practice of Dermatology, 2nd ed. New York: Churchill Livingstone; 1996.

Wolff K, Johnson RA, Suurmond R. Fitzpatrick's Color Atlas and Synopsis of Clinical Dermatology, 5th ed. New York: McGraw-Hill; 2005.

Review Articles

Bender TW. Cutaneous manifestations of disease in athletes (part 1). Skinmed. 2002;1:107-14.

Bender TW. Cutaneous manifestations of disease in athletes (part 2). Skinmed. 2003;2:34-40.

12

Diabetes Mellitus in Athletes

Balakrishnan (Balu) Natarajan, MD

P hysical activity can play a major role in the prevention and treatment of diabetes mellitus. Consistent exercise, combined with an appropriate diet, can delay or prevent the onset of type 2 diabetes mellitus. Among those who have the disease, exercise can produce short-term and long-term benefits, including improved metabolic control and reduced likelihood of end-organ damage (1).

Prevalence

Diabetes mellitus afflicts 150 million individuals in the world today and is expected to double in prevalence by 2025 (1). Sixteen million Americans are currently diabetic, but one-third remain undiagnosed. Consistent with its often-silent nature early in its course, diabetes mellitus is often not diagnosed until 5-8 years after its onset.

A number studies have analyzed the increasing prevalence of diabetes mellitus. For many, the major problem is the consistent use of high-fat foods; for others, sedentary lifestyle is at the root of the disease. With increasing urbanization, more individuals are sedentary, overweight, and at greater risk for developing diabetes. Research has shown that physical activity helps to prevent this endocrine disorder (2).

In the United States, the diabetes mellitus epidemic continues to expand (2). From 1990 to 1998, a 33% increase was seen in the prevalence of the disease across all ages, genders, and ethnic groups. Among those in the fourth decade of life, a 70% increase was noted, attributable in large part to weight gain often caused by high-fat, energy-dense diets (2).

Pathophysiology and Classification

Diabetes mellitus is characterized by an inability to regulate glucose levels. In patients with type 1 diabetes, autoimmune destruction of pancreatic beta-cells precludes the body from manufacturing insulin (3). In contrast, in type 2 diabetes, the pancreas is able to produce insulin. However, excess body fat leads to insulin resistance; thus, the body has to manufacture more insulin to regulate blood glucose levels. Due to a relative resistance to insulin, gestational diabetics have elevated blood sugar levels during pregnancy. While these abnormal levels resolve postpartum, afflicted mothers have a higher risk of developing type 2 diabetes mellitus later on in life.

Long-Term Complications

The long-term complications of diabetes mellitus are well known. Microvascular effects include retinopathy, nephropathy, peripheral and autonomic neuropathy, and peripheral vascular disease. Macrovascular effects include the development of coronary artery disease.

The Diabetes Control and Complications Trial (DCCT) revealed that tight control of blood sugars among type 1 diabetics significantly reduced the risk of developing microvascular complications (4). Tight blood glucose control also benefits type 2 diabetics, as determined by the UK Prospective Diabetes Study (5). Consequently, a regimen that leads to a reduction of blood sugars is desirable; this chapter will discuss the role of exercise in achieving this goal.

Energy Utilization During Exercise

During physical activity, muscle glycogen is broken down through an anaerobic process to produce ATP (6). After the first few minutes of exercise, glucose is mobilized from the liver, and free fatty acids are released from adipose tissue through lipolysis (Table 12-1). Thirty minutes into exercise, circulating blood glucose (obtained from dietary carbohydrates) is used. Sixty to ninety minutes into activity, free fatty acids provide the main source of energy.

When normal individuals exercise at moderate intensity, blood glucose levels are maintained within appropriate limits (6). This is managed by the complex interplay of insulin, glucagon, catecholamines, cortisol, and growth hormone. The hormonal regulation of blood glucose is altered in the diabetic athlete. Consequently, blood glucose, insulin, and diet have to be actively monitored while engaging in physical activity. This will be discussed later in this chapter.

Table 12-1   Energy Utilization in the Exercising Individual

Time after Initiation of Exercise	Principal Source of Energy
First few minutes	ATP produced from anaerobic breakdown of glycogen
After several minutes	Glucose produced from liver and free fatty acids (FFA) from adipose tissue
After 30 minutes	Circulating blood glucose from dietary carbohydrates
After 60-90 minutes	FFA from adipose tissue through lipolysis

Table 12-2   Benefits of Exercise in Diabetics

- Improved lipid profile
- Improved blood pressure
- Reduced cardiac risk
- Weight loss
- Improved psyche

Benefits of Exercise

Moderate exercise should be encouraged in diabetic patients for the same reasons that it is beneficial in persons without diabetes: it promotes weight loss, contributes to overall improvement in health and mood states, and prevents cardiovascular disorders, hypertension, and complications of obesity (Table 12-2). In nondiabetic persons, exercise may help prevent the development of type 2 diabetes. In addition, exercise may have benefits specific to diabetes mellitus.

Prevention of Diabetes

Many longitudinal studies have found that physical activity reduces the incidence of type 2 diabetes mellitus. Manson and colleagues followed more than 87,000 middle-aged women over an 8-year period and monitored physical activity. Women who exercised at least once weekly, and vigorously enough to produce sweat, had a 0.67 relative risk of developing diabetes compared to their inactive counterparts (7).

Helmrich and colleagues reported similar results among men who were at risk for the development of type 2 diabetes. After over nearly 100,000 man-years of follow-up, researchers found that those in the highest risk group experienced a 41% incidence reduction through physical activity (8). Overall, for each increment of 500 kcal expended weekly, a 6% decrease in the occurrence of type 2 diabetes was noted.

Other studies have reported similar results; some have found a dose-response, by which increased frequency of exercise provides a greater protective effect.

Exercise Benefits in Patients with Diabetes

Type 1 Diabetes

In the past, exercise was considered a "cornerstone" in the treatment of diabetes, but this is no longer the case. To date, studies have been unable to demonstrate that exercise leads to long-term metabolic control among type 1 diabetics. However, adverse effects have not been shown either. In addition, consistent engagement in moderate exercise has been associated with decreased illness and death (1).

Type 2 Diabetes

The positive effects of activity are consistently observed among type 2 diabetics. Recently, a randomized trial from Denmark, which included brisk walking at least 3 times weekly as part of a multidisciplinary treatment plan, revealed a 50% decrease in cardiovascular and microvascular events over an 8-year period (9). A few studies have found a mortality benefit to activity. Wei and colleagues studied 1263 men with type 2 diabetes for an average of 12 years. The low-fitness group had a 2.1-fold risk of death compared to fit men. Physical inactivity was associated with a 1.7-fold increase in mortality over this time period (10). Recently published articles have confirmed these findings. In study of 3,000 men with type 2 diabetes, Tanasescu and colleagues reported that total mortality was reduced 43% among those in the highest activity group (11).

While these studies have observed the long-term effects of exercise, other research has attempted to determine the basis for these positive findings. Most analyses have determined that physical activity leads to 1) reduction in blood sugars, 2) lowered blood pressure, and 3) enhanced insulin sensitivity (2). In the acute phase, exercise at moderate intensity leads to a decrease in blood glucose levels, improved insulin sensitivity, and reduced endogenous glucose production (12). With consistent exercise, glycosylated hemoglobin values tend to decline, and fasting insulin levels improve (2,12). In order to elucidate these observations further, some investigators have looked at glucose transport. Glucose transport activity in muscle is primarily mediated by the contraction of muscle fibers (2). Insulin is another significant mediator of glucose transport in skeletal muscle. Studies have revealed that these mediators act at two separate locations in the cell, such that exercise and insulin can have additive effects in the diabetic athlete (2). Many studies have revealed that physical training can lead to a reduction in insulin levels, with improvement in insulin sensitivity (2). Unfortunately, this improvement is lost after as little as 2.5 days of inactivity. The mechanism for the enhanced insulin sensitivity is not yet known.

Case Study 12-1

A 56-year-old female with type 2 diabetes visited her internist's office after poor glucose control with metformin, a sulfonylurea, and a thiazolinedione at maximal doses for 6 months. She was told she would need to initiate insulin therapy if her glucose levels did not improve.

Physical examination revealed a well-developed, well-nourished, obese female, 5 feet 3 inches, 160 pounds. Vitals were within normal limits, with no signs of orthostasis. Funduscopic exam was normal, heart exam was normal, abdomen was benign, and foot and joint exams were unremarkable. Peripheral pulses were strong.

Lab tests revealed normal chemistries, including renal and liver function tests. Hemoglobin A_{1C} was 11%; LDL was 115.

In an effort to avoid the initiation of insulin, the patient obtained an exercise prescription. Pre-exercise stress testing was negative for ischemia. Her exercise prescription called for walking 4 times weekly, 10 minutes each time to start. After 2 weeks, the duration was increased to 15 minutes, and one month after initiation, the duration was extended to 30 minutes.

After 12 weeks of activity, the patient weighed 154 pounds. After 20 weeks, her weight was 145, hemoglobin A_{1C} was 9%, and LDL was 99. Her internist recommended that she remain on the oral hypoglycemic regimen and that insulin use not be initiated.

Gestational Diabetes

The International Workshop-Conference on Gestational Diabetes Mellitus determined in 1991 that exercise is one therapy that would be beneficial in the management of blood glucose in gestational diabetes. Studies to substantiate this recommendation, however, are limited in number (13).

One Spanish study observed that light postprandial exercise among gestational diabetics was associated with decreased 1-hour postprandial glucose levels. This beneficial effect was not observed 2 hours after exercise. The women in this study averaged only a nine-beat-per-minute increase in heart rate during the exercise period (14).

Metabolic Complications

Exercise in the setting of hyperglycemia may actually cause worsening of glycemic control and lead to ketosis. This is due to: 1) dehydration due to increased urine production as a result of hyperglycemia, and 2) excessive secretion of counterregulatory hormones that may increase both serum glucose and ketones (3). Hypoglycemia, especially for insulin users, is a risk during exercise because the injected insulin is mobilized during exercise. Lower cortisol levels (which can lead to decreased blood glucose) in the evening can exacerbate this problem (3).

Pre-Exercise Screening

Before recommending an exercise program, the physician must perform a detailed preparticipation evaluation of the diabetic patient (6). This involves a history, physical examination, and, in some cases, diagnostic testing.

Table 12-3   Indications for Preparticipation Exercise Stress Testing

- Age > 35 years
- History of type 2 diabetes for 10 years or more
- History of type 1 diabetes for 15 years or more
- One additional risk factor for coronary artery disease
- Microvascular disease
- Peripheral-vascular disease
- Autonomic neuropathy

A detailed history pertinent to diabetes, along with answers to questions about blood sugar control, medication and insulin needs, and frequency of hyperglycemia and hypoglycemia, should be obtained. A history of diabetic complications is significant because these complications may preclude certain physical activities. A family history should also be obtained to determine the athlete's risk of cardiovascular damage and other complications.

Physical examination should include a thorough musculoskeletal survey to rule out capsulitis, joint disease, or skin breakdown. An eye examination should be performed to assess retinal damage. A neurological evaluation, with attention to the feet, should be performed to rule out autonomic or peripheral neuropathy. The cardiovascular system should be assessed with a focus on peripheral pulses, blood pressure, and abnormal cardiac findings.

If not recently performed, blood tests are necessary. A glycosylated hemoglobin will help to confirm the patient's history of blood sugar control and provide some insight into the diurnal variation of his or her glucose levels. A lipid profile will assist in cardiac risk assessment. Diabetic nephropathy can be ruled out by urine protein and serum creatinine levels (6).

Once the preparticipation examination is completed, a graded exercise test may be indicated (Table 12-3) (15).

Contraindications to Exercise

Those patients with existing end-organ disease may not be able to participate in all sports (Table 12-4). In patients with moderate nonproliferative diabetic retinopathy, power lifting and heavy Valsalva maneuvers should be avoided due to their association with elevated blood pressure (15). In those individuals with severe nonproliferative disease, active jarring, as may occur with boxing or certain competitive sports, should also be avoided. Among patients with proliferative disease, jogging, high-impact aerobics, scuba diving, and racquet sports should be discouraged, in addition to the aforementioned activities (15,16). In these patients, preferred

Table 12-4   Contraindications to Exercise Based on End-Organ Damage

Condition	Avoid
Diabetic retinopathy	
Moderate nonproliferative	Power lifting, heavy Valsalva
Severe nonproliferative	As above, plus active jarring
Proliferative	As above, plus jogging, high-impact aerobics, scuba diving, racquet sports
Peripheral neuropathy	Jogging, walking, long treadmill use, step exercise
Autonomic neuropathy	(Based on individual status)
Diabetic nephropathy	Very intense exercise

exercise involves low-impact movement that stresses cardiovascular conditioning (15). Swimming and cycling are appropriate activities (16).

Individuals with peripheral neuropathy have impaired sensation in their feet. Footwear is extremely important in these patients. They should assess their feet after exercise in an effort to identify blisters and calluses early. In addition, they should avoid jogging, walking, prolonged use of the treadmill, or step exercises, because these weight-bearing activities can lead to ulceration and fractures (15).

Autonomic neuropathy can have adverse effects on an athlete's exercise capacity (15). Cardiac autonomic neuropathy is associated with a resting tachycardia, orthostatic blood pressures, and autonomic regulatory deficiencies of other organ systems. Wide variations in blood pressure after exercise are common in these individuals. Because of the risk of silent ischemia, these patients may require stress testing with imaging to rule out coronary artery disease before the initiation of an exercise program.

Recommendations have not been proposed for athletes with diabetic nephropathy or microalbuminuria. The American Diabetes Association suggests that high-intensity exercise be avoided (15). In light of a lack of evidence in this area, it would be prudent to monitor renal function and proteinuria closely in a person who has just initiated an exercise program. The frequency of monitoring can be reduced once stable renal function has been confirmed during a consistent exercise regimen.

Initiating and Maintaining Exercise

Prior to initiating exercise, the diabetic should be able to answer questions about the duration and intensity of the intended exercise. The physician can assist by estimating the consequent caloric expenditure. Knowledge of caloric expenditure, insulin regimen, meal timing, and blood glucose levels are essential in determining the appropriate exercise prescription for the diabetic patient (17).

Specific glucose levels have been proposed as guidelines for the type 1 diabetic due to the associated risks of ketosis, hypoglycemia, and hyperglycemia. Particularly in type 1 diabetics, exercise should be avoided when blood glucose levels before activity are greater than 250 mg/dl, since levels tend to increase during exercise in such situations (16). When levels are less than 100 mg/dl, a carbohydrate snack is advised, and individuals may initiate activity 10 minutes thereafter (3). Those with levels between 100-250 mg/dl may proceed with exercise without any additional carbohydrate intake.

In individuals with type 2 diabetes, ketosis is rare, but caution should be employed when exercising at high glucose levels, as further hyperglycemia may still develop. The risk of hypoglycemia, while lower in the type 2 diabetic than in the type 1 individual, still exists if the athlete takes oral hypoglycemic medication or uses insulin. Therefore, a pre-exercise carbohydrate snack would be beneficial for those with glucose levels less than 100 mg/dl.

Investigators have found that carbohydrate ingestion during exercise maintains glucose levels in persons with diabetes. For each hour of intense exercise, 15-45 g of carbohydrate may be needed (Table 12-5). This is, however, simply a guideline on the basis of research; each individual will have to monitor his or her blood sugars before, after, and during exercise in the early stages of activity to determine the appropriate long-term interventions. Management of oral intake and insulin dosage is essential in maintaining euglycemia (Table 12-6).

Table 12-5   Calories in Various Foods and Beverages

Food	Grams of Carbohydrate
Energy drink—8 oz	12-20
Whole milk—8 oz	50
1% milk—8 oz	12
Mixed nuts—1 cup	35
Carrot—1 cup	12
Slice of bread	12-15
Pretzel	14
Fruit	20

Table 12-6   Maintaining Normal Blood Sugars with Activity

- Perform frequent glucose checks until a pattern is determined.
- Don't confuse pregame hypoglycemia and pregame anxiety; check a glucose level.
- Use some long-acting starches during exercise to prevent delayed hypoglycemia.
- Exercise in the morning if possible.
- Be consistent in the exercise regimen and make gradual modifications over time.

Table 12-7   Oral Intake Based on Pre-Exercise Blood Glucose

Glucose Before Exercise	Consume	For Every
<130 mg/dl	15-30 g of carbohydrate	30-45 min of light-moderate exercise
130-180 mg/dl	15 g of carbohydrate	30-45 min of light-moderate exercise
180-250 mg/dl	Nothing. Recheck blood sugar 30 minutes into exercise and follow above regimen.	
250 mg/dl or greater	Nothing. Avoid exercise.	

Appropriate oral intake based on blood glucose readings and intensity of exercise is indicated in Table 12-7 (16). Exercise in the morning is helpful in avoiding hypoglycemia, because cortisol levels are higher early in the day. Exercise should be avoided at night, because hypoglycemia can develop several hours after physical activity. Some athletes may need to wake up in the middle of the night to monitor blood glucose levels. Despite attention to insulin use and oral intake, some diabetics may still develop hypoglycemia. As a consequence, athletes should have carbohydrates easily accessible for use as needed.

Individuals on insulin need to engage in more of a balancing act than those who are controlled on oral medications or diet alone. Most insulin users find that they need to decrease their dose of short-acting insulin 30%-50% 2 to 3 hours before initiating exercise (3). For exercise longer than 90 minutes, some individuals must reduce their insulin by 80% (12). These athletes must monitor their blood glucose frequently when starting an exercise program, and they will be able to use the results to modify insulin dosage and oral intake before and during physical activity.

Appropriate warm-up and cool-down are essential in preventing injuries. Individuals who exercise consistently, 3 to 5 times weekly at a similar intensity each time, will have more stable blood sugar control and will be less prone to acute injury. Gradual alterations are preferable to sudden modifications when changes in an exercise regimen are made.

Glycemic Index

The glycemic index is a good indicator of how quickly a food or beverage can raise blood sugar levels. Foods with a high glycemic index, such as crackers or sports drinks, will raise blood sugars quickly. Foods with a low glycemic index, such as those that contain fructose or plain yogurt, will raise blood sugars more slowly. Athletes should use high glycemic index items during exercise to maintain blood sugar, but they can use items with a low glycemic index several hours before exercise to prevent hypoglycemia from occurring.

Case Study 12-2

A 22-year-old male soccer player with type 1 diabetes presented with recurrent bouts of hypoglycemia that tended to occur towards the end of the first half of the game. On several occasions, he experienced headache, tachycardia, and difficulty focusing while playing and had to leave the game to get glucose tablets or a sports drink.

The patient has had diabetes for 10 years. He uses NPH insulin in the morning and at bedtime, in addition to regular insulin 30-45 minutes before meals.

Physical examination after glucose administration was normal after each episode. Hemoglobin A_{1C} was 6.2%. Chemistries were within normal limits.

Further dietary history revealed that the patient ingested foods with a high glycemic index (such as bagels) at lunchtime, 30 minutes after using regular insulin. In addition, he avoided oral intake in the hour before games, which were typically held in the late afternoon and early evening.

The patient's insulin regimen was changed to include insulin lispro before lunch instead of regular insulin, and he was encouraged to eat an 8-oz cup of plain yogurt, which has a low glycemic index. The player reported fewer bouts of hypoglycemia and is now able to play consistently until halftime, when he has a sports drink and some pretzels before resuming play in the second half.

Education of the Athlete and Associated Individuals

Because hypoglycemia can have dire consequences, the diabetic patient should be clearly instructed in the prevention and management of blood glucose abnormalities. Teammates, coaches, and athletic trainers should also be aware of the issues surrounding a diabetic patient who engages in team sports. It is essential for those individuals to be able to identify a hypoglycemic reaction in order to respond to it appropriately.

On-Field Management of Hypoglycemia

When the blood glucose level cannot be measured, a questionable reaction should be treated as hypoglycemia until proven otherwise. The athletic trainer or team physician should stop the athlete from further activity immediately (1). Glucose tablets or half a cup of fruit juice can raise glucose levels rapidly, and the consumption of one starch exchange (1 slice of bread or $3/4$ oz of pretzels) is appropriate thereafter. After a minimum of 15 minutes rest to allow euglycemia, the athlete may return to activity if he or she reports symptom relief but must be monitored closely.

Intramuscular glucagon is indicated for the athlete who does not respond to the above measures. If the glucagon does not reverse the hypoglycemic reaction, the patient will need to be taken to a medical facility for intravenous glucose therapy.

The team trainer's or physician's "medicine bag" should contain appropriate food, drink, and medication if a known diabetic athlete is participating in an activity.

The Gestational Diabetic

The development of an exercise program for gestational diabetes is complicated but can have significant benefits for the mother and the fetus. The involvement of an obstetrician is essential to ensure the success of the exercise prescription and the safety of the mother and the child. Once the obstetrician has cleared the patient for exercise, a regimen can begin. Artal and colleagues have published a clinical protocol for the gestational diabetic (13). The program involves monitoring of blood glucose levels while fasting and 2 hours after meals, exercising at mild-to-moderate intensity, and monitoring of fetal activity. The patient is expected to maintain records of her exercise and is given clinical thresholds for contacting her obstetrician.

Options for Insulin Users

A number of insulin preparations are available and have different times of onset and duration. While dosing of some shorter-acting preparations may be cumbersome, they may be appropriate for some athletes depending on the activity (18,19). The insulin regimen that most simulates normal endocrine responses to exercise involves a continuous insulin infusion through a pump. Although long-term studies of athletes with type 1 diabetes are not available, early research demonstrates that the use of an insulin pump is associated with good metabolic control (18). Athletes should be screened appropriately for such therapy, given the risks of displacement during exercise and potential malfunction while sweating and during extremes of ambient temperature.

Pearls for the Exercise Prescription

While the benefits of exercise may be obvious to most diabetics, ensuring compliance with a program is difficult. Some concepts are helpful in staying with a regimen: setting realistic goals with associated rewards, exercising with a partner, setting a schedule, and cross-training (Table 12-8). The physician can help by identifying barriers and pitfalls specific to each patient. In

Table 12-8   Sticking with the Program

- Set realistic goals for activity frequency, intensity, and duration.
- Find an exercise partner.
- Set a schedule and follow it.
- Cross-train to avoid activity monotony.
- Plan rewards for various milestones.
- Arrange physician visits as needed to remain or get back on course.

some cases, frequent patient-physician visits may be needed at the beginning of the exercise program.

Hypoglycemia in the Nondiabetic Patient

Some authors have proposed mechanisms for the development of hypoglycemia in nondiabetic subjects (20,21). Further study is needed to elucidate the clinical significance of this transient finding. All athletes should monitor their food and beverage intake before and during exercise in order to determine their individually optimized energy intake and use during physical activity.

Conclusion

The last decade has provided substantial proof of the merits of exercise in the management of diabetes mellitus. With the availability of many oral medications and insulin preparations, medical providers can play a vital role in increasing the physical activity of their diabetic patients. Over time, this intervention will have measurable effects on the physical and emotional health of those individuals.

REFERENCES

1. **Birrer RB, Sedaghat VD.** Exercise and diabetes mellitus. Phys Sportsmed. 2003; 31(5):29-41.
2. **Hamdy O, Goodyear LJ, Horton ES.** Diet and exercise in type 2 diabetes mellitus. Endocrinol Metab Clin North Am. 2001;30(4):883-907.
3. **Colberg SR, Swain DP.** Exercise and diabetes control. Phys Sportsmed. 2000; 28(4):63-81.
4. **Diabetes Control and Complications Trial Research Group.** The effect of intensive treatment of diabetes on the development and progression of long-term complications in insulin-dependent diabetes mellitus. N Engl J Med. 1993;329(14): 977-86.

5. **Nasr CE, Hoogwerf BJ, Faiman C, Reddy SS.** United Kingdom Prospective Diabetes Study. Effects of glucose and blood pressure control on complications of type 2 diabetes mellitus. Cleve Clin J Med. 1999;66(4):247-53.

6. **Hough DO, Woods MJ.** Endocrinology. In: Safran MR, et al., eds. Manual of Sports Medicine. Philadelphia: Lippincott-Raven; 1998:216-25.

7. **Manson JE, Rimm EB, Stampfer MJ, et al.** Physical activity and incidence of non-insulin-dependent diabetes mellitus in women. Lancet. 1991;338:774-8.

8. **Helmrich SP, Ragland DR, Leung RW, Paffenberger RS.** Physical activity and reduced occurrence of non-insulin-dependent diabetes mellitus. N Engl J Med. 1991;325:147-52.

9. **Gaede P, Vedel P, Larsen N, et al.** Multifactorial intervention and cardiovascular disease in patients with type 2 diabetes. N Engl J Med. 2003;348:383-93.

10. **Wei M, Gibbons LW, Kampert JB, et al.** Low cardiorespiratory fitness and physical inactivity as predictors of mortality in men with type 2 diabetes. Ann Intern Med. 2000;132:605-11.

11. **Tanasescu M, Leitzmann MF, Rimm EB, Hu FB.** Physical activity in relation to cardiovascular disease and total mortality among men with type 2 diabetes. Circulation. 2003;107:2435-9.

12. **Zinker BA.** Nutrition and exercise in individuals with diabetes. Clin Sports Med. 1999;18(3):585-606.

13. **Artal R.** Exercise: An alternative therapy for gestational diabetes. Phys Sportsmed. 1996;24(3):54-66.

14. **Garcia-Patterson A, Martin E, Ubeda J, et al.** Evaluation of light exercise in the treatment of gestational diabetes. Diabetes Care. 2001;24(11):2006.

15. **American Diabetes Association.** Clinical Practice Recommendations 2000: diabetes mellitus and exercise. Diabetes Care. 2000;23:S50-4.

16. **Berg K.** The diabetic athlete. In: Mellion MB, et al., eds. Team Physician's Handbook, 3rd ed. Philadelphia: Hanley and Belfus; 2002:262-5.

17. **Horton ES.** Exercise and diabetes mellitus. Med Clin North Am. 1988;72(6):1301-21.

18. **Colberg SR, Walsh J.** Pumping insulin during exercise. Phys Sportsmed. 2002; 30(4):33-8.

19. **Draznin MB.** Type 1 diabetes and sports participation. Phys Sportsmed. 2000; 28(12):49-56.

20. **Brun JF, Dumortier M, Fedou C, Mercier J.** Exercise hypoglycemia in nondiabetic subjects. Diabetes Metab. 2001;27(11):92-106.

21. **Kuipers H, Fransen EJ, Keizer HA.** Pre-exercise ingestion of carbohydrate and transient hypoglycemia during exercise. Int J Sports Med. 1999;20(4):227-31.

13

Cardiac Conditions in Athletes

Stephanie M. Cooper, MD

Gary R. Cooper, MD

Athletic heart syndrome (AHS), a benign condition caused by prolonged, intense physical training, is characterized by an enlarged heart, altered cardiac rate and rhythm, and normal left ventricular systolic function. Identifying AHS and differentiating it from structural heart disease, in particular hypertrophic cardiomyopathy and dilated cardiomyopathy, is often difficult. However, our understanding of this syndrome, first described in 1897 by Henschen (1) on the basis of physical findings in cross-country skiers, has improved with advances in diagnostic imaging and identification of gene mutations that code for sarcomeric proteins.

Sudden cardiac death (SCD) in athletes is a rare complication of participation in competitive sports. When such a tragedy occurs, it creates headlines in the media, as well as the potential for litigation. Several of the cardiac abnormalities associated with SCD can be confused with AHS. Preparticipation screening is intended to reduce such untoward outcomes, but it can not entirely eliminate them.

This chapter describes the clinical and laboratory features of AHS, including the history, physical examination, ECG, chest X-ray, echocardiogram, and magnetic resonance imaging.

Cardiac Remodeling and Types of Exercise

Athletic heart syndrome is the adaptation of the structurally normal heart to regular, intense athletic training. The type, duration, and intensity of training affect the degree of cardiac remodeling. Changes in left ventricular internal dimensions and wall thickness have been well studied in participants in organized competitive sports. Few data are available, however, on anatomical changes in hearts of individuals who train at a lower frequency or intensity or only occasionally participate in sports. The polar extremes of training modalities have been defined as *strength training* (also called *power, static,* or *isometric training*) and *endurance training* (also termed *dynamic* or *isotonic training*). Training for many sports includes elements of both. Endurance-trained athletes have a more profound change in both left ventricular wall thickness and left ventricular end diastolic dimension than do strength-trained individuals.

Identification of Athletic Heart Syndrome

History and Physical Examination

Identifying AHS as a clinical entity is important, particularly to differentiate it from conditions such as hypertrophic or dilated cardiomyopathy. In obtaining the medical history, practitioners should always seek to exclude prior documentation of structural heart disease. There should be no past medical history of valvular heart disease, cardiomyopathy, angina, syncope, dyspnea, orthopnea, peripheral edema, atrial fibrillation, atrial flutter, or significant ventricular arrhythmia. The family history should be negative for sudden cardiac death, Marfan syndrome, hypertrophic cardiomyopathy, or ventricular arrhythmias.

Systolic and diastolic blood pressures are typically normal. The cardiac rate is slow and may be irregular because of sinus arrhythmia or other arrhythmias. The point of maximal impulse may be displaced laterally and may be slightly enlarged. The first heart sound is of normal intensity. The second heart sound splits physiologically. A third heart sound may be present. Less frequently, a fourth heart sound may be heard. Due to an increase in stroke volume, a soft systolic ejection murmur may be present at the base of the heart. The intensity of the murmur should be grade 1 or 2 and should not change with respiration. Louder murmurs or murmurs that radiate to the axilla or back are likely to be pathologic. The murmur should not intensify with maneuvers that reduce venous return, such as the Valsalva maneuver. Diastolic murmurs are always pathologic and should not be present in AHS.

Electrocardiogram

The 12-lead ECG has been proposed as a preparticipation screening tool for athletes because of its low cost, ease of acquisition, and virtually universal availability. Numerous changes may be present on the 12-lead ECG of trained athletes. Abnormalities of cardiac rate and rhythm, increased voltage suggesting ventricular hypertrophy, and changes in ST or T wave morphology are commonly seen on the ECGs of athletes with AHS. These changes can be minor, mildly abnormal, or distinctly abnormal and can mimic ECG changes associated with structural heart disease. The ECG is of little use in differentiating between left ventricular hypertrophy and repolarization changes due to training and pathologic ventricular hypertrophy of other etiologies.

However, ECGs have only approximately a 50% sensitivity and a 60% specificity. The positive predictive accuracy is < 10%, and the negative predictive accuracy is > 95%. Therefore, the usefulness of the 12-lead ECG alone as a preparticipation screening tool remains in doubt (2).

Cardiac Rate and Rhythm

Most athletes with AHS have normal sinus rhythm, sinus arrhythmia, or sinus bradycardia. At times, the sinus rate may be very slow and junctional, or ventricular escape rhythms may be detected. Sinus bradycardia and atrioventricular (A-V) block are common in athletes (3). These arrhythmias do not require intervention, provided they do not produce symptoms or manifest pauses longer than 4 seconds. Wandering atrial pacemaker, Mobitz type I second-degree A-V block, junctional rhythm, and first-degree A-V block are believed to be secondary to increased vagal tone and typically resolve with exercise.

Persistent Mobitz type II second-degree heart block and third-degree heart block are exceedingly rare in athletes and should be considered pathological if found. Supraventricular tachyarrhythmias are atypical in trained athletes and should be evaluated to exclude underlying structural heart disease. Premature ventricular contractions and ventricular couplets are present in athletes to the same degree seen in the general population and do not require further investigation. Accelerated idioventricular rhythm may be a normal consequence of AHS. There is no contraindication to training or competition if this arrhythmia disappears with activity. Ventricular tachycardia must be considered abnormal in athletes, as well as the general population. It is the responsibility of the physician evaluating such a patient to exclude structural heart disease before approving such participation.

There are two distinct types of ventricular tachycardia originating primarily from the right ventricle of interest to physicians caring for athletes. These are related to arrhythmogenic right ventricular dysplasia (ARVD) and right ventricular outflow tract (RVOT) tachycardia. The former is a pathologic condition in which there is a structural abnormality in a portion of the right ventricular myocardium that is replaced by a fibro-fatty tissue. This abnormal tissue, which can usually be seen on MRI, is frequently the origin of ventricular tachyarrhythmias. ARVD is one of the common causes of SCD in athletes.

Case Study 13-1

An 18-year-old female member of a university swim team suffered a cardiac arrest while walking to class. Passers by immediately began CPR, and EMS was called. CPR was continued for the five minutes that elapsed until the arrival of EMS. "Quick Look" paddles documented ventricular fibrillation (VF). A single defibrillation shock resulted in conversion to a slow idioventricular rhythm, which within 60 seconds converted to NSR.

The patient was admitted to the Coronary Care unit. Over the next 36 hours, she returned to her normal level of consciousness. There was no permanent neurological impairment.

No significant history other than her cardiac arrest was obtained. Specifically, she had no personal history of syncope or heart disease. There was no family history of sudden cardiac death, hypertrophic cardiomyopathy, or Marfan syndrome.

Physical examination revealed only tenderness of the anterior chest. Serial cardiac markers were minimally elevated. Initial and three follow-up 12-lead ECGs were all normal. Transthoracic echocardiogram was normal. No wall motion abnormalities, ventricular hypertrophy, ventricular dilation, or mitral valve prolapse was observed. Basic metabolic panel, serum magnesium, CBC, thyroid studies, and drug screen were all unremarkable. Cardiac catheterization demonstrated normal left ventricle function, no evidence of mitral valve prolapse, normal origin of the coronary arteries, and no fixed coronary artery narrowing. Pharmacologic stimulation did not produce coronary artery spasm. MRI demonstrated evidence of fibro-fatty infiltration of the right ventricle. The origin and course of the coronary arteries were found to be normal by this technique.

The patient had a normal electrophysiologic study. There was no evidence of a concealed accessory pathway. Multiple attempts to induce ventricular tachycardia before and after the administration of isoproterenol were unsuccessful.

In view of the fact that she had a documented VF arrest and MRI evidence of right ventricular dysplasia, an AICD was placed. The patient did well for the next 13 months. She discontinued competitive sports. Then, while running to class, her AICD documented an episode of rapid ventricular tachycardia and delivered a single appropriate, successful shock. She has been well ever since.

Ventricular tachycardia arising from RVOT is typically exercise-induced. There is usually no associated structural cardiac abnormality. Frequently, this arrhythmia can be successfully treated with either beta-blockers or verapamil. More definitively, radiofrequency ablation is curative. Seldom is an implantable defibrillator required. Since this arrhythmia occurs in structurally normal hearts, it is usually well tolerated. The 12-lead ECG obtained during an episode of tachycardia is often diagnostic. The QRS vector during episodes of this particular arrhythmia is directed inferiorly, creating a positive deflection in leads II, III, and AVF, as well as left bundle branch morphology in the precordial leads (4). Figure 13-1 illustrates the typical ECG from a patient with this arrhythmia.

Syncope, whether related to bradycardia, tachycardia, or neurocardiogenic vasovagal instability, heralds possible cardiovascular problems and requires further evaluation.

QRS Axis and Morphology

The mean QRS vector (axis) in trained athletes is usually between 0 and 90 degrees. However, both left-axis deviation and right-axis deviation may be present in elite athletes with structurally normal hearts.

A modest increase in the QRS duration is commonly seen in athletes. The so-called incomplete right bundle branch block has been reported in up to 50% of Olympic athletes (5). Both complete right bundle branch block and left bundle branch block are rare. Pre-excitation, the Wolff-Parkinson-White syndrome also causes an increase in the duration of the QRS complex. The initial depolarization of the QRS complex demonstrates the classical "delta" wave. Patients with this abnormality are prone to

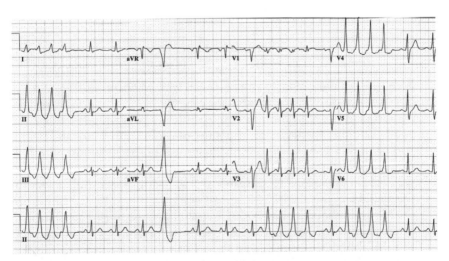

Figure 13-1 This ECG demonstrates nonsustained right ventricular outflow tract ventricular tachycardia. Characteristically, the inferiorly directed ectopic beats are conducted in a left bundle branch block configuration.

re-entrant tachycardia. Athletes with symptomatic Wolff-Parkinson-White syndrome should be evaluated by an electrophysiologist (6).

Fortunately, the accessory pathway responsible for both the ECG abnormalities and the re-entrant tachycardia are usually amenable to radiofrequency ablation. Atrial fibrillation in the presence of Wolff-Parkinson-White syndrome is of particular concern because the atrial fibrillation is conducted down the anomalous pathway in a brisk fashion and leads to a ventricular response so fast as to cause hemodynamic instability, ventricular fibrillation and SCD. Characteristically, the wide, complex tachyarrhythmia characteristic of atrial fibrillation in patients with Wolff-Parkinson-White syndrome is very irregular on the surface ECG and on rhythm strips. This irregularity may be the initial key to diagnosis.

Increases in QRS voltage can represent a normal persistence of a juvenile voltage pattern often seen in young athletes. Increased QRS voltage can also be seen in association with increased echocardiographic measurements of left ventricular wall thickness, left ventricular mass, and left ventricular end diastolic measurements. Athletes who demonstrate voltage criteria for left ventricular hypertrophy are predominantly men who engage in endurance-type athletic pursuits. Endurance sports such as cycling, cross-country skiing, rowing, and basketball have the greatest effect on the ECG, whereas wrestling, alpine skiing, and competitive equestrian activities have the least. Even in those sports in which ECG changes are most common, the ECG remains normal or minimally abnormal in roughly half the participants. Progressive increases in QRS voltage have been seen as a result of training. The increased voltage usually returns to normal with cessation of training.

Case Study 13-2

A 26-year-old professional football player, who had been working out during the off-season, was referred for evaluation of syncope. He experienced sudden loss of consciousness at rest. There was a prodrome of a rapid heart rate. There was no incontinence and no post-ictal state. He had been well prior to this event. There was no personal history of heart murmur, arrhythmia, abnormal ECG, or seizure disorder. There was no family history of sudden cardiac death, heart disease, or Marfan's syndrome.

Physical examination revealed a well-developed, well-nourished, healthy appearing, African American male. The heart was not enlarged. The apical impulse was medial to the mid-clavicular line. No murmur, gallop, or rub was appreciated. Femoral and distal pulses were normal. Chest examination was normal. Cranial nerves II-XII were intact. There was no sensory or motor deficit. Deep tendon reflexes were brisk. There were no cerebellar abnormalities. CBC, basic metabolic profile, and TSH were normal.

The patient's resting ECG is shown below:

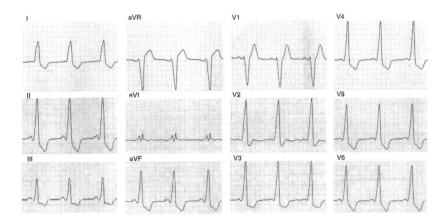

This tracing was interpreted as demonstrating sinus bradycardia, a short PR interval, and "delta," all of which are best appreciated in the inferolateral leads and are consistent with Wolf-Parkinson-White (WPW) syndrome.

An electrophysiology study confirmed the presence of an accessory pathway. With atrial stimulation, atrial fibrillation was initiated. Atrial fibrillation with rapid conduction over the accessory A-V pathway was observed on the second 12-lead ECG:

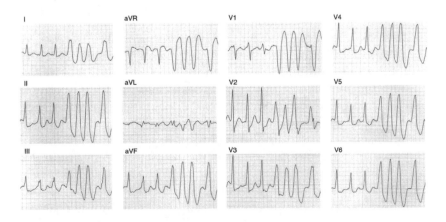

The patient underwent radiofrequency catheter ablation of his accessory pathway. An ECG revealed incomplete right bundle branch block but without pre-excitation:

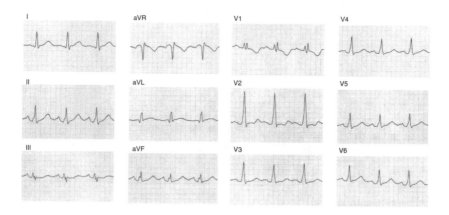

The patient had no further episodes of syncope. After 6 months, he was able to rejoin his team and play competitively.

Repolarization Abnormalities

The ST segment elevation of early repolarization commonly is seen in both endurance-trained and strength-trained individuals. The "J" point elevation and ST segment elevation of early repolarization are seen more commonly in the anterior leads than in the limb leads. The ST segment elevation of early repolarization often improves or resolves during exercise. This normalization of the ST segment elevation helps to differentiate between this benign condition and a pathologic epicardial current of injury.

These ST changes can be mistaken for the epicardial current of injury due to pericarditis or ST segment elevation myocardial infarction. The clinical setting is often useful in differentiating between similar ECG changes. The presence of pleuritic retrosternal pain suggests pericarditis. Classical oppressive retrosternal pain in association with ST segment elevation suggests myocardial infarction. In suspicious cases, transthoracic echocardiography is often useful. Echocardiographic evidence of a segmental wall motion abnormality is strongly suggestive of an ischemic cause. In pericarditis, a small pericardial effusion is often seen.

T wave abnormalities may represent the persistence of a juvenile electrocardiographic pattern most commonly seen in V1 through V4. Deep lateral T wave inversion, particularly in association with increased QRS voltage, is more likely to be related to increased left ventricular wall thickness, as seen in AHS. Compared with whites, blacks have a higher incidence of both early repolarization and the persistent juvenile pattern.

Exercise-induced ST segment depression in athletes is distinctly abnormal. This change must be viewed as a marker of subendocardial ischemia, and either cardiac catheterization or stress myocardial perfusion imaging is indicated. ST segment elevation occasionally can be seen with ischemic heart disease or exercise-induced coronary artery spasm. Once exercise-associated ST segment elevation or depression is identified, referral for further cardiovascular testing is indicated.

The ECG may be abnormal in well-conditioned athletes with structurally normal hearts who have AHS; however, an ECG abnormality may be the first clue to underlying cardiovascular abnormalities. Further investigation to exclude structural heart disease is indicated when ECG abnormalities are identified.

Noninvasive Imaging

Transthoracic echocardiography (TTE) and, more recently, MRI have yielded substantial understanding of the anatomical and physiologic changes associated with AHS. Of equal importance, these noninvasive techniques differentiate between AHS and pathologic states, particularly hypertrophic cardiomyopathy, with which AHS is often confused.

Transthoracic Echocardiography

Transthoracic echocardiography is a universally available noninvasive tool that reveals anatomical and physiologic data in patients with suspected structural heart disease. Measurements of cardiac chamber dimension, wall thickness, wall motion, estimated ejection fraction, valvular regurgitation, and intracardiac shunts are typically well documented in patients using this technique. Only in patients with significant pulmonary disease is the visualization of the heart difficult because of limited cardiac windows.

The TTE of an athlete may seem normal or show significant morphologic changes. Athletes who participate in endurance training, especially cycling and rowing, are the most likely to show these anatomical changes. Total cardiac mass may increase to 45% greater than normal (7). These changes are due to dilation and hypertrophy and have been well documented by TTE and cardiac MRI.

Elite athletes with left ventricular end-diastolic cavity measurements compatible with dilated cardiomyopathy but with normal systolic function most likely represent an extreme example of physiologic conditioning. The long-term consequences of cardiac remodeling are not well-studied. Usually, trained athletes who are documented to have dilated left ventricles do not develop systolic dysfunction, cardiac symptoms, impaired physical performance, or regional wall motion abnormalities.

Magnetic Resonance Imaging

With recent improvement in the quality and availability of MRI and magnetic resonance angiography, these noninvasive techniques have become adjunctive imaging modalities used for the study of heart disease. In particular, TTE evaluation of right ventricular size, morphology, and mass has proved difficult because of the chamber's bellows-type shape and heavy trabeculation. In a recent study of elite endurance-trained athletes, cardiac MRI was obtained (8). This study confirmed that right ventricular hypertrophy was a regular feature of AHS.

The origination of the left coronary artery from the right sinus of Valsalva or the right coronary artery from the left sinus of Valsalva, also called origination of the coronary artery from the "wrong sinus" of Valsalva, is a common cause of SCD in athletes. Compression of a vessel because of its abnormal course between the aorta and pulmonary artery can lead to ischemia and ventricular arrhythmias. The origin of the coronary arteries and the course of the coronary arteries relative to the great vessels is easily visualized using either magnetic resonance angiography or contrast computed tomography.

Natural History of Athletic Heart Syndrome

Increased left ventricular mass, wall thickness, and end-diastolic proportions of AHS are typically mild in most athletes. These changes, however, can be marked in elite athletes, particularly those who have trained for many years. The morphologic changes seen in AHS may be similar to those present in hypertrophic cardiomyopathy and, to a lesser extent, dilated idiopathic cardiomyopathy. AHS has long been considered a physiologic response to the rigors of an intense training regimen and is not thought to portend an adverse long-term prognosis. Indeed, individuals with AHS are asymptomatic and have not been shown to have a reduced life expectancy. On the other hand, hypertrophic cardiomyopathy and dilated cardiomyopathy are pathological conditions. Hypertrophic cardiomyopathy is the leading cause of SCD in young athletes in the United States. Both dilated cardiomyopathy and hypertrophic cardiomyopathy limit life expectancy and frequently are associated with symptoms. Return to normal morphology with the cessation of training had been considered the *sine qua non* of the diagnosis of the AHS.

In a prospective longitudinal study of trained athletes during and after the cessation of training, TTE abnormalities observed during training trended back toward normal. Left ventricular wall thickness returned to < 13 mm in all the deconditioned former athletes, whereas left ventricular end-diastolic dimensions fell from the training state but were typically still in the abnormal range. Although cessation of training may help differentiate between AHS and hypertrophic cardiomyopathy, left ventricular dilation can persist in elite athletes, even after termination of training. The long-term consequences of left ventricular cavity dilation associated with AHS have yet to be fully delineated (6).

Preparticipation Screening and Sudden Cardiac Death

Sudden cardiac death of elite athletes on the playing field or on the practice court arouses public curiosity and consternation. Hank Gathers, Reggie Lewis, Flo Hyman, Florence Joyner, Len Bias, Sergei Grinkov, and Pete Maravich are among the group of elite athletes who have died suddenly. All were or had been Olympic or professional competitors. There are approximately 4 million high school and 500,000 college athletes (8). The incidence of SCD in these athletes is in the range of 1 in 100,000 to 1 in 300,000 participants. Preparticipation screening is intended to reduce, but can not completely eliminate, such tragedies. Nevertheless, preparticipation screening for competitive high school and college athletes lacks uniformity, and many states do not require evidence of special expertise or training to perform preparticipation screening.

SCD before the age of 35 is typically congenital in origin. Among the most common etiologies of SCD in athletes of less than 35 years of age are hypertrophic cardiomyopathy, coronary artery anomalies, increased cardiac mass (without definite evidence of hypertrophic cardiomyopathy), ruptured aorta (particularly associated with Marfan syndrome), tunneled left anterior descending coronary artery, aortic stenosis, myocarditis, dilated cardiomyopathy, long QT syndrome, and arrhythmogenic right ventricular dysplasia. Table 13-1 lists the most common etiologies of SCD in young athletes.

Table 13-1   The Most Common Causes of Pathologic Conditions Associated with Sudden Cardiac Death in Young Athletes in the United States*

---

1. Hyperthrophic cardiomyopathy
2. Increased cardiac mass of uncertain cause
3. Anomalous origin of the coronary arteries
4. Other coronary anomalies
5. Aortic aneurysm with rupture-Marfan syndrome and medial necrosis
6. Tunneled left anterior descending coronary artery
7. Arrhythmogenic right ventricular dysplasia
8. Aortic valve stenosis
9. Myocarditis
10. Mitral valve prolapse
11. Congenital heart disease
12. Long QT syndrome
13. Ventricular arrhythmias not associated with structural heart disease

---

*Listed in descending order of frequency.

Several of these more common etiologies of SCD are inherited in autosomal dominant fashion.

After age 35, acquired forms of heart disease, especially coronary artery disease, are more common causes of SCD. Preparticipation screening is required of all high school, college, and professional athletes. In addition, screening is recommended for all patients older than 35 years of age who are beginning a recreational exercise program. SCD occurs most commonly in football and basketball, the team sports with the highest participation. The American Heart Association has published recommendations for preparticipation screening of competitive and recreational athletes (8-10). When a cardiovascular abnormality is suspected or documented, referral to a cardiovascular specialist is recommended. Once the diagnosis is confirmed, an athlete's participation in training and competition should be governed by the recommendations of the 36th Bethesda Conference (11).

Preparticipation screening consists primarily of a detailed history and focused physical examination (see Chapter 1). A family history with particular inquiry into a record of family members with SCD at a young age is mandatory. Diagnostic studies such as ECG, TTE, and Holter monitoring may be undertaken as indicated by the PPSE.

Given the large number of athletes to be screened, noninvasive testing is thought to be cost-prohibitive and troubled by both false-positive and false-negative results. It has been estimated that routine use of TTE would cost about $250,000 to identify one previously undiagnosed case of hypertrophic cardiomyopathy. Some have advocated the routine use of ECG in preparticipation screening. The vast majority of patients with hypertrophic cardiomyopathy have abnormal 12-lead ECGs. The ECG is frequently abnormal in patients with other common causes of SCD, such as coronary anomalies and the long QT syndrome. However, because of the ECG changes associated with the physiologic adaptation of training, the ECG has a relatively low sensitivity in large groups of athletes. The routine use of the ECG as a screening tool is not currently advocated due to the high false-positive rate.

Summary

Athletic heart syndrome is a benign condition in which cardiac remodeling is a prominent feature. This syndrome can mimic serious forms of structural heart disease. In AHS, abnormalities may be found in the patient's physical examination, ECG, TTE, and MRI. The magnitude of these changes is related to environmental (training) and genetic factors. Because AHS often mimics disease states associated with sudden cardiac death, an attempt to exclude structural heart disease by preparticipation screening (a carefully focused history and physical examination) is the first step. When indicated, appropriate diagnostic studies such as ECG, TTE, and Holter monitoring should be undertaken. The long-term consequences and natural history of AHS have yet to be fully delineated.

REFERENCES

1. **Bryan G, Ward A, Rippe JM.** Athletic heart syndrome. Clin Sports Med. 1992;11: 259-72.
2. **Pelliccia A, Maron BJ, Culasso F, et al.** Clinical significance of abnormal electro-cardiographic patterns in trained athletes. Circulation. 2000;102:278-84.
3. **Zehender M, Meinertz T, Keul J, Just H.** ECG variants and cardiac arrhythmias in athletes: clinical relevance and prognostic importance. Am Heart J. 1990;119: 1378-91.
4. **Lerman BB, Stein KM, Markowitz SM.** Idiopathic right ventricular outflow tract tachycardia: a clinical approach. Pacing Clin Electrophysiol. 1996;19(12 Pt 1):2120-37.
5. **Venerando A, Rulli V.** Frequency, morphology, and meaning of the electrocar diographic anomalies found in Olympic marathon runners and walkers. J Sports Med Phys Fitness. 1964;4:135-41.
6. **Al-Sheikh T, Zipes DP.** Guidelines for competitive athletes with arrhythmias. In: Bayes de Luna A, et al. Arrhythmias and Sudden Death in Athletes. Boston: Kluwer Academic; 2000.
7. **Maron BJ.** Structural features of the athlete heart as defined by echocardiography. J Am Coll Cardiol. 1986;7:190-203.
8. **Pelliccia A, Maron BJ, DeLuca R, et al.** Remodeling of left ventricular hypertro-phy in elite athletes after long-term deconditioning. Circulation. 2002:105:944-9.
9. **Maron BJ, Thompson PD, Puffer JC, et al.** Cardiovascular preparticipation screening in competitive athletes. Circulation. 1996;94:850-6.
10. **Maron BJ, Araujo CG, Thompson PD, et al.** Recommendations for preparticipa-tion screening and the assessment of cardiovascular disease in master athletes. Circulation. 2001;103:327-34.
11. **Maron BJ, Zipes DP.** 36th Bethesda Conference: eligibility recommendations for competitive athletes with cardiovascular abnormalities. J Am Coll Cardiol. 2005;45:1311-75.

SUGGESTED READING

Balady GJ, Chaitman B, Driscoll D, et al. Recommendations for cardiovascular screening, staffing, and emergency policies at health/fitness facilities. Circulation. 1998;97:2283-93.

Bayes de Luna A, Furlanello F, Marron BJ, Zipes DJ, eds. Arrhythmias and Sudden Death in Athletes. Boston: Kluwer Academic; 2000.

Williams RA, ed. The Athlete and Heart Disease: Diagnosis, Evaluation and Management. Philadelphia: Lippincott Williams & Wilkins; 1999.

WEB-BASED PATIENT INFORMATION SOURCES

American Heart Association. Physical Activity in Your Daily Life. Available from: www.americanheart.org/presenter.jhtml?identifier=2155

Gear K, Marcus F. Arrhythmogenic Right Ventricular Dysplasia/Cardiomyopathy. Available from: circ.ahajournals.org/

Maron BJ. Hypertrophic Cardiomyopathy. Available from: circ.ahajournals.org/

Myers J. Exercise and Cardiovascular Health. Available from: circ.ahajournals.org/

14

■ ■ ■

Hypertension in Athletes

Mark W. Niedfeldt, MD

ypertension is a major problem in our society; 50 million U.S. adults have hypertension (1). Athletes and active individuals are usually thought to be free of cardiovascular disease and hypertension owing to their often apparently high level of fitness, and it is true that the overall incidence of hypertension in this group is approximately 50% less than in the general population (2). However, some active people are at *increased* risk for hypertension, including blacks, the elderly, obese athletes, and those with diabetes, renal disease, or a family history of hypertension. Wheelchair athletes with spinal cord injuries may also have increased blood pressure due to loss of autonomic control of blood pressure (3).

Hypertension often begins in young adulthood and is progressive. Incidence increases with age, affecting 5%-10% of adults 20-30 years old, 20%-25% of middle-aged adults, and more than 50% of adults greater than age 60, with a residual lifetime risk of more than 90% (4-6). Almost 80% of adolescents found to have elevated blood pressure greater than 142/92 during a preparticipation physical examination have chronically elevated blood pressure (7). This is especially true in blacks, who have been shown to have significantly higher blood pressures starting before age 10 (8). This earlier onset of elevated blood pressure makes a substantial contribution to higher rates of cardiovascular and renal disease in the black population (9). Therefore, athletes should be screened for hypertension, and, if the condition is diagnosed, they must be treated appropriately to reduce risks of ilness and death associated with cardiovascular disease (10).

The Seventh Report of the Joint National Committee on Prevention, Detection, Evaluation, and Treatment of High Blood Pressure points out the progressive nature of hypertension and divides it into three classifications (Table 14-1) (10). Most active individuals with hypertension will fall into stage 1 or the lower range of stage 2. Active individuals and athletes with compelling indications, such as diabetes mellitus or renal disease, should

Table 14-1   Blood Pressure Classification (mm Hg)*

	Systolic	*Diastolic*
Normal	< 120	< 80
Prehypertension	120-139	80-89
Stage 1 Hypertension	140-159	90-99
Stage 2 Hypertension	≥160	≥100

*If the systolic blood pressure (SBP) and diastolic blood pressure (DBP) fall into different categories, the higher category should be used.
Adapted with permission from the Seventh Report of the Joint National Committee on Detection, Evaluation, and Treatement of High Blood Pressure (JNC-7). JAMA. 2003:289:2560-75.

be treated at the prehypertensive level. Secondary hypertension, seen in less than 5% of cases, tends to be found in younger patients, adults with a rapid onset of severe hypertension, or those with hypertension that responds poorly to routine therapies. The most common cause of secondary hypertension is renal disease, either vascular or parenchymal; however, the estrogen in oral contraceptives commonly taken by female athletes can lead to hypertension soon after starting treatment. Overall about 5% of women taking this medication will develop hypertension over a 5-year period (11).

Clinical Evaluation

The clinical evaluation of patients with documented hypertension has three objectives: 1) to assess lifestyle and other cardiovascular risk factors or disorders; 2) to look for identifiable causes of high blood pressure; and 3) to assess the presence of end-organ damage.

History

The history should focus on behaviors and risk factors. Cardiovascular risk factors include documented hypertension, smoking, family history of cardiac disease in men under 55 and women under 65, obesity, physical inactivity, diabetes mellitus, dyslipidemia, and age under 55 in men and 65 in women (10). Identifiable causes of hypertension include sleep apnea, chronic kidney disease, endocrine disorders such as adrenal dysfunction, thyroid or parathyroid disease, pheochromocytoma, and sex hormone excess or decrease, and coarctation of the aorta (10).

Additionally, the history should explore the athlete's diet and behaviors that may affect blood pressure, including high sodium and saturated fat intake from processed and fast foods, alcohol consumption, recreational drug abuse (specifically stimulants, which may be taken before workouts or competitions, as well as cocaine), smoking or chewing tobacco use, and anabolic steroid use. Many common over-the-counter medications used by active individuals, such as NSAIDs, caffeine, diet pills, and decongestants, also may lead to increased blood pressure. Athletes should be questioned about the use of herbs and other supplements, with special notice given to substances purchased for increased energy or weight control. These often contain "natural" substances such as guarana, ma huang, and ephedra, all of which are stimulants. Stress can also be a risk factor for hypertension in athletes, because chronic environmental or social stress may lead to higher circulating catecholamines and chronic neurogenic activation of the sympathetic nervous system (12).

Measurement of Blood Pressure

Proper measurement of blood pressure is essential (11). The screening blood pressure measurement should be performed in a standard measurement situation. This is often difficult to do with young athletes, whose blood pressure is often measured during a routine sports physical taking place outside a doctor's office (for example, a training room, where noise, anxiety, and other distractions may interfere with the accuracy of blood pressure measurement). Measurements should be performed in a seated position with the arm supported at heart level after 5 minutes of rest. Any high reading should be measured again at least two minutes after the first reading. It is important to use the appropriate blood pressure cuff size. The bladder of the cuff should encircle at least 80% of the arm, so many athletes will require a large cuff size. The cuff should be deflated at a rate of 2-3 mm Hg/second, and rapid deflation should be avoided (12). Verification should be performed in the contralateral arm (10).

Physical Examination

The physical exam focuses on ruling out secondary causes of hypertension and looking for end-organ damage. Body mass index (BMI) is a useful tool in the nonathletic population; however, it may not be useful in some athletes due to increased muscle mass. For example, a collegiate football running back may be 68 inches tall and weigh 191 lbs with 8% body fat. His BMI would be 29, which is considered overweight in the average population. The optic fundi are examined to rule out hypertensive retinopathy. The neck is examined for carotid bruits, jugular venous distention, or enlargement of the thyroid gland. Thorough examination of the heart and lungs focuses on abnormalities in cardiac rate, rhythm, and size; murmurs, extra heart sounds, and rales; or bronchospasm. The abdominal examination seeks to identify abdominal masses, enlarged kidneys, abnormal pulsations, or bruits, while the examination of the extremities evaluates edema, pulses, and femoral bruits.

Laboratory Studies

Laboratory studies are performed before initiation of treatment to determine the presence of target organ damage or causes of secondary hypertension. Studies include hematocrit, Na^+, K^+, BUN, creatinine, calcium, fasting glucose, total cholesterol, triglycerides, LDL and HDL cholesterol, urinalysis, and electrocardiogram (10). Other studies and further workup may be pursued if the clinician is suspicious of a secondary cause of hypertension or if blood pressure control is not achieved.

Treatment

Goals of Therapy

Treating systolic and diastolic blood pressure (BP) to a target less than 140/90 mm Hg is associated with a decrease in cardiovascular disease complications. In patients with diabetes or known renal disease, the goal is less than 130/80 mm Hg. The primary focus should be on achieving the systolic goal, as most patients with hypertension, especially those older than age 50, will reach the diastolic BP goal once systolic BP is at the goal level (13,14).

Nonpharmacologic Therapy

Active individuals are often more motivated than the general population to comply with nonpharmacologic treatment of hypertension, since treatment has virtually no side effects. These treatments depend on long-term adherence and lifestyle changes. Lifestyle modifications are recommended as an adjunct for patients with hypertension who are receiving pharmacologic treatment. Although such modifications cannot always be used as a substitute for medication, their adjunctive use may enable the medication dosage to be reduced, thus lessening the possibility of side effects.

Dietary Changes
A reduction of sodium in the diet can result in a significant decrease in blood pressure (15,16). Reducing intake of processed foods such as lunchmeats and fast food, common in the diets of adolescent athletes, is an important recommendation, as such food provides 75% of the sodium in the typical American diet. In general, blacks, older people, and diabetics seem to be more sensitive to dietary sodium (17), but all hypertensives can benefit from a low-sodium diet (18).

Foods such as bananas, potatoes, and many fruits that contain significant amounts of potassium (K^+) are a good addition to the athlete's diet, because high dietary potassium intake may protect against development of hypertension and improve blood pressure control (19), especially in endurance athletes who may tend to be hypokalemic (15). The blood-pressure-lowering effect of potassium supplementation appears greater in those with higher levels of sodium intake (20).

Increased calcium intake (1-2 g/day) may lower blood pressure in some hypertensive individuals, especially women who are calcium-deficient, but the overall effect is minimal (21). A lower magnesium level may lead to higher blood pressure, because magnesium is a vasodilator. There may be some benefit to supplementation in selected patients, especially those whose magnesium has been depleted by the use of diuretics (22). However, supplementation of calcium and magnesium for the sole purpose of improving blood pressure control is not routinely recommended in active individuals (15).

Fish oil supplementation with relatively high doses of omega-3 polyunsaturated fatty acids lowers blood pressure in hypertensive individuals, especially those with untreated hypertension (23,24). The effect seems to be small in normotensive individuals. However, an increased intake of fish oil may reduce the risk of coronary heart disease and stroke (25,26).

Excess body weight is correlated with increased blood pressure (10). Weight reduction has been shown to reduce blood pressure in overweight individuals with hypertension (27,28) and seems to enhance the blood-pressure-lowering effect of many medications (29). A weight-reduction plan should include a high-fiber diet with low saturated fat (18).

Special mention should be given to DASH (Dietary Approaches to Stop Hypertension), which has been shown to reduce blood pressure in hypertensives (18,30,31). This diet has reduced levels of total and saturated fat and cholesterol with increased potassium, calcium, magnesium, fiber, and protein. It emphasizes fruits, vegetables, low-fat dairy products, whole grains, poultry, fish, and nuts (18,32). A decrease of 11.4/5.5 mm Hg in hypertensive patients and 5.5/3.0 mm Hg in those with borderline BP was observed—as much as with some medications (18). DASH has been shown to be particularly effective in blacks (33).

There are few clinical reports to support the use of herbal and botanical supplements in the prevention or treatment of hypertension. Athletes should be asked about the use of herbal products and other supplements for risk and to consider the possibility of herb-drug interactions (20).

Lifestyle Changes

Excess alcohol can cause resistance to antihypertensive therapy. Adults who drink should limit alcoholic beverage intake to the equivalent of two beers daily. Women and lighter-weight individuals should consume no more than the equivalent of one beer daily (15).

Relaxation techniques, such as biofeedback, muscle relaxation, meditation, yoga, and stress management, are commonly used by some athletes and may have value as adjunct therapies.

Regular aerobic exercise adequate to achieve moderate fitness can lower blood pressure (20,34), enhance weight loss, and reduce the death rate of athletes who are not performing true aerobic exercise (35). The effect of exercise on hypertension is even more dramatic in those whose hypertension is secondary to renal dysfunction. An exercise prescription for hypertensive patients is shown in Table 14-2.

It has been documented that individuals with above-optimal BP and stage 1 hypertension can make multiple lifestyle changes, such as decreasing alcohol consumption, performing moderate physical activity, losing weight, and following the reduced-sodium DASH diet, to lower BP and control hypertension (20).

Pharmacologic Therapy

Management of hypertension in the active individual and athlete requires that certain factors, such as drug effects on athletic performance and the permissibility of certain drugs in competitive sports, be considered. Most individuals with hypertension will require two or more antihypertensive medications to achieve goal BP (10). Additionally, if initial BP is more than 20/10 mm Hg above the goal level, consideration can be given to initiating therapy with two agents, one of which is generally a thiazide diuretic (10).

Table 14-2   Exercise Prescription and Sports Participation for Hypertensive Patients

Exercise
- The recommended mode, frequency, duration, and intensity of exercise are generally the same as those for nonhypertensive individuals.

Sports Participation
- Hypertensive athletes should have their blood pressure controlled before returning to participation in vigorous sports, because both dynamic and isometric exercise can cause remarkable blood pressure increases.

Exercise Restrictions for Hypertensive Athletes

Prehypertensive	No restrictions
Controlled mild/moderate (< 140/90)	No restrictions on dynamic exercise; physicians may choose to limit isometric training or sports in some cases
Uncontrolled (> 140/90)	Limit to low-intensity dynamic exercise; avoid isometric sports.
Controlled with end-organ damage	Limit to low-intensity dynamic exercise; avoid isometric sports
Controlled severe hypertension	Low-intensity dynamic sports if blood pressure is under adequate control
Secondary hypertension (renal origin)	Low intensity sports are recommended; avoid "collision" sports, which could lead to kidney damage

Data from 36th Bethesda Conference: Recommendations for determining eligibility for competition in athletes with cardiovascular abnormalities. J Am Coll Cardiol. 2005;45:1311-75.

Exercising individuals and competitive athletes will need to monitor the effects of medications on their activities, because some medications have a potential influence on exercise tolerance. NSAIDs may decrease the action of several antihypertensives, including diuretics, beta-blockers, and angiotensin-converting enzyme (ACE) inhibitors (36). Be aware that the United States Olympic Committee (USOC) and the NCAA ban some medications (37). Pharmacologic therapies for hypertension are summarized in Table 14-3 and discussed below.

Diuretics

The diuretic antihypertensive drugs include both the thiazides and the loop inhibitors. These medications decrease plasma volume, cardiac output, and vascular resistance (38). Thiazide-type diuretics have been shown to result in a decrease in illness and death, mainly in the elderly, and are superior in preventing one or more major forms of cardiovascular disease (15,39). Thiazide diuretics are inexpensive and should be the preferred first step for antihypertensive therapy, especially for casual exercisers, active elderly, and black patients (39). They should be used in small doses, possibly combined with a potassium-sparing agent, and are also useful as a second-line therapy in salt-sensitive hypertensive athletes (33). Side effects of thiazide diuretics can include hypovolemia, orthostatic hypotension, and urinary loss of potassium and magnesium, which can lead to muscle cramps, arrhythmias, and rhabdomyolysis in individuals exercising intensely or competing in warm weather. The more potent loop diuretics magnify these effects and are therefore inappropriate for use in the treatment of hypertension in athletes. All diuretics are athletic-association banned substances because they dilute the concentration of steroids and drugs in the urine and cannot be used by elite athletes who are required to undergo drug testing (37).

ACE Inhibitors

ACE inhibitors block the conversion of angiotensin I to angiotensin II, a potent vasoconstrictor and source of sodium retention. There is an increase in stroke volume, a slight decrease in heart rate, and a decrease in total peripheral resistance with the use of ACE inhibitors (38). These antihypertensives have been shown to have beneficial effects in patients with heart failure, systolic dysfunction or nephropathy, and they have been shown to reverse ventricular hypertrophy and microalbuminuria and to preserve renal function. In exercise, ACE inhibitors have no major effect on energy metabolism, no impairment of maximum oxygen uptake (Vo_{2max}), and, in general, no deleterious effects on training or competition (38). The major side effect is a dry, nonproductive cough. There are also anecdotal reports of postural hypotension after intense exercise; therefore, an adequate cooldown period after intense exercise is recommended. This class of antihypertensives is excellent for mild-to-moderate hypertension and is often a first-line agent for hypertension in active patients, especially those with

Table 14-3   Pharmacologic Treatments for Hypertension

Drug Class	Heart Rate Effects on Training	Stroke Volume Side Effects	Cardiac Output Recommended for	Avoid In	Plasma Volume Banned Status
Diuretics	No effect No effect or decreased endurance	Decrease Hypovolemia, orthostatic hypotension, urinary loss of potassium and magnesium, muscle cramps, arrhythmias, rhabdomyolysis in warm weather	Decrease Elderly, African-American, CHF	Endurance athletes, college athletes	Significant decrease Banned by USOC and NCAA
ACE-I/ARB	Slight decrease No effect	Increase Dry, nonproductive cough (ACE-I)	Increase Diabetics, renal insufficiency, CHF, asthma, hyperlipidemia	Women not using contraception	No effect None
Alpha-blockers	No effect No effect	No effect First-dose effect; central acting may cause drowsiness, dry mouth, impotence, and rebound hypertension	No effect Hyperlipidemia, BPH	Men older than 55	No effect None
Beta-blockers	Significant decrease Significant decrease	No effect Increased perceived exertion ratings, impairment of cardiac output and VO_{2max}, earlier fatigue and lactate threshold, exercise-induced bronchospasm; asthma may be exacerbated	Significant decrease Coronary artery disease	Asthmatics, endurance athletes, college athletes	No effect Banned in precision sports (rifle, archery, diving, ice skating)

| Calcium channel blockers | Decrease, increase, or no effect No effect | No effect or decrease Nondihydropyridines (for example, verapamil, diltiazem) can cause heart rate suppression and minor impairment of maximal heart rate, decreased left ventricular contractility, and constipation; dihydropyridines (for example, amlodipine, nifedipine) can cause reflex tachycardia, fluid retention, and vascular headaches | No effect or decrease Asthma, African-Americans | None | No effect or increase None |

diabetes (10). Effectiveness may be improved with addition of a low-dose thiazide diuretic, either taken separately or in combination. The concomitant use of NSAIDs and ACE inhibitors may increase the potassium-sparing effect of the medication (40).

Case Study 14-1

History

A 47-year-old "ironman" triathlete presented with new-onset hypertension. He had had readings of 148/94, 150/92, and 148/94 over the past 6 months. He exercised approximately 15-20 hours weekly and had no other medical problems. He took no medications outside of occasional ibuprofen, his daily multivitamin, vitamin E 400 IU, and vitamin C 250 mg. Family history was remarkable for hypertension in his father and myocardial infarction in his paternal grandfather at age 62. He did not smoke; he drank a glass or two of wine weekly; he drank 3-4 cups of coffee daily; and he worked as an attorney. Review of systems was unremarkable.

Physical Examination

The patient was 72 inches tall and weighed 179 lbs. Blood pressure was 146/94, and resting pulse was 58. Observation showed a lean male who appeared younger than his stated age. Physical examination was otherwise unremarkable. Lab results, including basic metabolic panel, CBC, UA, and EKG, were all normal. His lipid profile was excellent.

Discussion

The patient's major concern about medication was the effect it could have on his performance. He was training for an upcoming competition in Florida. He was started on enalapril 10 mg daily since this would not affect his exercise tolerance. He returned 4 weeks later and had a blood pressure reading of 126/82. He experienced no ill effects from the medication and had not noticed any problems with his training performance or race times. The patient also cut his caffeine intake to 1-2 cups of coffee daily. He was continued on his dose of medication. The interaction between NSAIDs and ACE inhibitors was also discussed. The patient stated he generally only used ibuprofen 400 mg once a week or less. He was instructed that chronic use of NSAIDs may increase his blood pressure.

Angiotensin Receptor Blockers

The angiotensin II receptor blockers (ARBs) block the renin-angiotensin system by preventing angiotensin II from binding to its subtype 1 receptor and produce effects similar to those of the ACE inhibitors but avoid the most common side effect (dry cough) due to their action at the receptor level (41). The effects of ARBs are similar to or identical to those of the ACE inhibitors, and these agents generally are recommended for the same patient populations as the ACE inhibitors, since the ARBs have been shown to slow the rates of progression of nephropathy and proteinuria (41). The likelihood of hyperkalemia is relatively low with this class of antihypertensive (42). Women of childbearing age should use contraception if taking ACE inhibitors or ARBs, as they are contraindicated in pregnancy.

Alpha-Blockers

Alpha 1 receptor blockers competitively block postsynaptic alpha-1 arteriolar smooth muscle receptors. They decrease systemic vascular resistance with no reflex increase in heart rate or cardiac output. There can be a first-dose effect, especially in the elderly. There are no major changes in energy metabolism during exercise, and the VO_{2max} is preserved; therefore, there are no major effects on training or sports performance (38). These agents have been used in hypertensive athletes who have diabetes and hypercholesterolemia, since they will not exacerbate those conditions (11). The ALLHAT (Antihypertensive and Lipid-Lowering Treatment to Prevent Heart Attack Trial) study discontinued the doxazosin arm of the study due to an increased incidence of congestive heart failure as compared to a diuretic (43). This should be taken into consideration, especially in master athletes greater than age 55.

Central Alpha-Agonists

The central alpha-agonists have no major effect on training or sports performance, (38) but are rarely used due to side effects, including mild-to-moderate drowsiness, dry mouth, impotence, and rebound hypertension, which can occur with abrupt discontinuation of oral clonidine (44).

Beta-Blockers

Beta-blockers are of two main types: noncardioselective and cardioselective. The noncardioselective agents decrease contractility of the heart and decrease heart rate by 20%-30%. Lipolysis and glycogenolysis are inhibited, so hypoglycemia may occur after intense exercise. Athletes perceive greater exertion while using beta-blockers, which may affect adherence (38). Additionally, there is potential to exacerbate bronchoconstriction in predisposed athletes. An increased total cholesterol and decreased HDL cholesterol may also be noted (11). Nonselective beta-blockers are therefore not desirable in athletes.

Cardioselective agents lead to fewer side effects but still impair cardiac output and VO_{2max}. Well-trained athletes have a greater drop in maximal oxygen uptake than sedentary patients. These agents are not recommended in active patients, unless there is an underlying condition requiring their use, such as coronary artery disease (38).

When combined alpha- and beta-blocker agents are used, the beta-effects are greater than the alpha-effects. There is a decreased systemic vascular resistance but less impairment of muscle blood flow and Vo_{2max}. These agents may be the best choice if beta-blockade is necessary (44). Beta-blockers are banned by the USOC in precision events such as archery, shooting, diving, and ice-skating, as they reduce tremors and heart rate, which increases accuracy (37).

Calcium Channel Blockers

Calcium channel blockers inhibit calcium slow-channel conduction, reducing calcium concentration in vascular smooth muscle cells and resulting in decreased systemic vascular resistance with generalized vasodilatation (38). These agents are effective in reversing ventricular hypertrophy. Dihydropyridines (for example, amlodipine, nifedipine) can cause reflex tachycardia, fluid retention (pedal edema), and vascular headaches. The nondihydropyridines (for example, verapamil, diltiazem) can cause heart rate suppression, minor impairment of maximal heart rate, decreased left ventricular contractility, and constipation (verapamil) (15). During exercise, there is no major effect on energy metabolism, and Vo_{2max} is generally preserved (38). There is the potential for competitive "steal" of muscle blood flow due to vasodilatation and earlier onset of lactate threshold (45); however, this class of antihypertensives, especially the dihydropyridines, is generally well-tolerated and effective for active patients. They are often used as the first-line monotherapy in black athletes (10).

Case Study 14-2

History

A 20-year-old black male collegiate athlete presented for his preparticipation physical examination. He was a junior linebacker on the football team and had no physical symptoms. His past medical history was remarkable for an anterior cruciate ligament reconstruction. He took no medication and had no known drug allergies. Family history was remarkable for hypertension in both parents and an obese brother (age 32). He did use smokeless tobacco (chew) and often binge-drank on weekends. He used an "energy drink" supplement along with creatine in the off-season to give him more energy during weight-training workouts. Review of systems was otherwise unremarkable.

Physical Examination

The patient was 74 inches tall and weighed 240 pounds. His blood pressure was initially 164/96, with a pulse of 72. He was a muscular male in no acute distress. Physical examination was unremarkable.

Discussion

The athlete was instructed to report to the training room the next day for a repeat blood pressure reading. At that time, a reading of 144/90 was obtained using a large cuff. The patient was advised to discontinue the use of the "energy drink," decrease alcohol intake, and stop using smokeless tobacco. Additional dietary changes were discussed, including decreasing salt load from fast food and making better choices at the training table. The patient was rechecked 4 weeks later. He had stopped using the "energy drink" supplement and had attempted to reduce his salt intake. He had continued using smokeless tobacco but had decreased his alcohol intake. His blood pressure at that time was 136/86. He was advised to continue his interventions, have his blood pressure monitored regularly, and avoid supplements containing stimulants.

This case illustrates some of the considerations when dealing with younger athletes. Binge drinking, use of smokeless tobacco, and supplement use are important to ascertain during the history. Many energy pills and drinks contain ephedra (ma huang), high levels of caffeine (guarana), or both. Using the proper blood pressure cuff size is also important; many athletes will require a large size cuff. Given his family history, this athlete is at high risk of developing chronic hypertension, especially if he stops exercising and gains weight. If medication must be started, one should consider using an ACE inhibitor or calcium channel blocker. Diuretics should be avoided because they are banned by the NCAA and because he exercises in the heat.

When to Refer

Athletes with hypertension may be referred to a hypertension specialist when first- and second-line medications are ineffective. Patients with secondary hypertension may need referral for treatment and management of the underlying condition.

Exercise in Hypertensive Patients

Aerobic Exercise

During aerobic exercise, several physiologic changes occur. An increased cardiac output occurs due to increases in heart rate, stroke volume, and contractility. Decreased vascular resistance occurs, resulting in increased systolic blood pressure with little change in diastolic blood pressure. In the athlete with stage 1 hypertension, the normal increased cardiac output is accompanied by a higher vascular resistance, which results in increased systolic and diastolic blood pressure. In the higher level of stage 2 hypertension, the increased vascular resistance is accompanied by decreased stroke volume, which can lead to a lower cardiac output (45).

Resistance Exercise

Resistance exercise shows a different physiological response. A rapid increase in systolic and diastolic pressure (pressor response) occurs with a reflex increased heart rate and resultant increased cardiac output. No change in vascular resistance is seen. In the hypertensive athlete, the relative increase in blood pressure is similar to that in the normotensive athlete, but the starting point is higher. Thus, the end blood pressure is higher than in normotensive individuals (45). The American College of Sports Medicine recommends resistance exercise for major muscle groups twice weekly for the average healthy adult (46,47). Resistance training should serve as an adjunct to an aerobic-based exercise program (48).

Exercise Prescription and Competition

The recommended modes, frequency, duration, and intensity of exercise are generally the same as those for the nonhypertensive person. Recommendations about athletic participation are based on the 36th Bethesda Conference guidelines (49). Athletes with high normal blood pressure have no restrictions. Athletes with controlled stage 1 and controlled lower stage 2 hypertension—that is, BP lowered below 140/90—have no restriction for dynamic exercise. Physicians may choose to limit isometric training or sports, however. Keep in mind that patients taking diuretics may be at risk for dehydration.

Athletes with uncontrolled blood pressure should be limited to low-intensity dynamic exercise. This restriction also applies to athletes with controlled hypertension with end-organ involvement; these athletes should avoid isometric sports.

Athletes with severe hypertension with no end-organ involvement may be limited to low-intensity dynamic sports if the blood pressure is under adequate control.

In secondary hypertension of renal origin, low-intensity sports are recommended. These athletes should avoid "collision" sports, which could lead to kidney damage.

REFERENCES

1. **Munter P, He J, Roccella EJ, Whelton PW.** The impact of the JNC-VI guidelines on treatment recommendations in the US population. Hypertension. 2002;39:897-902.
2. **Lehmann M, Durr H, Meikelbach H, Schmid A.** Hypertension and sports activity: institutional experience. Clin Cardiol. 1990;13:197-208.

3. **Swain R, Kaplan B.** Treating hypertension in active patients: which agents work best with exercise? Phys Sportsmed. 1997;25(9):47-64.

4. **Gifford RW, Kirkendall W, O'Connor DT, Weidman W.** Scientific Council Special Report: Office evaluation of hypertension. Circulation. 1989;79:721-31.

5. **Burt VL, Whelton P, Roccella EJ, et al.** Prevalence of hypertension in the US adult population: results from the Third National Health and Nutrition Examination Survey, 1988-1991. Hypertension. 1995;25:305-13.

6. **Vasan RS, Beiser A, Seshadri S, et al.** Residual life-time risk fro developing hypertension in middle-aged women and men: the Framingham Heart Study. JAMA. 2002;287:1003-10.

7. **Tanji JL.** Tracking of elevated blood pressure values in adolescent athletes at 1-year follow-up. Am J Dis Child. 1991;145(6):665-7.

8. **Harshfield GA, Treiber FA.** Racial differences in ambulatory blood pressure monitoring-derived 24 h patterns of blood pressure in adolescents. Blood Press Monit. 1999;4:107-10.

9. **Levine RS, Foster JE, Fullilove RE, et al.** Black-white inequalities in mortality and life expectancy, 1993-1999: implications for healthy people 2010. Public Health Rep. 2001;116:474-83.

10. **Joint National Committee on Detection, Evaluation, and Treatment of High Blood Pressure.** The Sixth Report of the Joint National Committee on Detection, Evaluation, and Treatment of High Blood Pressure (The JNC 7 Report). JAMA. 2003;289:2560-75.

11. **Kaplan NM.** Clinical Hypertension, 7th ed. New York: Williams & Wilkins; 1997.

12. **Julius S, Nesbitt S.** Sympathetic overactivity in hypertension: a moving target. Am J Hypertension. 1996;9(11):113S-120S.

13. **American Diabetes Association.** Treatment of hypertension in adults with diabetes. Diabetes Care. 2003;26(Suppl 1):S80-82.

14. **National Kidney Foundation Guideline.** K/DOQI clinical practice guidelines for chronic kidney disease. Kidney Disease Outcome Quality Initiative. Am J Kidney Dis. 2002;39(Suppl 2):S1-246.

15. **Joint National Committee on Detection, Evaluation, and Treatment of High Blood Pressure.** The Sixth Report of the Joint National Committee on Detection, Evaluation, and Treatment of High Blood Pressure (JNC-VI). 1997; NIH Publication No. 98-4080.

16. **Whelton PK, Appel LJ, Espeland MA, et al., for the TONE Collaborative Research Group.** Sodium reduction and weight loss in the treatment of hypertension in older persons: a randomized controlled trial of non-pharmacologic intervention in the elderly (TONE). JAMA. 1998;279:839-46.

17. **Weinberger MH.** Salt sensitivity of blood pressure in humans. Hypertension. 1996;27(Pt 2):481-90.

18. **Appel LJ, Moore TJ, Obarzanek E, et al., for the DASH Collaborative Research Group.** A clinical trial of the effects of dietary patterns on blood pressure. N Engl J Med. 1997;336:1117-24.

19. **Whelton PK, HE J, Cutler JA, et al.** Effects of oral potassium on blood pressure: meta-analysis of randomized controlled trials. JAMA. 1997;277:1624-32.

20. **Whelton PK, He J, Appel LJ, et al., for the National High Blood Pressure Education Program Coordinating Committee.** Primary prevention of

hypertension: clinical and public health advisory from the National High Blood Pressure Education Program. JAMA. 2002;288:1882-8.

21. **Cappuccino FP, Elliot P, Allender PS, et al.** Epidemiologic association between dietary calcium intake and blood pressure: a meta analysis of randomized clinical trials. Ann Intern Med. 1996;124:825-31.

22. **Stamler J, Caggiula AW, Grandits GA.** Relation of body mass and alcohol, nutrient, fiber, and caffeine intakes to blood pressure in the special intervention and usual care groups in the Multiple Risk Factor Intervention Trial. Am J Clin Nutr. 1997;65 (Suppl):338S-365S.

23. **Trials of Hypertension Prevention Collaborative Research Group.** Effects of weight loss and sodium reduction intervention on blood pressure and hypertension incidence in overweight people with high-normal blood pressure: the Trials of Hypertension Prevention, phase II. Arch Intern Med. 1997;157:657-67.

24. **Appel LJ, Miller ER III, Seidler AJ, Whelton PK.** Does supplementation of diet with "fish oil" reduce blood pressure? A meta-analysis of controlled clinical trials. Arch Intern Med. 1993;153:1429-38.

25. **Morris MC, Sacks F, Rosner B.** Does fish oil lower blood pressure? A meta-analysis of controlled trials. Circulation. 1993;88:523-33.

26. **Dehmer GJ, Popma JJ, vanden Berg EK, et al.** Reduction in the rate of early restenosis after coronary angioplasty by a diet supplemented with n-3 fatty acids. N Engl J Med. 1988;319:733-40.

27. **Ascherio A, Rimm EB, Stampfer MJ, et al.** Dietary intake of marine n-3 fatty acids, fish intake, and the risk of coronary disease among men. N Engl J Med. 1995;332:977-82.

28. **Miller ER III, Erlinger TP, Young DR, et al.** Results of the diet, exercise, and weight loss intervention trial (DEW-IT). Hypertension. 2002;40:612-8.

29. **Neaton JD, Grimm RH Jr, Prineas RJ, et al., for the Treatment of Mild Hypertension Study Research Group.** Treatment of Mild Hypertension Study: final results. JAMA. 1993;270:713-24.

30. **Writing Group of the PREMIER Collaborative Research Group.** Effects of comprehensive lifestyle modification on blood pressure control: main results of the PREMIER clinical trial. JAMA. 2003;289:2083-93.

31. **Sachs FM, Swetkey LP, Vollmer WM, et al., for the DASH-Sodium Collaborative Research Group.** Effects on blood pressure of reduced dietary sodium and the Dietary Approaches to Stop Hypertension (DASH) diet. N Engl J Med. 2001;344:3-10.

32. **Karanja NM, Obarzanek E, Lin PH, et al.** Descriptive characteristics of the dietary patterns used in the Dietary Approaches to Stop Hypertension trial. J Am Diet Assoc. 1999;99(Suppl):S19-27.

33. **Douglas JG, Bakris GL, Epstein M, et al.** Management of high blood pressure in African Americans: consensus statement of the hypertension in African Americans working group of the International Society on Hypertension in Blacks. Arch Intern Med. 2003;163:525-41.

34. **Whelton SP, Chin A, Xin X, He J.** Effect of aerobic exercise on blood pressure: a meta-analysis of randomized, controlled trials. Ann Intern Med. 2002;136:493-503.

35. **Petrella LS.** How effective is exercise training for the treatment of hypertension? Clin J Sports Med. 1998;8:224-31.

36. **Brook RD, Kramer MB, Blaxall BC, Bisognano JD.** Nonsteroidal anti-inflammatory drugs and hypertension. J Clin Hypertens. 2000;2:319-23.

37. **United States Anti-Doping Agency (USADA).** 2005 USADA Guide to Prohibited Substances and Prohibited Methods of Doping. [cited 2005 Feb]. PDF available from: www.usantidoping.org

38. **Chick TW, Halperin AK, Gacek EM.** The effect of antihypertensive medications on exercise performance: a review. Med Sci Sports Exerc. 1988;20:447-54.

39. **ALLHAT Officers and Coordinators for the ALLHAT Collaborative Research Group.** Major outcomes in high-risk hypertensive patients randomized to angiotensin-converting enzyme inhibitor or calcium channel blocker vs diuretic: the Antihypertensive and Lipid-Lowering Treatment to Prevent Heart Attack Trial (ALLHAT). JAMA. 2002;288:2981-97.

40. **Gifford RW.** Antihypertensive therapy: angiotensin-converting enzyme inhibitors, angiotensin II receptor antagonists, and calcium antagonists. Med Clin North Am. 1997;81:6;1319-34.

41. **Toto R.** Angiotensin II subtype 1 receptor blockers and renal function. Arch Intern Med. 2001;161:1492-9.

42. **Bakris GL, Siomos M, Richardson D, et al.** ACE inhibition or angiotensin receptor blockade: impact on potassium in renal failure. Kidney Int. 2000;58:2084-92.

43. **ALLHAT Collaborative Research Group.** Major cardiovascular events in hypertensive patients randomized to doxazosin vs chlorthalidone: the antihypertensives and lipid-lowering treatment to prevent heart attack trial (ALLHAT). JAMA. 2000;283(15):1967-75.

44. **Freis ED.** Current status of diuretics, β-blockers, α-blockers, and α-β-blockers in the treatment of hypertension. Med Clin North Am. 1997;81(6):1305-18.

45. **Lund-Johansen P.** Hemodynamics in essential hypertension. Clin Sci. 1980;59: 3435-45.

46. **Pate RR, Pratt M, Blair SN, et al.** Physical activity and public health: a recommendation from the Centers for Disease Control and Prevention and the American College of Sports Medicine. JAMA. 1995;273:402-7.

47. **Pollock ML, Gaesser GA, Butcher JD, et al.** ACSM position stand: The recommended quantity and quality of exercise for developing and maintaining cardiorespiratory and muscular fitness and flexibility in healthy adults. Med Sci Sports Exer. 1998;30(6):975-91.

48. **Pescatello LS, Franklin BA, Fagard R, et al.** American College of Sports Medicine position stand: Exercise and hypertension [Review]. Med Sci Sports Exer. 2004;36:533-53.

49. **Maron BJ, Zipes DP.** 36th Bethesda Conference: eligibility recommendations for competitive athletes with cardiovascular abnormalities. J Am Coll Cardiol. 2005;45:1311-75.

15

■　■　■

Exercise-Induced Asthma, Urticaria, and Anaphylaxis

Philip H. Cohen, MD

For many people, exercise is a vital and enjoyable part of a healthy lifestyle. However, in certain individuals, exercise can trigger pathologic pulmonary and/or systemic reactions, ranging from the subclinical, to the uncomfortable, to the potentially fatal. This spectrum of pathology is represented by three main conditions: exercise-induced asthma, exercise-induced urticaria, and exercise-induced anaphylaxis. In this chapter, we examine these entities and review current understanding of their pathogenesis, diagnosis, and treatment.

Exercise-Induced Asthma

Exercise-induced asthma (EIA) is generally defined as reversible airway obstruction that is caused by and occurs during, or up to 30 minutes after, moderate-to-intense exercise (1,2). EIA and EIB (exercise-induced bronchoconstriction) are often used interchangeably in the literature. Healthy lungs respond to exercise by bronchodilation and increases in minute ventilation mediated by increased tidal volume and respiratory rate (1). In EIA, however, after transient bronchodilation, subsequent bronchoconstriction occurs, with obstruction peaking 5-10 minutes after the end of exercise. Up to 30% of patients with EIA also exhibit a "late response," consisting of a second decline in pulmonary function 6 to 8 hours after the initial episode. It is not well-characterized, but it is believed to be caused by delayed inflammatory mediators and/or perhaps circadian variation (3).

Patients with EIA typically experience symptoms such as wheezing, shortness of breath, cough, and chest tightness or discomfort. However, some athletes may have only subtle symptoms such as "feeling out of shape." Athletes may also seek evaluation due to poor sports performance, especially in cold, dry conditions.

Symptoms usually begin after 5 to 8 minutes of strenuous exercise and peak 5 to 10 minutes after completion of exercise. They generally dissipate by 30 minutes after cessation of exercise (1). Approximately 50% of individuals with EIA may experience a "refractory period" that lasts for up to 2 hours after exercise. During this time, repeated bouts of exercise produce little-to-no airway constriction (1,2,4-7); this phenomenon may be exploited by athletes who use a specialized warm-up before activities.

Epidemiology

EIA has been found to occur in up to 90% of patients with underlying asthma (8), in up to 40% of nonasthmatic patients with allergic rhinitis, and in up to 10% of the general population without known asthma (9). Athletes competing in cold-weather sports seem to be at highest risk, with overall prevalence rates of 22.4% among US Olympians competing in the 1998 Winter Games.

Pathophysiology

The pathophysiology of exercise-induced asthma is a topic of much debate. Two main hypotheses have been put forth, the osmotic and the thermal. Details of these hypotheses can be found elsewhere; however, there are multiple inconsistencies in the thermal hypothesis, and, therefore, the majority of data support the osmotic hypothesis (10).

It is known that, during inspiration of dry air, the nose, pharynx, and the first seven to twelve generations of bronchi warm and humidify the air before it reaches the alveoli. EIA severity is proportional to the humidity of inspired air, and is prevented when a patient inhales humidified air regardless of the temperature (11,12). Thus, the humidity of the inspired air seems to be a key factor. This would explain the observation of many patients that their asthma is worse with dry conditions and better with moist conditions. Other factors, such as underlying inflammation in patients with baseline asthma, atopy, and allergic diatheses, probably also contribute to the pathophysiology of EIA. Therefore, EIA is likely a multifactorial phenomenon, whose various manifestations and exact mechanisms are not yet fully understood.

Diagnosis

Physical exam at rest is typically unrevealing for the athlete with isolated EIA. Therefore, an objective diagnosis of EIA usually rests on spirometry showing a postexercise decrease in FEV_1 of at least 10%-15% from baseline (1,12a). Many authors have used the less restrictive criteria of a 10% drop in

FEV_1 (13-15), whereas others have required a drop of at least 20% in FEV_1 (16,17). For the 2002 Winter Olympic Games, the IOC required athletes who claimed to have asthma or EIA to provide the following proof: 1) an increase in the predicted FEV_1 of at least 12% after administration of an inhaled β_2-agonist; 2) a reduction in FEV_1 of at least 10% in response to exercise or eucapnic voluntary hyperpnea (EVH); or 3) a PD_{20} (provocative dose) to methacholine or histamine of less than 200 µg, or less than 1320 µg in athletes taking inhaled corticosteroids for 3 months. Peak expiratory flow rates and written notes from physicians were deemed unacceptable for documentation (17). Based on these new requirements, only 5.2% of athletes (79% of those who requested permission) at the 2002 Winter Olympic Games were permitted to use inhaled β_2-agonists (17,18).

The most common form of testing for EIA is exercise challenge, which is usually carried out on a treadmill or exercise bike, with rapid incremental increases in intensity to attain at least 90% of predicted maximum heart rate for 5 to 8 minutes. Testing should not involve strenuous exercise lasting greater than 10 minutes, as longer duration of activity can attenuate drops in FEV_1 (1,19). Failure to attain high enough intensity may lead to a false negative result, especially in a well-trained athlete. Spirometry typically is performed before exercise and at 5-minute increments from the cessation of exercise until 30 minutes into recovery (19). Post-exercise FEV_1 decrements of 10%-15%, up to 30%, are considered positive for mild EIA (19,20). Decreases of 30%-40% are considered moderate EIA, and decreases of greater than 40% are considered severe (20).

Field testing is a variation of exercise challenge, in which the testing is performed with portable spirometry equipment in the setting in which the athlete competes or experiences symptoms. This "real world" approach may be more accurate than isolated formal testing in a PFT lab; one study (21) showed that 78% of elite cold-weather athletes who tested positive "in the field" had negative tests in the lab. These findings underscore the importance of exercise intensity and environmental stress in determining physiologic response.

Bronchial provocation testing can also be performed chemically, usually with methacholine or histamine inhalation. These agents bind to specific receptors on bronchial smooth muscle, resulting in bronchoconstriction. Methacholine is generally preferred over histamine, as it is safer and gives more reproducible results (1,22). The protocol involves the patient inhaling the agent from a nebulizer, with doses titrated upward until there is a 20% decline in FEV_1. These provocation tests may be more sensitive than exercise challenge but are less specific; therefore, they are best reserved as second-line tests in an athlete with a highly suggestive history but a nondiagnostic exercise challenge test (1,19,20,22). Cold, dry air; aerosolized hypertonic saline; nebulized distilled water; inhaled powdered mannitol; and other provocative agents may also be used in some settings.

The EVH test involves the patient hyperventilating a dry gas to maintain eucapnia. A 20% or greater decline in FEV_1 is considered a positive test. It is a well-studied, potent, and standardized method for provoking bronchoconstriction in patients with EIA (16,23). However, EVH still misses some patients who test positive by exercise challenge (13). Thus, there is no perfect objective test for EIA. As previously mentioned, subjective symptoms either may be too subtle or denied by the patient, making symptom-based diagnosis unreliable; therefore, it is recommended that clinicians maintain a high index of suspicion for EIA, especially for high-risk individuals (history of asthma, atopy, participant in a high-risk sport). Testing may begin with exercise challenge; if inconclusive, second-line testing may be undertaken. With institution of appropriate therapy, subjects who truly have EIA should demonstrate positive diagnostic testing, appropriate improvements in test results, and possibly improvements in symptoms and performance.

In some cases, physicians may attempt to diagnose isolated EIA on the basis of history alone and prescribe an empiric course of a short-acting inhaled β_2-agonist without definitive testing. Although not recommended, if this approach is taken then close follow-up must occur to evaluate treatment response, side effects, and the possibility of incorrect diagnosis.

Differential Diagnosis

Vocal cord dysfunction (VCD) is a syndrome in which upper airway obstruction occurs due to inappropriate adduction of the vocal cords. This condition is often mistaken for EIA because it may present with exertional wheezing and shortness of breath.

It is extremely important not to miss underlying chronic asthma in a patient with EIA. Occurrence of symptoms at rest, worsening of symptoms during viral infections, and lack of complete response to β_2-agonists should prompt a thorough evaluation. A careful history (including assessment for tobacco use or occupational exposure to noxious chemicals) and physical exam must be performed to evaluate for other pulmonary or cardiac etiologies, such as pulmonary embolism, pneumothorax, coronary artery disease, congestive heart failure, cardiomyopathy, exercise-induced anaphylaxis, and so forth. Gastroesophageal reflux disease (GERD), chronic sinusitis, postnasal drip, and postviral airway hyperreactivity may cause cough and chest discomfort. Infections, tumors, aspiration, medication reaction (e.g., ACE-inhibitors, NSAIDs), and a host of other disorders must be considered, especially in the patient with atypical features or lack of response to treatment.

Treatment

Nonpharmacologic Treatment

Patients with underlying asthma must first gain good baseline control of their asthma in order to properly manage their EIA. For patients with or without underlying asthma, development and maintenance of a good cardiorespiratory fitness level is extremely important. Endurance training increases the capacity for aerobic exercise by enhancing oxygen delivery and skeletal muscle utilization. In addition, such training raises the anaerobic threshold, effectively decreasing minute ventilation for a given level of exercise (1); this subsequently decreases the evaporative and hyperosmolar effects of increased ventilation during exercise. In other words, being in good shape does not cure asthma, but it can improve performance and raises the threshold at which symptoms develop.

As previously mentioned, some athletes with EIA may be able to induce a refractory period during a warm-up session, thereby enabling them to exercise for up to 2 hours with little or no bronchoconstriction (1,2,4-7,24). There is no one standardized regimen for inducing this refractory period. It appears that the degree of refractoriness may depend, in part, on the extent of the bronchoconstriction response provoked by the warm-up (6). However, other work has shown that a 30-minute run at moderate intensity may provide similar protection to a 6 minute run at high intensity without inducing significant bronchoconstriction (7). Similarly, another study showed that a series of 30-second sprints produced a refractory period without inducing bronchoconstriction (25). A subsequent study using moderately trained asthmatics found no significant difference between the improvements in pulmonary function after either a 15-minute low-intensity running warm-up or a set of 8-second sprints with 1.5 minutes of rest between sprints (5).

Maintenance of proper hydration status is recommended, as is avoidance of known airway irritants. Therefore, outdoor exercise should be performed when ambient pollution and allergen levels are at their lowest. Control of related disorders, such as allergic rhinitis, is important. Similarly, learning to inhale through the nostrils will aid in humidifying inspired air, although, as exercise intensity increases, mouth breathing becomes inevitable. Some researchers have advocated the use of a face mask or scarf to warm and humidify the inspired air (1,20).

Choice of activity and environment should be considered. Sports that involve brief, intense efforts (short sprints, baseball) or low intensity but longer duration (golf) present little problem, whereas activities that involve prolonged periods of high minute ventilation (distance running, cross-country skiing) are more likely to provoke symptoms. Moist and warm air conditions are the most favorable, so an indoor pool may be an ideal place to train, whereas a cold and dry setting (for example, winter endurance sports) will be more problematic. Overall, athletes should be encouraged to participate in the activities that they enjoy, but they and their health care providers need to be mindful of these factors.

One activity that deserves special mention is scuba diving. Asthma and EIA were formerly considered absolute contraindications to scuba diving due to concerns over the risk of air-trapping, pulmonary barotrauma, arterial gas embolism (AGE), and decompression illness (DCI). In addition, inhaling a cold, dry gas mixture while being subjected to the high physiologic stresses of diving can precipitate an asthma attack. An asthma attack during a dive obviously would be life threatening; thus, active bronchospasm is clearly an absolute contraindication to diving. However, the available evidence suggests that for patients whose EIA is mild and well-controlled, scuba diving appears to pose no greater risk of DCI or death than to individuals without EIA. A small and statistically insignificant increased risk of AGE has been found. Medical clearance is still controversial, so expert consultation should be pursued, and potential risks must be fully explained to the patient. Divers must strictly follow safe diving guidelines, must adhere to their appropriate medical regimen, and must not dive if they are experiencing current asthma symptoms. Before they are cleared for scuba participation, it is recommended that athletes undergo pre- and postprovocational spirometry to document that their regimen does indeed prevent EIA (26-28).

Pharmacologic Treatment

β_2-Agonists

Inhaled β_2-agonists are the mainstay of prevention and treatment for EIA. As a class, their main effect is relaxation of bronchial smooth muscle, which leads to bronchodilation and improved pulmonary function. They also decrease vascular permeability (which may reduce mucosal edema), enhance mucociliary clearance, and inhibit release of inflammatory mediators, including histamine from mast cells and basophils (29). Short-acting agents, such as albuterol, begin acting within minutes, peak at 30-60 minutes, and last 4 to 6 hours. The recommended dose is two puffs 30 seconds apart, taken 15-20 minutes before exercise. This may prevent asthmatic symptoms in up to 90% of athletes with EIA (3,30).

Common side effects of the short-acting β_2-agonists include tremor, tachycardia, palpitations, and jitteriness, although these are usually transient and mild. Q_{Tc} prolongation may occur. With regular use of these agents, tolerance may develop. Tolerance takes the form of shortened duration of action but does not decrease the immediate bronchodilator effect. Mechanisms may include receptor down-regulation and desensitization (20,29).

Long-acting β_2-agonists, such as salmeterol, begin to exert bronchodilatory effects after 10-15 minutes and reach peak effect at 1-3 hours. The effects last for approximately 12 hours. This makes these agents unsuitable for rescue use but excellent for prevention of EIA symptoms, especially for athletes engaged in long-duration activities. However, as with the short-acting agents, regular use can lead to tolerance, which may begin to develop after only two doses (29,31-33).

The NCAA and IOC ban all oral forms of β_2-agonists due to their stimulant and potential ergogenic and anabolic effects. In particular, oral clenbuterol has been used by athletes attempting to obtain anabolic benefits

(3,20,33a). However, no inhaled β_2-agonists have been shown to confer a performance advantage to athletes without asthma or EIA, and most experts agree that the legitimate use of these agents by athletes with asthma or EIA is appropriate and does not confer any unfair advantage (3,20,30,34). As mentioned previously, Olympic athletes must meet strict criteria to obtain permission to use inhaled β_2-agonists.

Inhaled Corticosteroids

Inhaled corticosteroids are recommended as first-line therapy for patients with chronic asthma (1,20,35). By decreasing inflammation, they subsequently decrease airway hyperreactivity, including in response to exercise. They have been shown to decrease EIA symptoms in patients with underlying chronic asthma and allow a higher level of exertion before the onset of symptoms (1,3,30). However, their use in patients with isolated EIA is less well studied. Due to their slow onset of action, they are not useful on an as-needed basis. Side effects are typically mild and include local irritation and candidiasis. Rinsing out the mouth after medication use may lessen these risks. Long-term use of inhaled corticosteroids may increase the risk of osteoporosis and adrenal suppression (36,37). These medications may be most useful as second-line therapy in EIA, in combination with β_2-agonists and/or other agents, for patients with refractory symptoms.

Mast Cell Stabilizers

Mast cell stabilizers, such as nedocromil and cromolyn, may also be effective choices for EIA prophylaxis, especially in conjunction with β_2-agonists. Cromolyn sodium appears to inhibit calcium entry into cells, thereby decreasing mast cell degranulation. Although not as effective as the β_2-agonists, cromolyn blocks EIA symptoms in approximately 40%-70% of patients and is extremely well tolerated (1,30). However, duration of protection is relatively short. Optimal dosing is 1600 µg four times per day, plus 15 to 20 minutes before exercise (1,3,30). Nedocromil sodium has shown similar properties, although many patients find it to have a most unpleasant taste (30). A recent meta-analysis (38) found that nedocromil decreased the fall in FEV_1 among patients with EIA by 15.6% and that post-exercise lung function returned to baseline levels faster than in patients given placebo. The effects were noted to be greater in patients with more severe disease. A meta-analysis (39) found no difference in effectiveness when comparing nedocromil to cromolyn.

Leukotriene Modifiers

The leukotriene modifiers represent a major advance in the treatment of asthma and EIA. Cysteinyl leukotrienes, initially termed "slow reacting substances of anaphylaxis" (40), are inflammatory mediators formed by the interaction between 5-lipoxygenase and arachidonic acid. Eosinophils, mast cells, basophils, monocytes, and macrophages appear to be the main cells involved in their production. Leukotriene production is greatly elevated in asthmatics as compared to nonasthmatics, and these compounds exert their effects by binding to specific receptors (especially CysLT1) on the bronchial smooth muscle cells. Leukotrienes are the most powerful bronchoconstrictors known, being 1000 times more potent than histamine. In addition to bronchoconstriction, they cause increased airway hyperresponsiveness, increased mucus secretion, airway edema, and influx of eosinophils. Over time, they also cause smooth muscle hypertrophy (41). Clinically, leukotriene administration has been shown to cause increased airway resistance, impaired pulmonary function, wheezing, and chest tightness in asthmatics (42). Thus, these compounds are clearly key components in the inflammatory cascade that occurs in asthma and EIA.

Although inhaled corticosteroids exert a powerful anti-inflammatory effect, they do not suppress leukotriene production or release (41). Therefore, leukotriene modifiers have been used in an effort to block this powerful part of the inflammatory response. Currently, three of these agents are available in the United States; zileuton is a 5-lipoxygenase inhibitor, whereas zafirlukast and montelukast are leukotriene receptor antagonists (LTRAs). All three are taken orally and have been found to attenuate EIA symptoms, but differences do exist. In one study, compared with the LTRAs, zileuton provided equal protection against EIA for 4 hours after a single dose but was less effective at 8 hours and no better than placebo at 12 hours. Zafirlukast and montelukast provided excellent EIA prophylaxis, equivalent to that seen with salmeterol, for 12 hours after a single dose but showed a slower onset of action than salmeterol (43).

Two separate 8-week trials comparing montelukast to salmeterol in patients with asthma and EIA found montelukast to be superior in protecting against EIA, especially as time went on (44,45). Overall, it is clear that the leukotriene modifiers, especially the LTRAs, have an excellent therapeutic effect on EIA, but data in high-level athletes are still lacking.

Case Study 15-1

A 19-year-old female soccer player presented to the office with a chief complaint of fatigue with exercise. She noted that her fatigue had been associated with a decrease in exercise capacity over the last 6 weeks and a mild cough. Her past medical history was significant only for allergic rhinitis, for which she used intermittent antihistamines. After further questioning and a physical exam, EIA is suspected and an empriric albuterol inhaler is prescribed. After she returned 3 weeks later with continued symptoms, an exercise challenge test was performed. After exercising on the treadmill for 10 minutes, a decrease in peak flow from 400 to 325 units was noted, confirming the diagnosis. Montelukast was added to the patient's regimen, and she was asked to perform several

8-second sprints before each practice and game. The patient reported
near normal activity levels 3 weeks later.

Miscellaneous Agents

Theophylline, a methylxanthine with bronchodilatory, mucolytic, and anti-
inflammatory properties, may be useful in the EIA patient with chronic
asthma and refractory symptoms; however, more effective and safer
choices exist. Ipratropium, a muscarinic antagonist that blocks the cholinergic contribution to asthma, has shown only variable clinical benefit as prophylaxis against EIA (20,30). Antihistamines have been found to provide a
small-to-medium amount of protection against EIA. In particular, terfenadine (no longer available in the United States due to safety concerns) had
shown promise, although there was significant variability in its effectiveness. However, terfenadine blocks not only histamine receptors but also
prevents leukotriene release (46). Loratadine, which does not have the
same ability to block leukotriene release, has been shown to be moderately
beneficial in children with EIA (47) but not in adults with milder cases of
asthma (48). Thus, it appears that antihistamines may have a limited role in
the management of EIA, perhaps especially in patients with an underlying
allergic diathesis.

Recommendations

For individuals with isolated EIA, inhaled β_2-agonists are front-line therapies and offer excellent protection in most cases. Mast cell stabilizers may
be added to the β_2-agonists or substituted for them if side effects are
prominent. Leukotriene modifiers can be added in refractory cases or used
in place of a long-acting β_2-agonist. Inhaled corticosteroids may be needed
in patients with severe EIA. For individuals with chronic asthma, inhaled
corticosteroids should be the keystone of their regimen; usually combination therapy is required to obtain optimal results in these patients. Athletes
with an allergic diathesis may benefit from adding an antihistamine and
treating associated conditions (e.g., allergic rhinitis).

   Athletes with EIA also should use the aforementioned nonpharmacologic options and should discuss their particular goals and concerns with
their physicians. As the large number of Olympic athletes with EIA would
attest, EIA does not have to limit performance or enjoyment of sports.
Appropriate diagnosis and treatment should allow athletes with EIA to
reach their full potential safely.

Exercise-Induced Anaphylaxis and Urticaria

Exercise-induced anaphylaxis (EIAn) is a potentially fatal physical allergy
to exercise or strenuous exertion. Since it was first systematically described

in 1980 (49), more than 1000 cases have been reported in the literature (50). The true prevalence of EIAn is unknown, although a Japanese junior high school survey estimated the prevalence at 0.031% (51). The average age at onset is 24-26 years of age, and, although not found in all reports, there appears to be an approximately 2:1 female to male ratio (52,53). Up to 71% of patients with EIAn have reported a personal or family history of atopic conditions (53).

In the classic form, symptoms begin with a generalized sensation of warmth, flushing, and pruritus, followed by the development of urticaria ("hives"). The urticarial lesions tend to be large (1-2 cm or larger) and may become confluent, but a rare, variant form of EIAn does exist, in which the urticarial lesions are only 2-5 mm in size (50,54). Angioedema of the palms, soles, larynx, and face may also occur (49,52). Impending vascular collapse may be heralded by tachycardia and hypotension, but many patients abort this development by stopping their activity (52,55). An epidemiologic study found that during attacks, 51% of patients with EIAn experienced shortness of breath; 33% had chest tightness; 32% lost consciousness; 28% had nausea, diarrhea, or colicky abdominal pain; 28% had a headache; and 25% had signs of upper respiratory tract obstruction such as stridor (53). Similar findings were noted in an earlier study (55).

Exercise or strenuous activity is the only stimulus which provokes EIAn; the symptoms do not occur with other stimuli, such as emotional stress or passive warming. A recent case report raises the possibility of a distinct entity, cold-dependent EIAn, in which EIAn only develops during exercise in a cold environment but not in a warm one (56). Episodes of EIAn are sporadic and poorly reproducible within subjects (49,52). Frequency of attacks has also been reported to decrease over time, dropping from an average of 14.5 attacks per year to 8.3 attacks per year over an average of 10 years in one study; 93% of patients reported either a decrease or stabilization in attack frequency over time. It is not clear whether this change represents disease remission or, perhaps more likely, activity modification by the subjects to avoid precipitating factors (53). Many different activities have been reported to cause EIAn, with jogging and other aerobic activities being the most commonly identified sports. However, this may reflect the popularity of certain exercises rather than actual risk by sport. Among subjects for whom jogging was the primary trigger, 90% had onset of symptoms within 30 minutes of beginning exercise. In general, EIAn symptoms last from 30 minutes to 4 hours after cessation of exercise, but vascular headaches have been noted to persist for up to 3 days (49,53,54).

The pathophysiology of EIAn has not been clearly elucidated. In an early study, seven subjects with a history of EIAn were given an exercise challenge on a treadmill. Four subjects demonstrated signs of EIAn; compared with those who remained asymptomatic, the serum histamine levels in symptomatic subjects were significantly higher from baseline (57). A subsequent study showed that, after exercise, cutaneous mast cells obtained from subjects with EIAn exhibited marked alterations consistent with degranulation. A concomitant increase in serum histamine levels was noted in these subjects, whereas such changes did not occur in controls (58). A more recent case report has shown that tryptase, an enzyme associated with mast cell activation, is markedly elevated during EIAn (59). Thus, it seems clear that mast cell activation and histamine are involved in the pathogenesis of EIAn. Other inflammatory mediators, such as leukotrienes, and activation of the complement system also may be involved (1,50,52,60). In addition, it has been suggested that neurologic factors, such as heightened α-adrenergic and autonomic tone during exercise, may stimulate mast cell degranulation (52). Menstrual cycle phase, concomitant use of medications (NSAIDs), hot or humid weather, cold weather, and high pollen counts have been identified by patients with EIAn as possible triggers (52-55), but, with the exception of NSAIDs, no data are available to support these contentions.

Food-Dependent Exercise Induced Anaphylaxis

Etiology and Pathophysiology

A discrete subtype of EIAn is known as food-dependent, exercise-induced anaphylaxis (FDEIAn). In this disorder, exercise must be preceded by food ingestion to cause symptoms; neither the food itself, nor exercise without the food, provokes the symptoms. In most cases, a specific food or food substance must be consumed to produce symptoms (61,62).

Diagnosis

A presumptive diagnosis of EIAn or FDEIAn can be made by taking a complete history. Physical exam findings at rest typically are unremarkable, although evidence of atopy or allergic rhinitis may be present. Confirmation of the diagnosis requires an exercise challenge with appropriate medical supervision and emergency equipment on hand. However, as EIAn attacks are sporadic, a negative test does not rule out the disorder. Patients with suspected FDEIAn should undergo an exercise challenge, as well as a simple challenge with the suspected offending food. If these are negative, the patient should undergo an exercise challenge shortly after ingesting the food in question. RAST and skin testing with specific food extracts may be helpful in identifying triggers (52). Consultation with an allergist is recommended to assist in appropriate diagnosis and management.

Differential Diagnosis

Patients with EIA often have exercise-associated wheezing, which is less common in EIAn, and they do not develop the urticaria, upper airway obstruction, vascular collapse, or gastrointestinal signs seen in EIAn. Similarly, patients with VCD may exhibit signs of upper airway obstruction but do not manifest the other findings of EIAn. Cardiac arrhythmias may be precipitated by exercise and can cause vascular collapse and syncope, but arrhythmias are not associated with the cutaneous, gastrointestinal, or respiratory findings seen in EIAn. The diagnosis most commonly confused with EIAn is cholinergic urticaria (see below). Although the urticarial reaction in variant EIAn closely resembles that seen in cholinergic urticaria, anaphylaxis only develops in the former. Bronchospasm actually may be more common in cholinergic urticaria, whereas in EIAn, primarily the larynx and upper airways are involved. Unlike cholinergic urticaria, EIAn only occurs with exertion and does not occur with passive warming, emotional stress, or fever (50,52,54).

Treatment and Prevention

It is essential that athletes with any form of EIAn be taught how to recognize early symptoms and to discontinue exercise and seek medical attention immediately if these symptoms occur. These patients should also carry with them at all times (and know how to use) an epinephrine auto-injector and wear a medical alert bracelet or identification tag. Exercise modifications, such as avoiding known triggers, not exercising in hot or humid conditions, and limiting exercise during allergy season, may be of benefit. These individuals should never exercise without a "buddy," who can administer epinephrine and summon help if needed. Aspirin and NSAIDs should be avoided before exercise, and food should be avoided for 4-6 hours before exercise. In patients with specific triggers for FDEIAn, these foods must be strictly avoided for at least 4-6 hours before exercise. A gluten-free diet has been reported to be beneficial in some cases of wheat- or gluten-specific FDEIAn (63,64).

In the acute setting, immediate administration of epinephrine is crucial, along with standard supportive measures to ensure cardiovascular and respiratory stability. Typical dosage is 0.1-0.5 mg epinephrine 1:1000 solution subcutaneously every 10-15 minutes. Endotracheal intubation or emergency cricothyrotomy may be required to ensure a patent airway. Antihistamines and glucocorticoids may also be of benefit once the above measures have been instituted. Appropriate observation is warranted after an attack to ensure symptoms do not rebound.

Pharmacologic prevention of EIAn has been attempted with various agents. Antihistamines, with or without the addition of H_2 blockers, have often been reported to confer a moderate level of protection (52-54). However, neither antihistamines nor other medications, such as sodium bicarbonate, mast cell stabilizers, or corticosteroids, have been shown to be consistently protective (52,53,59). The use of leukotriene modifiers for preventing EIAn has been suggested but has not yet been objectively studied. With the development of omalizumab, it is possible that other monoclonal anti-IgE therapies may become available, perhaps specifically targeting the food antigens responsible for FDEIAn.

Patients with EIAn should avoid the use of β-blockers, because these drugs may blunt the receptor-mediated response to epinephrine during attempted emergency treatment. ACE-inhibitors may also be problematic, because angiotensin II inactivates bradykinin, a potential factor in the anaphylactic cascade. ACE-inhibitors and angiotensin receptor blockers may also prevent angiotensin II-mediated pressor effects during anaphylaxis (52).

Cholinergic Urticaria

Cholinergic urticaria is a type of physical urticaria in which punctuate (2-5 mm), pruritic, urticarial papules, surrounded by an erythematous flare, develop on the skin of the neck, thorax, or other body parts, in response to elevation of the body temperature. These lesions are very similar to those seen in variant EIAn. In some cases, a large (up to 20 cm), confluent area of pruritic erythema may be the main manifestation. Some patients also exhibit other signs of cholinergic activation, such as lacrimation, salivation, and diarrhea. The symptoms may be caused by exercise, passive warming (hot bath or shower, environmental heat), or other factors (fever, emotional stress). It is perhaps the most common of the physical urticarias, representing 4%-7% of cases of urticaria, and typically has its onset in the 26-28 year old age group (54,65,66).

In severe cases, patients with cholinergic urticaria may exhibit bronchospasm, but they do not develop the vascular collapse seen in EIAn. Symptoms usually begin within 10 minutes of initiating exercise, peaking after 20-30 minutes. After the inciting stimulus is removed, symptoms usually resolve within 15 minutes (mild reactions) to 4 hours (more severe reactions) (50,52,54). Unlike EIAn, cholinergic urticaria seems to be very reproducible and consistent. However, it has been suggested that these afflictions may actually represent two ends of the spectrum of a similar disorder, with "heat rash" representing the mildest form of cholinergic urticaria and full-blown EIAn marking the most severe manifestation (65).

Pathophysiology

The pathologic basis of cholinergic urticaria is not fully understood, but it seems to be related to an abnormal cholinergic response in reaction to a rapid increase in body temperature by at least 1°C. This may lead to an inappropriate release of acetylcholine, which may subsequently trigger mast cell degranulation. This is supported by findings of elevated plasma histamine levels in patients with cholinergic urticaria. Neurovascular factors may also be involved, but the exact mechanisms are unclear (54). It has recently been hypothesized that occlusion of superficial sweat ducts may lead to anhidrosis, temperature elevation and subsequent urticaria in certain patients (65,67).

Diagnosis

A careful history will suggest the diagnosis. Provocative testing, such as passive warming, will usually produce a urticarial response, along with an elevated serum histamine level. Such testing will be negative in cases of EIAn. Intradermal methacholine injection will result in a localized urticarial reaction in only a third of patients with cholinergic urticaria but is highly specific. Exercise challenge is the most reliable test, but appropriate personnel and emergency equipment must be in place in case a severe reaction occurs (50,54). As with EIAn, consultation with an allergist is recommended.

Differential Diagnosis

EIAn must be ruled out by history and confirmatory testing. Other types of physical urticaria, such as aquagenic, solar, cold, and vibratory, also should be considered. Again, a thorough history should lead the clinician in the appropriate direction. For patients with cholinergic urticaria that does not seem to fit the pattern of a physical urticaria, clinicians should consider chronic idiopathic urticaria, autoimmune disease, underlying malignancy, parasite infestation, mastocytosis, and other systemic disorders.

Treatment

Treatment of cholinergic urticaria begins with patient education. Patients must learn to cease the offending activity as soon as symptoms begin, and should modify their activities to avoid onset of symptoms in the first place. Patients should warm up slowly, exercise in cooler ambient conditions, and wear appropriate clothing. Hydroxyzine is often effective, but its sedative effects may not be well-tolerated by active people. Therefore, use of the nonsedating antihistamines may be attractive; in particular, cetirizine, at 20 mg/day, has shown effectiveness in treating this condition (68). The addition of H_2-blockers may be of benefit if a satisfactory result is not obtained (69,70). Doxepin and the tricyclic antidepressants have also shown some success, likely due to their antihistaminergic and anticholinergic properties. However, these medications may not be well tolerated in athletes. Serotonin-specific reuptake inhibitors have also shown benefit, suggesting that serotonin may play a role in this disorder (70). In patients with severe and recalcitrant symptoms, immunosuppressive therapy may be needed (69).

Case Study 15-2

A 38-year-old female runner presented with a neck rash. The rash began several months ago and was almost universally associated with exercise. The rash was mildly puritic. She denied any change in her activity and did not have wheezing with exercise. Her past history was remarkable for asthma as a child. She did not smoke, was married, and had one child at home. She took no regular medication and had not changed her diet recently.

Based on this history, the patient was asked to place a warm, moist towel on her neck at home, wait an hour or so, and to report any symptoms. The patient phoned back several hours later and said that the rash was reproduced with the warm towel. This confirmed a diagnosis of cholinergic urticaria. She was instructed to take cetirizine daily and to immediately report any breathing difficulty with exercise.

REFERENCES

1. **Truwit J.** Pulmonary disorders and exercise. Clin Sports Med. 2003;22:161-80.

2. **Anderson SD.** Exercise-induced asthma: the state of the art. Chest. 1985;87S:191S-5S.

3. **Lacroix VJ.** Exercise-induced asthma. Phys Sportsmed. 1999;12:75.

4. **Anderson SD, Holzer K.** Exercise-induce asthma: is it the right diagnosis in elite athletes? J Allergy Clin Immunol. 2000;106:419-28.

5. **McKenzie DC, McLuckie SL, Stirling DR.** The protective effects of continuous and interval exercise in athletes with exercise-induced asthma. Med Sci Sports Exerc. 1994;26:951-6.

6. **Nowak D, Jorres R, Magnussen H.** Influence of exercise-induced bronchoconstriction on refractoriness. Lung. 1992;170:75-84.

7. **Reiff DB, Choudry NB, Pride NB, Ind PW.** The effect of prolonged submaximal warm-up exercise on exercise-induced asthma. Am Rev Respir Dis. 1989;139:479-84.

8. **McFadden ERJ, Gilbert IA.** Exercise-induced asthma. N Engl J Med. 1994;330:1362-7.

9. **Mellman MF, Podesta L.** Common medical problems in sports. Clin Sports Med. 1997;16:635-62.

10. **Anderson SD, Daviskas E.** The mechanism of exercise-induced asthma is . . . . J Allergy Clin Immunol. 2000;106:453-9.

11. **Strauss RH, McFadden ER, Ingram RH, et al.** Influence of heat and humidity on the airway obstruction induced by exercise in asthma. J Clin Invest. 1978;61:433-40.

12. **Anderson SD, Schoeffel RE, Follet R, et al.** Sensitivity to heat and water loss at rest and during exercise in asthmatic patients. Eur J Respir Dis. 1982;63:459-71.

12a. **Sonna LA, Angel KC, Sharp MA, et al.** The prevalence of exercise-induced bronchospasm among US Army recruits and its effects on physical performance. Chest. 2001;19:1676-84.

13. **Mannix ET, Manfredi F, Farber MO.** A comparison of two challenge tests for identifying exercise-induced bronchospasm in figure skaters. Chest. 1999;115:649-53.

14. **Mannix ET, Farber MO, Palange P, et al.** Exercise-induced asthma in figure skaters. Chest. 1996;109:312-5.

15. **Provost-Craig MA, Arbour KS, Sestili DC, et al.** The incidence of exercise-induced bronchospasm in competitive figure skaters. J Asthma. 1996;33:67-71.

16. **Holzer K, Anderson SD, Douglass J.** Exercise in elite summer athletes: challenges for diagnosis. J Allergy Clin Immunol. 2002;110:374-80.

17. **Anderson SD, Fitch K, Perry CP, et al.** Responses to bronchial challenge submitted for approval to use inhaled β_2-agonists before an event at the 2002 Winter Olympics. J Allergy Clin Immunol. 2003;111:45-50.

18. **Weiler JM.** Why must Olympic athletes prove that they have asthma to be permitted to take inhaled β_2-agonists? J Allergy Clin Immunol. 2003;111:36-7.

19. **Crapo RO, Casaburi R, Coates AL, et al.** Guidelines for methacholine and exercise challenge testing. 1999 ATS statement. Am J Respir Crit Care Med. 2000;161:309-29.

20. **Nichols AW.** Exercise-induced bronchospasm. In: Puffer JC, ed. Twenty Common Problems in Sports Medicine. New York: McGraw-Hill; 2002:287-301.

21. **Rundell KN, Wilber RL, Szmedra L, et al.** Exercise-induced asthma screening of elite athletes: field versus laboratory exercise challenge. Med Sci Sports Exerc. 2000;32:309-16.

22. **Cain H.** Bronchoprovocation testing. Clin Chest Med. 2001;22:651-9.

23. **Anderson SD, Argyros GJ, Magnussen H, Holzer K.** Provocation by eucapnic voluntary hyperpnoea to identify exercise-induced bronchoconstriction. Br J Sports Med. 2001;35:344-7.

24. **Rundell KW, Spiering BA, Judelson DA, Wilson MH.** Bronchoconstriction during cross-country skiing: is there really a refractory period? Med Sci Sports Exerc. 2003;35:18-26.

25. **Schnall RP, Landau LI.** Protective effects of repeated short sprints in exercise-induced asthma. Thorax. 1980;35:828-32.

26. **Dillard TA, Ewald FW Jr.** The use of pulmonary function testing in piloting, air travel, mountain climbing, and diving. Clin Chest Med. 2001;22:795-816.

27. **Strauss MB, Borer RC Jr.** Diving medicine: contemporary topics and their controversies. Am J Emerg Med. 2001;19:232-8.

28. **Van Hoesen KB, Neuman TS.** Asthma and scuba diving. Immunol Allergy Clin North Am. 1996;16:917-28.

29. **Dutta EJ, Li JT.** β-agonists. Med Clin North Am. 2002;85:991-1008.

30. **Smith BW, LaBotz M.** Pharmacologic treatment of exercise-induced asthma. Clin Sports Med. 1998;17:343-63.

31. **Nelson HS.** Clinical experience with levalbuterol. J Allergy Clin Immunol. 1999;104:S77-84.

32. **Bhagat R, Kalra S, Swystun VA, Cockroft DW.** Rapid onset of tolerance to the bronchoprotective effect of salmeterol. Chest. 1995;108:1235-9.

33. **Nelson JA, Strauss L, Skowronski M, et al.** Effect of long-term salmeterol treatment on exercise-induced asthma. N Engl J Med. 1998;339:141-6.

33a. **Prather ID, Brown DE, North P, Wilson JR.** Clenbuterol: a substitute for anabolic steroids? Med Sci Sports Exerc. 1995;27:1118-21.

34. **Carlsen KH, Hem E, Stensrud T, et al.** Can asthma treatment in sports be doping? The effect of the rapid onset, long-acting inhaled β_2-agonist formoterol upon endurance performance in healthy well-trained athletes. Respir Med. 2001;95:571-6.

35. **Staresinic AG, Sorkness CA.** The use of inhaled corticosteroids in adult asthma. Med Clin North Am. 2002;86:1035-47.

36. **Israel E, Banerjee TR, Fitzmaurice GM, et al.** Effects of inhaled glucocorticoids on bone density in premenopausal women. N Engl J Med. 2001;345:941-7.

37. **Zimmerman B, Gold M, Wherrett D, Hanna AK.** Adrenal suppression in two patients with asthma treated with low doses of the inhaled steroid fluticasone propionate. J Allergy Clin Immunol. 1998;101:425-6.

38. **Spooner C, Rowe BH, Saunders LD.** Nedocromil sodium in the treatment of exercise-induced asthma: a meta-analysis. Eur Respir J. 2000;16:30-7.

39. **Kelly K, Spooner CH, Rowe BH.** Nedocromil sodium vs. sodium cromoglycate for preventing exercise-induced bronchoconstriction in asthmatics. Cochrane Database Syst Rev. 2000;4:CD002731.

40. **Murphy RC, Hammarstrom S, Samuelson B.** Leukotriene C: a slow-reacting substance from murine mastocytoma cells. Proc Natl Acad Sci USA. 1979;76:4275-9.

41. **Salvi SS, Krishna MT, Sampson AP, Holgate ST.** The anti-inflammatory effects of leukotriene-modifying drugs and their use in asthma. Chest. 2001;119:1533-46.

42. **Peters SP.** Leukotriene receptor antagonists in asthma therapy. J Allergy Clin Immunol. 2003;111:S62-70.

43. **Coreno A, Skowronski M, Kotaru C, McFadden ER Jr.** Comparative effects of long-acting β_2-agonists, leukotriene receptor antagonists, and a 5-lipoxygenase inhibitor on exercise-induced asthma. J Allergy Clin Immunol. 2000;106:500-6.

44. **Villaran C, O'Neill SJ, Helbling A, et al.** Montelukast versus salmeterol in patients with asthma and exercise-induced bronchoconstriction. Montelukast/Salmeterol Exercise Study Group. J Allergy Clin Immunol. 1999;104:547-53.

45. **Edelman JM, Turpin JA, Bronsky EA, et al.** Oral montelukast compared with inhaled salmeterol to prevent exercise-induced bronchoconstriction. A randomized double blind trial. Exercise Study Group. Ann Intern Med. 2000;132:97-104.

46. **Anderson SD, Brannan JD.** Exercise-induced asthma: is there still a case for histamine? J Allergy Clin Immunol. 2002;109:771-3.

47. **Baki A, Orhan F.** The effect of loratadine in exercise-induced asthma. Arch Dis Child. 2002;86:38-9.

48. **Dahlén B, Roquet A, Inman M, et al.** Influence of zafirlukast and loratadine on exercise-induced bronchoconstriction. J Allergy Clin Immunol. 2002;109:789-93.

49. **Sheffer AL, Austen KF.** Exercise induced anaphylaxis. J Allergy Clin Immunol. 1980;66:106-11.

50. **Hosey RG, Carek PJ, Goo A.** Exercise-induced anaphylaxis and urticaria. Am Fam Physician. 2001;64:1367-72.

51. **Aihara Y, Takahashi Y, Kotoyori T, et al.** Frequency of food-dependent, exercise-induced anaphylaxis in Japanese junior-high-school students. J Allergy Clin Immunol. 2001;108:1035-9.

52. **Horan RF, DuBuske LM, Sheffer AL.** Exercise-induced anaphylaxis? Immunol Allergy Clin North Am. 2001;21:769-82.

53. **Shadick NA, Liang MH, Partridge AJ, et al.** The natural history of exercise-induced anaphylaxis: survey results from a 10-year follow-up study. J Allergy Clin Immunol. 1999;104:123-7.

54. **Sweeney TM, Dexter WW.** Cholinergic urticaria in a jogger: ruling out exercise-induced anaphylaxis. Phys Sportsmed. 2003;31:32-6.

55. **Wade JP, Liang MH, Sheffer AL.** Exercise-induced anaphylaxis: epidemiologic observations. Prog Clin Biol Res. 1989;297:175-82.

56. **Ii M, Sayama K, Tohyama M, Hashimoto K.** A case of cold-dependent exercise-induced anaphylaxis. Br J Dermatol. 2002;147:368-70.

57. **Sheffer AL, Soter NA, McFadden ER Jr, Austen KF.** Exercise-induced anaphylaxis: a distinct form of physical allergy. J Allergy Clin Immunol. 1983;71:311-6.

58. **Sheffer AL, Tong AK, Murphy GF, et al.** Exercise-induced anaphylaxis: a serious form of physical allergy associated with mast cell degranulation. J Allergy Clin Immunol. 1985;75:479-84.

59. **Schwartz HJ.** Elevated serum tryptase in exercise-induced anaphylaxis. J Allergy Clin Immunol. 1995;95:917-9.

60. **Denzlinger C, Haberl C, Wilmanns W.** Cysteinyl leukotriene production in anaphylactic reactions. Int Arch Allergy Immunol. 1995;108:154-64.

61. **Maulitz RM, Pratt DS, Schocket AL.** Exercise-induce anaphylactic reaction to shellfish. J Allergy Clin Immunol. 1979;63:433-4.

62. **Tilles S, Schocket A, Milgrom H.** Exercise-induced anaphylaxis related to specific foods. J Pediatr. 1995;127:587-9.

63. **Palosuo K, Alenius H, Varjonen E, et al.** A novel wheat gliadin as a cause of exercise-induced anaphylaxis. J Allergy Clin Immunol. 1999;103:912-7.

64. **Palosuo K, Varjonen E, Nurkkala J, et al.** Transglutaminase-mediated cross-linking of a peptic fraction of omega-5 gliadin enhances IgE reactivity in wheat-dependent, exercise-induced anaphylaxis. J Allergy Clin Immunol. 2003;111:1386-92.

65. **Greaves M.** Chronic urticaria. J Allergy Clin Immunol. 2000;105:664-72.

66. **Zuberbier T, Althaus C, Chantraine-Hess S, Czarnetzki BM.** Prevalence of cholinergic urticaria in young adults. J Am Acad Dermatol. 1994;31:978-81.

67. **Kobayashi H, Aiba S, Yamagishi T, et al.** Cholinergic urticaria, a new pathogenic concept: hypohydrosis due to interference with delivery of sweat to the skin surface. Dermatology. 2002;204:173-8.

68. **Zuberbier T, Münzberger C, Haustein U, et al.** Double-blind crossover study of high-dose cetirizine in cholinergic urticaria. Dermatology. 1996;193:324-7.

69. **Grattan CEH, Sabroe RA, Greaves MW.** Chronic urticaria. J Am Acad Dermatol. 2002;46:645-57.

70. **Gupta MA, Gupta AK.** Psychodermatology: an update. J Am Acad Dermatol. 1996;34:1030-46.

16

■ ■ ■

Neurological Conditions
in Athletes

Kyle J. Cassas, MD

A thorough understanding of neurological conditions sustained in sports, such as concussion and brachial plexus injuries, is a vital aspect in the care of athletes. Many, if not most, of these injuries are mild but may have both short and long term sequelae if not detected early and treated properly. Many of these injuries may not be preventable, but the secondary consequences or morbidities associated with these injuries may be diminished by the proper care of these athletes. This chapter reviews some of the common neurological conditions encountered in athletes.

Concussion

The recognition and management of the concussed athlete is one of the most challenging and controversial areas in sports medicine (1). Concussion is the most common of all head injuries occurring in sports (2). Sports associated with concussions include football, soccer, boxing, ice hockey, and basketball (Table 16-1) (2). It has been estimated that up to 20% of high-school football players sustain a concussion each season (2-4). However, the true incidence of concussions in sports is difficult to determine because of the underreporting of symptoms by athletes. Once an athlete has sustained a concussion he or she is at increased risk for sustaining another, with an even higher risk if the athlete returns to play without completely recovering from the prior concussion (2,5). It is therefore important for the physician caring for athletes to have a thorough understanding of the nature of traumatic brain injury, including its accurate diagnosis and proper management.

Table 16-1   Sports Associated with Concussions

• Football	• Martial arts	• Ice hockey	• Basketball	• Soccer
• Lacrosse	• Boxing	• Rodeo	• Wrestling	• Gymnastics

Definition and Risk Factors

The word *concussion* is derived from the Latin verb "concussus," meaning "to shake violently" (6). A concussion may occur either from a direct blow or secondary to indirect rotational forces transmitted to the brain. Despite extensive research in the area of traumatic brain injury, there continues to be no universal agreement on the definition of concussion.

Concussion may be defined as "a trauma-induced alteration in mental status that may or may not involve loss of consciousness" (3). A current definition of concussion can be found in the 2001 Summary and Agreement Statement of the First International Conference on Concussion in Sport. This Concussion in Sport Group (CISG) defines concussion as a "complex pathophysiological process affecting the brain, induced by traumatic biochemical forces" (7).

Risk factors for concussion may include improper and unsafe tackling technique, such as leading with the head ("spearing," which may also lead to cervical spine injuries), or using a helmet as a weapon. There is also evidence that some athletes with polymorphism of the gene apolipoprotein E (a gene also responsible for the late onset and sporadic cases of Alzheimer's disease) may have a genetic predisposition to traumatic brain injuries (5).

Signs and Symptoms

The signs and symptoms of concussion often can be subtle and difficult to detect. The hallmark signs of concussion are confusion and amnesia (3). Table 16-2 lists the early and late signs of concussion. Common early signs and symptoms include a "dazed" feeling, confusion, disorientation, memory disturbances, and headaches. Later signs and symptoms may include chronic headaches, fatigue, mood or sleep disturbances, poor attention, and difficulty concentrating.

Concussion Grading and Guidelines

Concussion grading guidelines are listed in Table 16-3. Concussion grading and return-to-play guidelines are based only on expert opinion, with no universal agreement or scientific evidence-based data to support the use of one guideline over another.

Most concussions are considered mild and fall into the grade 1 category; grade 1 concussions account for up to 90% of cases. Athletes with mild concussions have symptoms that resolve very quickly and are often

Table 16-2   Concussion Signs and Symptoms

Early (minutes to hours)	Late (days to weeks)
• Headache	• Poor attention and concentration
• Confusion	• Blurry vision or double vision
• Feeling "dazed"	• Persistent low-grade headaches
• Vacant stare	• Light sensitivity
• Disorientation	• Feeling sluggish or "foggy"
• Dizziness	• Altered sleep habits
• Balance disturbance	• Difficulty concentrating
• Nausea and or vomiting	• Memory problems
• Tinnitus	• Irritability
• Fatigue	
• Anxiety	
• Depression	

Table 16-3   Concussion Grading Guidelines

Evidence-Based Cantu Grading System for Concussion, 2002

Grade 1 (mild)	No LOC*; PTA* < 30 minutes, PCSS* < 30 minutes.
Grade 2 (moderate)	LOC < 1 minute, PTA or PCSS > 30 minutes < 24 hours.
Grade 3 (severe)	LOC > 1 minute, PTA 24 hours or more, PCSS > 7 days.

*AAN** Practice Parameter Grading System for Concussion, 1997*

Grade 1	Symptoms < 15 minutes
Grade 2	Symptoms > 15 minutes
Grade 3	Any LOC

Colorado Medical Society Grading System for Concussion, 1991

Grade 1	Confusion without amnesia
Grade 2	Confusion with amnesia
Grade 3	Any LOC

* LOC, loss of consciousness; PTA, post-traumatic amnesia (retrograde and anterograde), PCSS, postconcussion signs and symptoms.
** American Academy of Neurology
Republished with permission from Cantu R. Posttraumatic retrograde and anterograde amnesia: pathophysiology and implications in grading and safe return to play. J Athl Train. 2001:36:244-8.

the most difficult for the team physician or athletic trainer to detect. These injuries are often referred to as "dings" or "bell ringers."

A true loss of consciousness (LOC) occurs in only a small percentage of athletes (less than 10% of concussions) (2). Any athlete who sustains LOC should be withheld from his or her sport and evaluated by medical personnel, who will make a decision about the need for transfer to the nearest medical facility.

Concussion and return-to-play guidelines truly are only guidelines used to provide insight into the management of these injuries. The team physician and athletic trainer must always use their individual clinical judgment when evaluating these athletes and making return-to-play decisions.

Sideline Evaluation

The initial evaluation of the head-injured athlete should begin with the basic ABCs (Airway, Breathing, and Circulation), followed by an evaluation of the cervical spine. It should be assumed that any athlete with loss of consciousness may have a cervical spine injury, until proven otherwise. Proper precautionary measures, including cervical stabilization and a complete neurological evaluation, should be performed in all athletes sustaining LOC. Transportation to the nearest hospital for further evaluation should be considered for those athletes with abnormal neurological examinations to rule out intracranial hemorrhage.

The systematic approach to the concussed athlete should include a detailed history about the events surrounding the injury, along with a complete cervical spine and neurological evaluation. Pupils must also be examined for symmetry and reaction to light.

The concussion history may include the features listed in Table 16-4. Mental status testing should include checking orientation, concentration, and memory. The evaluation for amnesia may be one of the most important aspects of the sideline evaluation and should include checking for both retrograde (before the injury) and anterograde or posttraumatic amnesia (after the injury). Retrograde amnesia can be assessed by asking questions about the play that led to the injury, the score of the game, or the name of opponent. To assess anterograde amnesia, the examiner should ask the athlete to recall three words, both immediately and in 5 minutes later. Other tests to assess concentration and memory could include reciting digits backwards, serial sevens, or months of the year in reverse order. Noting the duration of anterograde or posttraumatic amnesia is an important aspect of the clinical evaluation and has been found to correlate with concussion severity and outcome (8). The importance of LOC in predicting concussion severity, neuropsychological impairment, and abiltity to return to play is believed to be less accurate and reliable when managing athletes with concussions (8-10).

Table 16-4   Concussion History

• Prior head, face, or neck injuries	• Bilateral symptoms
• Number of prior concussions	• Mood alterations
• Any loss of consciousness	• Sleep disturbances
• Neck pain	• School or memory problems
• Numbness	• Acute or chronic headaches
• Paresthesias	• Visual difficulties
• Weakness	

Return-to-Play Criteria

Tables 16-5, 16-6, and 16-7 describe current guidelines for returning an athlete to play after he or she has suffered a concussion. The safest and most logical way to return the athlete to full participation is through a gradual and step-wise approach, as defined in Table 16-6. It is important that, during this time, functional activities are simulated in order to determine if concussion symptoms will return. Any athletes with concussion signs and

---

Table 16-5   Return-to-Play Guidelines: General Principles

1. No player should return to participation while symptomatic.
2. Any athlete who sustains a LOC should not return to competition, and considerations should be made about transport to the nearest medical facility.
3. Return-to-play decisions should not be game or situational dependent.
4. Return-to-play decisions should only be made by medical personnel, not by players, parents, or coaches.
5. "Star" players should not get special treatment.

Adapted with permission from Aubrey M, Cantu R, Dvorak J, et al. Summary and agreement statement of the First International Conference on Concussions in Sport, Vienna, 2001. Clin J Sport Med. 2002;12:6-11.

Table 16-6   Return-to-Play Protocol of the First International Conference on Concussion in Sport

Level One	Complete rest with no activity until asymptomatic
Level Two	Begin light aerobic activity or exercise (e.g., stationary bike, walking)
Level Three	Sport-specific training and activities (e.g., running, jumping, skating)
Level Four	Noncontact training and drills
Level Five	Full participation

Adapted with permission from Aubrey M, Cantu R, Dvorak J, et al. Summary and agreement statement of the First International Conference on Concussions in Sport, Vienna, 2001. Clin J Sport Med. 2002;12:6-11.

Table 16-7   Guidelines for Return to Play after Concussion Based on Concussion Severity and Number of Previous Concussions*

	First Concussion	*Second Concussion*	*Third Concussion*
Grade 1 (mild)	May RTP if asymptomatic for 1 week	May RTP in 2 weeks if asymptomatic for 1 week	Terminate season; may RTP next season if asymptomatic
Grade 2 (moderate)	May RTP if asymptomatic for 1 week	No RTP for at least 1 month; may then RTP if asymptomatic for 1 week; consider season termination	Terminate season; may RTP next season if asymptomatic
Grade 3 (severe)	No RTP for at least 1 month; may RTP if asymptomatic	Terminate season; may RTP next season if asymptomatic	—

*Asymptomatic in all cases means no postconcussion symptoms, including retrograde or anterograde amnesia, at rest or with exertion.
Adapted with permission from Cantu R. Posttraumatic retrograde and anterograde amnesia: pathophysiology and implications in grading and safe return to play. J Athl Train. 2001;36:244-8.

symptoms during activity or strenuous exercise should not be allowed to participate until all symptoms have cleared, both at rest and with exertion. The athlete who does return to competition should be made aware of the increased risk of sustaining another concussion, as well as the possibility of postconcussion syndrome or even second-impact syndrome. The athlete also needs to understand the importance of accurately reporting any post-concussion symptoms to medical personnel (see the section "Postconcussion Syndrome" later in this chapter). Other considerations include when to recommend discontinuation of collision or contact sports after sustaining multiple concussions.

Case Study 16-1

A 16-year-old football player was evaluated by the team physician after coming off the field complaining of nausea and headache. He had a vacant stare and looked "dazed" on questioning, but denied visual changes, ringing ears, and vomiting. There was no loss of consciousness, and he denied neck pain or stiffness.

The initial ABCs were within normal limits, pupils were equal and reactive, and initial neurological examination, including gross sensation and strength, were within normal limits. He was able to recall the opponent, the play called, and the score at the time of the injury. The athlete was able recall three words both immediately and within 5 minutes without difficulty. He was able to perform serial sevens easily, as well as the months of the year in reverse order. He was orientated to person, place, time, and situation. All symptoms, such as headache and nausea, cleared within 10 minutes of the injury.

It was felt that the athlete had suffered a grade 1 concussion. The athlete was asked to perform sideline push-ups, sit-ups, and a thirty-yard dash. His symptoms quickly returned with exertion; therefore, the athlete was held from further competition. After the game, he and his parents were given head injury warnings and precautions. He was evaluated the following day. Upon repeat evaluation, all symptoms had cleared both at rest and with exertion and there were no new findings. The athlete was then allowed to return to competition one week after all symptoms had cleared. He had no further concussion episodes the remainder of the season.

Currently, there are no scientific data to determine how many concussions are too many; however, the following guidelines may provide some guidance when making these return-to-play decisions.

1. Any athlete who sustains repeated concussions secondary to minimal or no contact should be very cautious in returning to his or her sport.

2. Any athlete who requires longer periods of recovery (either longer than anticipated, or for increasingly longer periods) in between concussion episodes may also be at risk when returning to collision sports.
3. Any athlete in whom the risk of continuing to play collision sports clearly outweighs the benefits should not be allowed to continue in collision or contact sports.

   [NOTE—Recently, some experts have moved away from the use of grading systems for concussion. They advocate the use of clinical signs and symptoms and, at times, neuropsychological testing and diagnostic tests. The editors of this book, however, feel that the grading systems presented herein help to build a good educational foundation and also serve as a practical guide for primary care physicians.]

Prevention

One of the most important aspects of concussion prevention is education of athletes in proper tackling techniques and enforcement of rules to protect athletes from activities such as spearing in football. All athletes, parents, coaches, athletic trainers, and team physicians should undergo education about the identification of concussion signs and symptoms, with an emphasis placed on immediate reporting of symptoms. Concussion education and outreach programs may also play an important role in the prevention of traumatic brain injury.

Postconcussion Syndrome

Most athletes recover from mild concussions quickly and without complications; however, there are a smaller number of athletes who may have postconcussion syndrome (PCS). The true incidence of this disorder is unknown (11). PCS may be defined as a constellation of symptoms, including persistent fatigue, dizziness, irritability, headaches (often with exertion), memory impairment, difficulty concentrating, and mood and sleep disturbances (11,12). PCS can last weeks to months. Any athlete with prolonged symptoms (i.e., PCS greater than one week) should have further evaluation with diagnostic imaging. Athletes showing signs of PCS should not be allowed to participate in athletics until further work-up has been completed and all symptoms have fully resolved (9).

Second Impact Syndrome

This rare but often ominous syndrome occurs when an athlete sustains a concussion and, before all symptoms from the initial injury have cleared, sustains a second traumatic brain injury (often a minor blow to the head or body). During the initial injury period, the central nervous system is often more vulnerable to repeat injury, leading to massive and often irreversible cerebral edema on the second insult. This cascade of events may then lead to brain stem herniation and imminent death, often before medical care has arrived. Those few athletes who survive this condition may have significant neurological illness secondary to permanent and irreversible brain injury (1,13).

Neuropsychological Testing

The use of neuropsychological testing in athletes is an exciting aspect of the management of sports-related head injury (14). Neuropsychological testing of athletes in sports began in the mid-1980s by Barth and colleagues (8,14). Neuropsychological testing can objectively measure persistent neuropsychological deficits that may occur in athletes after a traumatic brain injury. Variables measured include impaired attention and concentration, reaction time, processing speed, and memory. With the development of computerized testing, using programs such as ImPACT(c) (Immediate Postconcussion Assessment and Cognitive Testing, UPMC Sports Concussion Program, Pittsburgh, PA) or CogSport (CogState Ltd., Australia), the tests now can be performed quickly and easily.

For athletes and physicians to use these tools, a preseason baseline neuropsychological assessment is performed, with subsequent testing at various intervals after the athlete sustains a concussion. This information may be used to help determine if an athlete has returned to a baseline or preinjury level of cognitive function. This information then can be used as an adjunctive tool when determining concussion recovery and making return-to-play decisions.

Neuropsychological testing is being performed and being used as a concussion-management tool at numerous high schools, colleges, and professional teams from the National Football League and the National Hockey League (14,15).

There is no universal agreement among experts about the usefulness of neuropsychological testing, but many studies attest to its clinical value. Its precise role in the management of sports-related concussions, however, has not been defined.

When to Refer

Many uncomplicated concussions can be managed safely. Table 16-8 lists some situations in which a referral to a specialist may be indicated.

Table 16-8   Conditions or Situations for Possible Referral to a Specialist in Concussions

- Athletes suffering from postconcussion syndrome or persistent symptoms such as headache
- Athletes who suffer repeated concussions
- Concussions occurring with minimal or no contact
- Athletes with prolonged (lasting minutes) loss of consciousness
- Abnormal findings on neurological examination

Brachial Plexus Injuries

Brachial plexus injuries are common in sports such as football, ice hockey, wrestling, basketball, and water sports. The most common injury of the brachial plexus is the transient brachial plexopathy, often referred to a "burners" or "stingers" (16-18). The mechanism of injury is usually secondary to either a traction or compression injury, which may occur during tackling with sudden shoulder depression and lateral cervical spine flexion to the opposite side (16-18) (Figure 16-1). Because of the

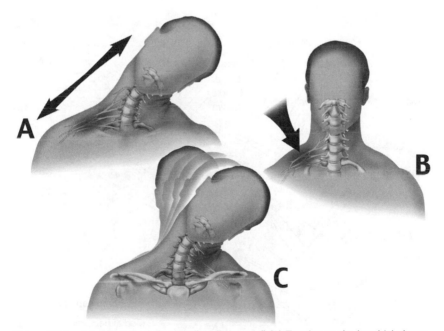

Figure 16-1   Mechanism of "burners" or "stingers." (A) Traction to the brachial plexus from ipsilateral shoulder depression and contralateral lateral neck flexion. (B) Direct blow to the supraclavicular fossa at Erb's point. (C) Compression of the cervical roots or brachial plexus from the ipsilateral lateral flexion and hyperextension. (From Kuhlman GS, McKeag DB. The "burner": a common nerve injury in contact sports. Am Fam Physician. 1999;60:2035-42; by permission of Renee L. Cannon.)

underdevelopment of neck musculature, brachial plexus injuries are common in the high school athlete. Up to 65% of football players report prior "burners" during their career, with a large number of players experiencing recurrent episodes (16,18).

The brachial plexus is formed from the ventral rami of C5 to T1 (16, 18), with the C5 and C6 nerve roots most commonly being affected (Figure 16-2) (18). Brachial plexus injuries can be classified into three categories: neuropraxia, axonotmesis, and neurotmesis. Focal demyelination without disruption of the axon occurs in neuropraxia. These mild injuries usually result in full recovery within minutes to days. Axonotmesis refers to damage or loss of axons, with symptoms lasting weeks to months. In neurotmesis the nerve is either torn or lacerated, with spontaneous recovery unlikely.

Most cases of brachial plexus injuries can be diagnosed from a careful history and physical examination, with nerve conduction studies performed to help differentiate between cervical radiculopathy, thoracic outlet syndrome, and brachial plexus injuries. Table 16-9 lists the differential diagnosis of athletic brachial plexus injuries. Signs and symptoms include weakness of the deltoid (C5), biceps (C5, C6) and wrist flexors (C6), along

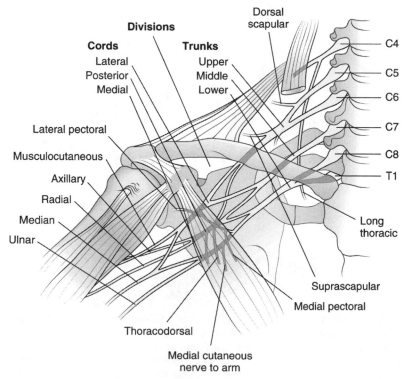

Figure 16-2   Anatomy of the brachial plexus.

with unilateral burning pain or numbness of the lateral arm (C5), thumb, and index finger (C6) (16,18).

The sideline evaluation should include careful evaluation of the cervical spine (along with Spurling's test [Figure 16-3] and axial compression test [Figure 16-4]), shoulder and upper extremity, and a complete neurological evaluation. Those athletes complaining of bilateral or lower extremity

---

Table 16-9   Differential Diagnosis of Athletic Brachial Plexus Injuries

- Acute brachial neuropathy/brachial neuritis
- Occult cervical spine fracture
- Cervical disc herniation
- Transient quadriplegia (Cord Contusion)

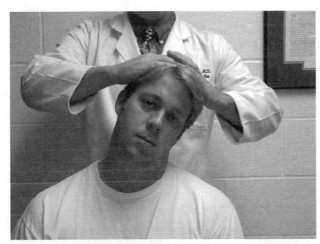

Figure 16-3
Spurling's test is performed by rotating and extending the neck to the involved side with gentle axial compression. A positive test reproduces radicular pain in the involved extremity (cervical nerve root compression).

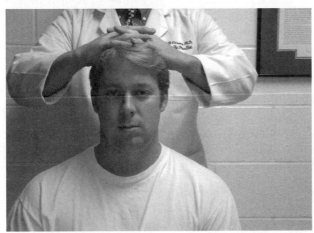

Figure 16-4   Axial compression test. Gentle downward pressure is placed on the head to evaluate for reproduction of symptoms.

Table 16-10   Indications for Further Work-Up in Athlete with Brachial Plexus Injury*

- Recurrent "stingers" (three or more)
- Persistent unilateral weakness or sensory loss (more than 1-2 weeks)
- Lower extremity symptoms (motor or sensory)
- Bilateral upper extremity symptoms ("burning" hands)
- Localized neck tenderness, stiffness, or apprehension

*Cervical spine series, electromyogram (EMG), or MRI.

Table 16-11   Return-to-Play Criteria after Brachial Plexus Injury

- Full and painless neck range of motion
- Complete symptom resolution
- Negative Spurling's test
- Negative axial compression test
- Normal neurological examination (e.g., strength, sensation, reflexes)

symptoms should be considered to have a spinal cord injury until proven otherwise. Proper spinal immobilization procedures should be performed, leaving the helmet and shoulder pads in place (unless there is airway compromise), and the athlete should be transported to the nearest medical facility (16).

Athletes with any of the symptoms listed in Table 16-10 should be withheld from play until further evaluation is performed for possible nerve root impingement, congenital spinal stenosis, cervical disk disease, or spinal cord injury (16,18,19). Criteria for return to play after a brachial plexus injury are listed in Table 16-11 (16).

Treatment of brachial plexus injuries includes relative rest, NSAIDs, and physical therapy. Preventive measures may include education on proper tackling techniques, proper fit of equipment, neck strengthening and flexibility programs, and cervical orthoses (protective collars, neck roll, or "cowboy collar"; Figure 16-5) (16,19).

Case Study 16-2

A team physician evaluated a young hockey player during the third period after the player complained of a "burning" sensation and weakness of his dominant arm. He believed he had a "stinger." He was able to recall the injury and reported someone hitting him in the shoulder with immediate onset of pain and burning in the supraclavicular region, radiating down the arm. He denied bilateral or lower extremity involvement and had no concussion signs or symptoms.

Upon initial examination, he had full, active cervical motion without pain or bony tenderness, along with a negative Spurling's test. Upon strength testing there was marked weakness of shoulder abduction along with decreased sensation of the lateral arm in the axillary nerve distribution. There was mild tenderness of the supraclavicular fossa but no other acute findings.

All symptoms gradually resolved within about five minutes as the game was ending.

He was evaluated the following week and continued to have no complaints and a normal examination. Return to play was discussed with the athlete and his family, and he was instructed in the use of protective padding and equipment, along with neck flexibility and strengthening exercises. The patient returned to competition without further episodes of transient brachial plexopathy.

Athletic Nerve Entrapment Syndromes

The evaluation and management of athletic nerve entrapment syndromes can be a challenging problem for the clinician and the patient suffering from these conditions. This section will discuss some of the entrapment neuropathies encountered in athletes. Athletes participating in overhead sports, such as baseball and volleyball, are at risk for these syndromes. Other sports, such as cycling, may encounter these conditions as well. Most entrapment syndromes can be treated with conservative measures, including relative rest, activity modification, NSAIDs, and physical therapy. Surgical intervention often is reserved for those cases not responding to conservative measures.

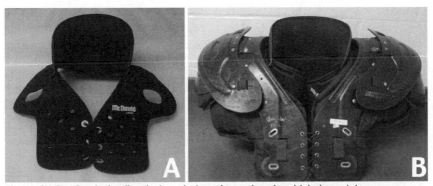

Figure 16-5   Cervical collar devices designed to reduce brachial plexus injury.

Ulnar Nerve Entrapment

Compression of the ulnar nerve in athletes may occur at the elbow (cubital tunnel syndrome) or wrist (Guyon canal syndrome). Cubital tunnel syndrome (ulnar neuropathy) may occur in the throwing athlete secondary to the significant valgus forces placed on the elbow during the throwing motion. This condition is the second most common entrapment neuropathy of the upper extremity (20). Carpal tunnel syndrome, the most common entrapment neuropathy, is discussed in Chapter 20.

The athlete may present with a constellation of injuries, which may include medial epicondylitis, ulnar collateral ligament injury, or cubital tunnel syndrome symptoms such as paresthesias, dysesthesias, and pain in the ulnar nerve distribution (ring and little fingers) (21). The athlete may also report decreased throwing velocity, elbow or hand weakness, pain, or a popping sensation on the medial aspect of the elbow.

On examination, the athlete may have a positive Tinel's sign over the cubital tunnel or pain along the distribution of the ulnar nerve with radiation to the ring and little fingers. Diagnosis often can be made with a detailed history and physical; however, nerve conduction studies may be necessary in difficult cases or to exclude cervical radiculopathy and brachial plexopathy (20). Treatment consists of relative rest, activity modification, NSAIDs, physical therapy, and correction of any underlying disorder (medial epicondylitis, ulnar collateral ligament injury) or poor throwing mechanics. Brief periods of immobilization, such as splinting, may be necessary for patients not responding to initial therapies.

Patients not responding to 3 to 6 months of conservative measures should be referred to a sports medicine physician or orthopedic surgeon to evaluate the need for surgery.

Suprascapular Nerve Entrapment

Suprascapular nerve entrapment occurs in athletes involved in overhead activities, such as baseball, volleyball, and weightlifting (20). The suprascapular nerve arises from the upper portion of the brachial plexus (C5, C6) (see Figure 16-2) passing through the scapular notch (the most common area of entrapment), giving off motor branches to the supraspinatus and infraspinatus muscles and sensory branches leading to the acromioclavicular joint and posterior shoulder.

Athletes with this disorder may report an insidious onset of poorly localized posterolateral shoulder pain and exhibit atrophy and weakness of the supraspinatus and infraspinatus muscles. Nerve conduction studies can be performed to aid in the diagnosis and to exclude a C5-C6 radiculopathy or brachial plexopathy (20).

Initial treatment should consist of conservative measures, including relative rest, NSAIDs, and rotator cuff and scapular stabilizing exercises.

Surgical exploration may be indicated for those cases failing to respond to conservative measures (20).

Piriformis Syndrome

First coined by Robinson in 1947 (20,22,23), piriformis syndrome, often overlooked by physicians, accounts for up 6% of sciatica cases seen in clinical practice (23). This syndrome is considered to be secondary to either a hypertrophied piriformis muscle or prior blunt pelvic or buttock trauma (a prior history of trauma to the buttock region may be found in up to 50% of cases) (22).

Patients will present with posterior buttock or thigh pain and paresthesias secondary to compression or irritation of the sciatic nerve as it passes through the piriformis muscle (Figure 16-6). The differential diagnosis of this syndrome includes L5-S1 radiculopathy, lumbosacral plexopathy, sacroiliac dysfunction, myofascial pain syndrome, and trochanteric bursitis (20,22). The pathognomonic sign on physical examination is a tender mass over the piriformis region, with reproduction of the patient's symptoms (24). Passive stretch of the piriformis (hip internal rotation and adduction)

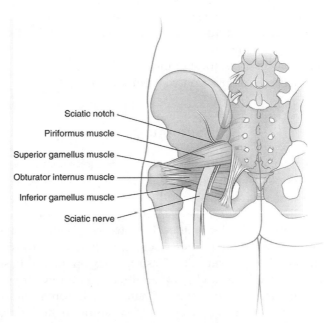

Sciatic notch
Piriformus muscle
Superior gamellus muscle
Obturator internus muscle
Inferior gamellus muscle
Sciatic nerve

Figure 16-6   Sciatic nerve as it passes through the sciatic notch and beneath the piriformis muscle—a site of possible nerve compression.

may also reproduce the patient's symptoms. Patients may also exhibit a positive Pace sign (weakness of resisted hip abduction and external rotation) or Freiberg sign (pain on forced hip internal rotation) (23). Back pain and neurological findings usually are not encountered in this condition. Plain films and MRI can be used to exclude other etiologies. Nerve conduction studies typically are unremarkable.

Treatment of piriformis syndrome consists of correction of any biomechanical hip and leg abnormalities (such as leg length discrepancy), stretching exercises and physical therapy, corticosteroid injection, or surgical decompression (20,22-24).

Peroneal Nerve Entrapment

The most common nerve entrapment of the lower extremity is that of the superficial peroneal nerve (25). The superficial peroneal nerve is a branch of the common peroneal nerve (L4,5, S1,2) on the anterior and lateral aspect of the leg. This nerve provides motor innervation to the peroneus longus and brevis muscles, along with sensation to the lower/lateral leg and dorsum of the foot (sparing the first dorsal web space). This nerve may be compressed with tight fitting casts, athletic taping, or secondary to direct trauma from repetitive ankle injuries.

Patients usually present with pain, numbness, and paresthesias along the distribution of the superficial peroneal nerve. Other findings include weakness of resisted ankle eversion and dorsiflextion. In severe or chronic cases, patients may exhibit a foot drop. Nerve conduction studies may be useful for diagnostic purposes.

Treatment consists of removal of the offending agent, NSAIDs, physical therapy, or surgical decompression when indicated (20,25).

Summary

Concussion is a common sports injury. All concussions should be regarded as potentially serious injuries and treated accordingly. Any athlete with concussion signs and symptoms should be removed from competition and evaluated closely by medical personnel. Athletes should not be allowed to return to their sport until all symptoms have cleared, both at rest and with exertion. There is need for further research to find ways to reduce the number of traumatic and potentially catastrophic brain injuries in sports.

Brachial plexus injuries and peripheral nerve entrapment syndromes are not uncommon in sports. Accurate diagnosis relies on a careful history and physical examination. These syndromes can be treated initially with conservative measures. Patients not responding to these measures should be referred for further work-up and evaluation.

REFERENCES

1. **Wojtys EM, Hovda D, Landry G, et al.** Current concepts: concussion in sports. Am J Sports Med. 1999;27(5):676-87.

2. **Harmon KD.** Assessment and management of concussion in sports. Am Fam Physician. 1999;60(3):887-94.

3. **Kelly JP, Rosenberg JH.** Diagnosis and management of concussion in sports. Neurol. 1997;48:575-9.

4. **Kushner DS.** Concussion in sports: minimizing the risk for complications. Am Fam Physician. 2001;64(6):1007-14.

5. **McCrory P, Johnston K, Mohtadi N.** Evidence-based review of sport-related concussion: basic science. Clin J Sport Med. 2001;11:160-5.

6. **Cantu R.** Posttraumatic retrograde and anterograde amnesia: pathophysiology and implications in grading and safe return to play. J Athl Train. 2001;36(3):244-8.

7. **Aubrey M, Cantu R, Dvorak J, et al.** Summary and Agreement Statement of the First International Conference on Concussion in Sport, Vienna, 2001. Clin J Sport Med. 2002;12:6-11.

8. **Johnston K, McCrory P, Mohtadi N, Meeuwisse W.** Evidence-based review of sport-related concussion: clinical science. Clin J Sport Med. 2001;11:150-9.

9. **Cantu RC.** Head injuries. In: Delee JC, Drez D, Miller MD, eds. Delee and Drez's Orthopaedic Sports Medicine: Principles and Practice, 2nd ed. Philadelphia: WB Saunders; 2003:769-75.

10. **Lovell MR, Iverson GL, Collins MW, et al.** Does loss of consciousness predict neuropsychological decrements after concussion? Clin J Sport Med. 1999;9:193-8.

11. **Cantu R.** Head and spine injuries in youth sports. Clin Sports Med. 1995;14:517-32.

12. **Cantu R.** Return to play guidelines after a head injury. Clin Sports Med. 1998; 17:45-60.

13. **Maroon J, Lovell M, Norwig J, et al.** Cerebral concussion in athletes: evaluation and neuropsychological testing. Neurosurg. 2000;47:659-72.

14. **Lovell MR.** The relevance of neuropsychological testing for sports-related head injuries. Curr Sports Med Reports. 2002;1:7-11.

15. **Collins MW, Hawn KL.** The clinical management of sports concussion. Curr Sports Med Reports. 2002;1:12-21.

16. **Koffler KM.** Neurovascular trauma in athletes. Orthop Clin North Am. 2002:33; 523-34.

17. **Evans RW, Wilberger JE.** Traumatic disorders. In: Goetz CG, Pappert EJ, eds. Textbook of Clinical Neurology. Philadelphia: WB Saunders; 1999:1052-3.

18. **Sallis RE.** Brachial plexus injuries. In: Sallis RE, Massimino F, eds. ACSM's Essentials of Sports Medicine. St. Louis: Mosby-Yearbook; 1997:258-89.

19. **Moore J, Rice EL, Moore J.** Neck injuries. In: Mellion MB, Walsh WM, Madden C, Putukian M, Shelton GL, eds. Team Physician's Handbook, 3rd ed. Philadelphia: Hanley & Belfus; 2002:372, 573.

20. **Shapiro BE, Preston DC.** Entrapment and compressive neuropathies. Med Clin North Am. 2003;87:663.

21. **Grana W.** Medial epicondylitis and cubital tunnel syndrome in the throwing athlete. Clin Sports Med. 2001;20:541-8.

22. **Benzon HT, Katz JA, Benzon IIA, Iqbal M.** Piriformis syndrome: anatomic considerations, a new injection technique, and a review of the literature. Anesthesiology. 2003;98:1442.

23. **Parziale JR, Hudgins TH, Fishman LM.** The piriformis syndrome. Am J Orthop. 1996;25:819-23.

24. **Nuccion SL, Hunter DM, Finerman GA.** Hip and pelvis: adult. In: Delee JC, Drez D, Miller MD, eds. Delee and Drez's Orthopaedic Sports Medicine: Principles and Practice, 2nd ed. Philadelphia: WB Saunders; 2003:1452.

25. **Andrish JT.** The leg: nerve entrapment. In: Delee JC, Drez D, Miller MD, eds. Delee and Drez's Orthopaedic Sports Medicine: Principles and Practice, 2nd ed. Philadelphia: WB Saunders; 2003:2177-8.

SUGGESTED READING

Aubrey M, Cantu R, Dvorak J, et al. Summary and agreement statement of the first International Conference on Concussion in Sport, Vienna, 2001. Clin J Sport Med. 2002; 12:6-11.

Koffler KM. Neurovascular trauma in athletes. Orthop Clin North Am. 2002:33;523-34.

Shapiro BE, Preston DC. Entrapment and compressive neuropathies. Med Clin North Am. 2003;87:663-96.

SECTION III

MUSCULOSKELETAL INJURIES

17

■   ■   ■

Neck Injuries

Kevin Eerkes, MD

David S. Ross, MD

Neck injuries are common during sports participation, but, fortunately, most are mild. On rare occasions, they can be devastating. Injuries can involve the vertebrae, intervertebral discs, ligamentous structures, muscles, spinal cord, nerve roots and peripheral nerves, or any combination of these structures. The physician must perform a thorough assessment to identify significant injuries that require specific care. The focus of this chapter is on neck injuries encountered in a general medical practice.

Relevant Anatomy and Biomechanics

There are seven cervical vertebrae, with a nerve exiting the left or right neuroforamena between each vertebra. Each nerve is named by corresponding vertebra below, except nerve root C8, which goes below the C7 vertebra; T1 vertebra is below. A disc is present between the vertebrae to provide cushioning and allow motion. The spinal cord is protected within the spinal canal. Motion in three planes allows flexion/extension, rotation, and side bending. One half of flexion/extension of the cervical spine occurs at the articulation between the occiput and the first cervical vertebrae (atlantooccipital joint). One half of rotation occurs between the first and second vertebrae (atlantoaxial joint). The remainder of rotation, as well as lateral bending, occurs between the second and seventh cervical vertebrae. While the cervical spine has a large range of motion (ROM), this comes at the cost of stability. Ligaments and muscles provide stability to make up for the relative lack of intrinsic bony stability in the cervical spine.

History

Knowing the mechanism of injury can be helpful in identifying the nature and extent of the injuries. Inquiry should be made about any preexisting neck problems. The athlete should be asked about neck pain, either at rest or with motion. Presence of limb numbness, paresthesias, weakness, or bowel/bladder dysfunction is also important.

Physical Examination

The physical exam begins with inspection for posterior neck swelling, ecchymosis, or obvious deformity. Next, the neck is palpated. Point tenderness over a spinous process may indicate fracture or ligament injury. Muscle spasm on palpation is a nonspecific finding. It may occur with any neck injury and functions as a protective mechanism. The patient may be asked to perform active ROM of the neck, except in cases of significant trauma, for fear of causing or worsening neurologic damage if a fracture or instability were present. In this case, appropriate x-rays must be performed before ROM testing. In acute insult to the cervical spine, appropriate assessment, including a neurogical exam, should be performed to rule out significant C-spine pathology. This is described later in the chapter.

The neurologic exam includes sensory, motor, and reflex testing. Patterns of sensory or motor deficit suggest injury of specific nerve roots (Table 17-1). The Spurling test is performed by extending, rotating, and side-bending the head to the involved side while applying an axial load to the head (Figure 17-1). This narrows the neuroforamen through which the nerve root passes. If the neuroforamen is narrowed by a herniated disc, bone spur, or congenital anomaly, then this maneuver will often exacerbate the neuritic symptoms down the arm. A variation of the Spurling test that

Table 17-1   Patterns of Sensory or Motor Deficit Suggesting Injury of Specific Nerve Roots

Nerve Root	Sensation	Muscle	Reflex
C4	Back of the neck, top of the shoulder	None	None
C5	Lateral arm	Deltoid, biceps brachii, spinati	Biceps
C6	Lateral forearm, thumb, and index finger	Wrist extensors	Brachioradialis
C7	Middle finger	Triceps, wrist flexors, finger extensors	Triceps
C8	Ring and little fingers	Finger flexors, hand intrinsics	None

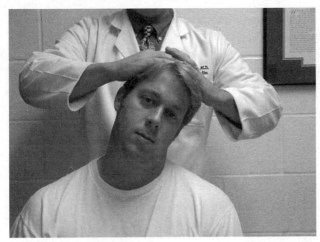

Figure 17-1
Spurling's test is performed by rotating and extending the neck to the involved side with gentle axial compression. A positive test reproduces radicular pain in the involved extremity (cervical nerve root compression).

Table 17-2   Indications for Immobilization of the Neck and Radiographic Evaluation

- Midline posterior neck tenderness
- Reduced cervical motion
- Motor deficits or altered mental status (high-grade concussion)

may also be effective in narrowing the neuroforamen is the "compression test." In this simpler test, an axial load is applied to the top of the head to determine if neuritic symptoms are elicited.

X-ray examination of the cervical spine should be performed in certain circumstances. The indications for obtaining x-rays and the particular views required in specific disorders are discussed later in the chapter. See Table 17-2 for indications for obtaining radiographs and Table 17-3 for information about interpretation of x-rays.

Specific Disorders

Neck Strain/Sprain

A *strain* is a stretch injury or tear of the muscle/tendon unit. A *sprain* is a tear of the ligament. These injuries occur when the structures are stressed beyond physiologic loads. Neck strains and sprains are the most common neck injury encountered in sports. It is often difficult to determine the specific ligament(s) or muscle/tendon(s) injured; however, in general, this does not change the treatment plan.

Typically, the patient's chief complaint will be that he "jammed" his neck and has subsequent localized pain. "Jamming" is a vague term and

---

Table 17-3   Checklist when Reading Cervical Spine Radiographs after Acute Injury

Lateral View

- Vertebral alignment (anterior or posterior subluxation > 3.5 mm may be pathological) (16)
- Intervertebral distance (increase or decrease)
- Prevertebral soft tissue space. Normal: C2, < 7 mm; C6, < 22 mm
- Space between facet joints and spinous processes
- Fracture: vertebral bodies, posterior elements, dens
- Atlantodens interval (no greater than 3 mm)
- Vertebral angulation (no angulation between 2 vertebrae that is 11 degrees greater than angulation between adjacent vertebra)
- Alignment of occipital condyles with the lateral masses of C1
- Alignment of the odontoid process with the clivus
- Pavlov ratio no less than 0.8

Anteroposterior View

- Spinous process alignment and distance
- Lateral angulation
- Fracture

Odontoid View

- Fracture: odontoid, atlas, occipital condyles
- Lateral overhang of the lateral masses of C1 (increase suggests fracture of C1)
- Atlantooccipital dissociation
- Asymmetry of lateral masses of C1 relative to the odontoid

---

may imply a hyperflexion or hyperextension injury, perhaps combined with rotation or lateral bending. There may be a delay in the onset of neck pain of up to several hours after the injury. Pain may be referred to the upper trapezius, periscapular, or proximal upper extremity areas on one or both sides. There may be a vague sense of heaviness, numbness, or tingling in a nonradicular pattern. Symptoms are generally not present below the elbow. ROM usually is restricted.

Physical exam may reveal tenderness or muscle spasm in the neck. Muscle spasm feels like a tight or knotted muscle on palpation and is a protective response to muscle injury. Painful and reduced ROM of the neck is usually present. Strength, gross sensation, and deep tendon reflexes in the upper extremities should be tested but will be normal with a simple strain/sprain. If the patient complains of any lower extremity symptoms, such as weakness or gait disturbance, consider the possibility of a cervical cord injury. In this case, one should also do a complete neurologic exam, including checking for long tract signs with the Babinski sign in the lower extremities and the Hoffman sign in the upper extremities (Figure 17-2).

Deciding when to get cervical spine x-rays after a neck injury can be difficult. Definite indications for x-rays include dangerous mechanism of

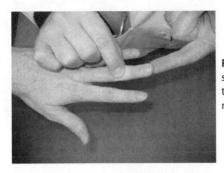

Figure 17-2   Hoffman's test. Rapid extension of the fingers leads to reflex flexion of the fingers. This is a sign of upper motor neuron dysfunction.

injury (for example, an axial load to the crown of the head), any neurologic abnormalities (paresthesias or weakness in the extremities), tenderness over the spinous processes, or less than 45 degrees active rotation of the neck in either direction. In addition, guidelines such as the Canadian C-Spine Rule have been published to aid the physician in deciding if radiographs are warranted (Figure 17-3) (1).

Initial x-rays after trauma should include anteroposterior, lateral, and open-mouth odontoid views. Table 17-3 outlines the protocol for reading cervical spine x-rays in the setting of acute neck injury. "Clearing" neck x-rays can be difficult, so if one is not experienced at reading these films it is best to review them with a radiologist or other appropriate specialist. Abnormalities to look for include fracture, dislocation, or subluxation of vertebra.

If neck pain continues or if the clinician is suspicious of spinal instability and initial films are negative, lateral flexion and extension views may then be obtained. This can be done when the acute paracervical muscle spasm subsides, allowing for ROM. One looks for abnormal anterior or posterior movement of vertebra with flexion and extension. Advanced imaging studies can be obtained if there is suspicion of injury not appearing on x-ray or to further assess x-rays abnormalities. CT scan is best at imaging bony abnormalities, such as fracture or malalignment. MRI is best at imaging soft tissue abnormalities, such as injuries to neural tissue or discs.

Treatment can begin after cervical spine films have been "cleared" and neurologic exam is found to be normal. Control of pain is achieved with rest, NSAIDs and/or acetaminophen, ice, and perhaps brief use of a soft cervical collar if there is marked pain with motion. Narcotic analgesics can be used cautiously in appropriate situations. Muscle relaxants may be prescribed in athletes with overt muscle spasm. With marked pain, muscle relaxants may be used with NSAIDs, but may have an additive effect.

Once acute symptoms have passed (usually within several days), rehabilitation can commence. Initially, this involves gentle active ROM exercises of the neck in flexion/extension, rotation and side bending, within limits of comfort. Gentle isometric strengthening exercises may begin when full, pain-free ROM has been achieved. Isometric exercise involves contraction

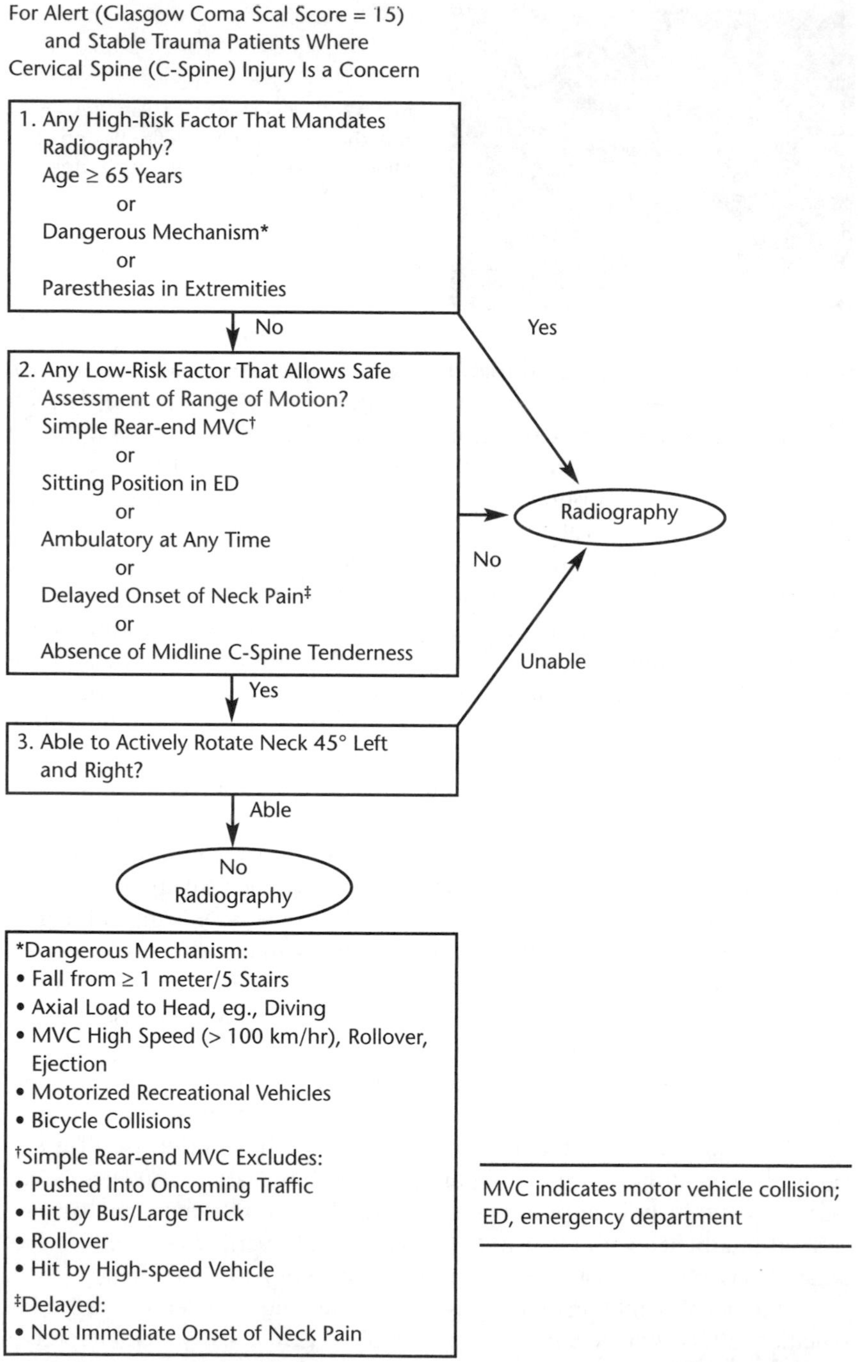

For Alert (Glasgow Coma Scal Score = 15)
    and Stable Trauma Patients Where
Cervical Spine (C-Spine) Injury Is a Concern

1. Any High-Risk Factor That Mandates
   Radiography?
   Age ≥ 65 Years
        or
   Dangerous Mechanism*
        or
   Paresthesias in Extremities

No   Yes

2. Any Low-Risk Factor That Allows Safe
   Assessment of Range of Motion?
   Simple Rear-end MVC†
        or
   Sitting Position in ED
        or
   Ambulatory at Any Time   Radiography
        or
   Delayed Onset of Neck Pain‡   No
        or
   Absence of Midline C-Spine Tenderness

                                            Unable

Yes

3. Able to Actively Rotate Neck 45° Left
   and Right?

Able

No
Radiography

*Dangerous Mechanism:
• Fall from ≥ 1 meter/5 Stairs
• Axial Load to Head, eg., Diving
• MVC High Speed (> 100 km/hr), Rollover,
  Ejection
• Motorized Recreational Vehicles
• Bicycle Collisions

†Simple Rear-end MVC Excludes:
• Pushed Into Oncoming Traffic   MVC indicates motor vehicle collision;
• Hit by Bus/Large Truck   ED, emergency department
• Rollover
• Hit by High-speed Vehicle

‡Delayed:
• Not Immediate Onset of Neck Pain

Figure 17-3   Canadian C-Spine Rule. (From Stiell IG, Wells GA, Vandemheen KL, et al.
                   The Canadian C-Spine Rule for radiography in alert and stable trauma pa-
                   tients. JAMA. 2001;286:1841-8; with permission.)

of the neck muscles without movement of the head, which is stabilized by the hand. Eventually, more aggressive stretching and strengthening exercises may be employed to correct any strength or flexibility deficits. Rehabilitation can be performed by the athlete on his or her own with an informational handout or under the supervision of a physical therapist or athletic trainer. Significant improvement occurs in most individuals by 2 weeks, and 90% recovery occurs by 4 weeks.

Return to play is allowed when the symptoms have resolved, no pain is present with axial compression, and there is full, painless ROM and strength of the neck. Additionally, the athlete should be able to perform sport-specific drills fully without pain. The recurrence rate of strains and sprains is fairly high, so athletes should allow adequate time for healing and rehabilitation before returning to activities and should continue the neck exercises for the remainder of the season.

Brachial Plexus Neurapraxia

Brachial plexus neurapraxia (BNP) is fairly common among contact-sport athletes. Up to 50% of college football linemen, linebackers, and defensive ends have one or more episodes per season (2). The terms "stingers" and "burners" describe what the athlete feels in the shoulder and upper limb as the nerve is compressed or stretched. In general, BNP is thought to involve the C5-C6 nerve distribution; this would imply a lesion of the upper brachial plexus or cervical nerve root. Two mechanisms of injury are thought to cause the clinical syndrome of the "stinger" (Figure 17-4). With the traction mechanism, the shoulder is pushed down and/or the head is pushed to the opposite side, stretching the upper trunk of the brachial plexus. This can occur if the athlete falls on the side of the head and/or on the top of the shoulder in sports such as football or wrestling. With the compression mechanism, the C5 or C6 nerve root is compressed at the neuroforamen when the head is forcefully rotated and laterally flexed toward the affected arm.

The athlete describes pain and burning in the shoulder and arm region. Dysesthesias often radiate down the arm and even to the fingertips in a dermatomal pattern. Dysesthesia usually resolves in seconds or minutes, although it may, in some instances, last for a few hours. There may be mild transient extremity weakness, usually lasting less than 10 minutes. Only one of the upper extremities is involved. On examination, strength of the deltoid, biceps, spinati, triceps, wrist flexors, and extensors should be tested, since usually these are innervated by the nerve(s) involved (C5-C7 roots and upper truck of the brachial plexus). Deep tendon reflexes and neck ROM should be normal, and the neck should be nontender.

Athletes are allowed to return to play when symptoms have resolved and exam is normal. There should be normal strength, sensation, and reflexes in the extremity. The ROM of the neck should be full and painless.

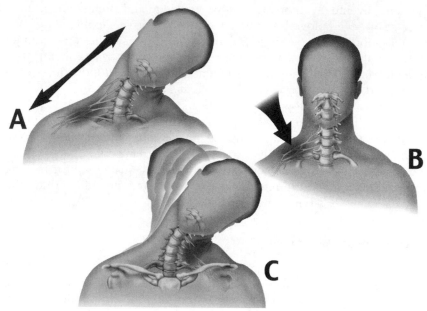

Figure 17-4   Mechanism of "burners" or "stingers." (A) Traction to the brachial plexus from ipsilateral shoulder depression and contralateral lateral neck flexion. (B) Direct blow to the supraclavicular fossa at Erb's point. (C) Compression of the cervical roots or brachial plexus from the ipsilateral lateral flexion and hyperextension. (From Kuhlman GS, McKeag DB. The "burner": a common nerve injury in contact sports. Am Fam Physician. 1999;60:2035-42; by permission of Renee L. Cannon.)

Table 17-4   "Red Flags" for Further Evaluation in Patients with Brachial Plexus Neuroapraxia

- Recurrent "stingers" (three or more)
- Persistent unilateral weakness or sensory loss (more than 1-2 weeks)
- Lower extremity symptoms (motor or sensory)
- Bilateral upper extremity symptoms (burning hands)
- Localized neck tenderness, stiffness, or apprehension

Some authors (3) recommend performing the Spurling maneuver before return to play. "Red Flags" that indicate need for x-ray evaluation of the neck are listed in Table 17-4. In these situations, diagnostic possibilities include occult cervical spine fracture, nerve disruption, disc herniation, transient quadriplegia (cord contusion), and cervical spinal stenosis.

Case Study 17-1

A 17-year-old football player landed on top of his right shoulder and head after being upended by an opponent when going up for a pass. He came out of the game holding his right upper extremity and complained of a burning pain running down the extremity. The neurological exam was normal, and the cervical ROM was full and painless. Spurling's maneuver produced discomfort in the right upper extremity, and the neurological exam was significant only for minor strength deficit. His symptoms quickly resolved following the insult, and within 5 minutes all exam maneuvers proved to be unremarkable. He was diagnosed with a "stinger" and allowed to return to play without further incident.

The incidence of stingers may be reduced with strengthening of the neck and shoulder muscles. In sports where shoulder pads are used, it is important that the pads fit properly. A U-shaped neck roll or cowboy collar may also be helpful in preventing the extreme neck deviation that may cause stingers. Evidence-based research on the use of neck roll devices to prevent these injuries is lacking.

Neurapraxia of the Cervical Cord

Neurapraxia of the cervical cord (transient quadriplegia) is a temporary injury to the spinal cord caused by compression or stretching of the spinal cord. This frightening condition may present similar to a major spinal cord injury, with a temporary paralysis in which the athlete is unable to move or feel their extremities. In other cases, transient quadriplegia may manifest as mild weakness. The typical pathology is a narrow spinal canal that may be either congenital or acquired (4). The injury occurs when there is an axial load applied to the head with the neck in maximal flexion or extension. It occurs most commonly in football. With hyperextension injuries of the neck, the canal narrows further, leading to compression of the cord. Infolding of the ligamentum flavum with hyperextension contributes to this narrowing. With hyperflexion injuries, the cord becomes stretched. The athlete experiences burning pain or numbness in the extremities. Varying degrees of weakness often occurs, ranging from mild weakness to complete paralysis. The symptoms may involve one or all four extremities. The symptoms are usually transient, with complete recovery usually within seconds or minutes. Occasionally, symptoms and signs may persist for 48 hours.

On-the-field evaluation and management are described later in this chapter. If symptoms and signs resolve promptly, the diagnosis of transient quadriplegia is suggested. Imaging tests should be performed. Neck x-rays should include posterior-anterior (PA), lateral, oblique, open-mouth odontoid, and flexion/extension views. The radiographs should be reviewed for spinal canal narrowing, osteophytes, vertebral fracture, and instability, all of which could cause the symptoms of transient quadriplegia. Traditionally, spinal canal narrowing was measured by the ratio of spinal canal diameter to the width of the vertebral body (Torg ratio). More recent studies have found x-rays unreliable in identifying spinal stenosis (5). Nonetheless, a Torg ratio of < 0.08 in an athlete with a history of transient quadriplegia should raise suspicion of spinal canal narrowing. MRI is the imaging test of choice and should be done in all athletes with transient quadriplegia. It will determine if the spinal canal is narrow relative to the cord (Figure 17-5) and may spot other conditions that could cause transient quadriplegia, such as an extruded disc or a ligament injury.

The decision to allow the athlete to return to contact sports after an episode of transient quadriplegia is controversial and probably best made with a specialist. Recurrence of symptoms is common in half of athletes

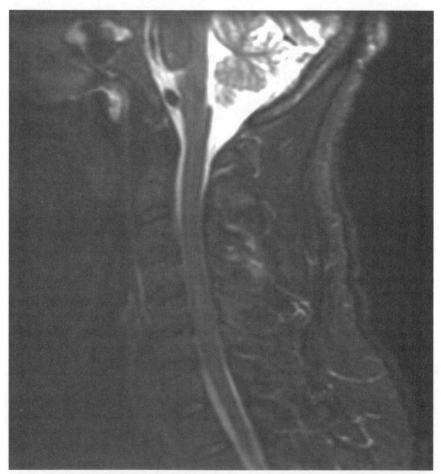

Figure 17-5   MRI of congenital cervical spinal stenosis. Note diminished cerebrospinal fluid around the upper cervical region, increasing the risk of cord compression.

who return to contact sports, but there is no evidence that this will cause permanent cord damage (6). An episode of transient quadriplegia does not seem to be a risk factor for catastrophic cord injury (7). If the MRI shows no spinal stenosis (adequate space between the cord and wall of the spinal canal), the athlete generally is allowed to return to contact and collision sports. If the MRI shows mild-to-moderate functional spinal stenosis, contact and collision sports are discouraged. Severe spinal stenosis with cord displacement and edema, along with disc herniation, is an absolute contraindication to contact and collision sports (8).

Acute Disc Herniation

Athletic injury may cause an acute disc herniation, although many disc herniations occur in the absence of demonstrable trauma. Acute trauma resulting in disc injury usually occurs in individuals more than 40 years old with some preexisting disc degeneration. Disc herniation in younger populations is rare because of their resilient discs. The mechanism of injury is similar to that described in the section on Neck Strain/Sprain. Injury most commonly occurs to the C6-C7 disc, irritating or compressing the seventh cervical nerve root. Most disc herniations occur intraforamenally (Figure 17-6, *B*). Symptoms may include localized neck pain, radicular pain in a dermatomal distribution,

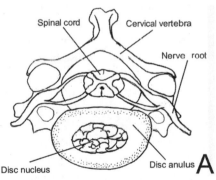

Figure 17-6   (A) Normal disc. (B) Lateral disc herniation impinging on nerve root. (C) Midline disc herniation compressing the spinal cord.

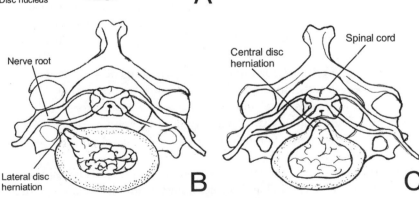

and/or weakness. Rarely, the disc may herniate posteriorly in the midline (Figure 17-6, C). In this situation, an acute myelopathy (cord compression) may develop. Preexisting bone spurs may narrow the canal so that a disc herniation, which further narrows the canal, would be more likely to be symptomatic.

The physical exam in a patient with acute disc herniation will reveal reduced neck range of motion and occasionally muscle spasm and mild tenderness. Sensation, strength, and deep tendon reflexes in the upper extremity may be diminished. The Spurling test is often positive. As mentioned earlier, another, simpler test that narrows the neuroforamen (to elicit the neuritic symptoms that suggest a herniated disc) is the "compression test." If cord involvement is suspected, a lower extremity neurologic exam and evaluation for long tract signs must also be performed. Signs of long tract dysfunction are positive Hoffman and Babinski tests (dorsiflexion of great toe and plantar flexion and splaying of lesser toes in response to plantar foot stimulation).

X-rays, if performed, are normal or show degenerative changes consistent with age. Occasionally narrowed disc space may be seen at the level of the herniation. It should be noted that athletes with a long history of being involved in collision sports have been shown to have a higher rate of x-ray abnormalities. These include "occult" fracture, vertebral compression fractures, disc-space narrowing, or other degenerative changes (9). Therefore, x-rays in these individuals must be interpreted with caution. An MRI may be done if there is a progressive or disabling deficit or no improvement in 4-6 weeks. The MRI is a very accurate test for disc herniation; however, one should be cautious in interpreting MRI in contact athletes and older individuals, as they have a high frequency of disc abnormalities, many of which can be asymptomatic. The patient's clinical findings must be correlated with MRI results.

Treatment for isolated acute disc herniation is usually nonoperative; 80% of isolated disc herniations will resolve with conservative therapy. A soft collar may be used for a few days. NSAIDs are used to reduce the inflammatory reaction around the herniated disc. If this fails and a neurologic deficit is present, oral steroids may be used. An epidural steroid injection, which deposits a high concentration of steroid at the site of inflammation, can be considered if motor findings are persisting despite conservative treatment. Physical therapy typically should start 10-14 days after the injury when acute symptoms have subsided. Progressive ROM exercises and isometric and, later, isotonic exercises are typically employed. Table 17-5 lists the indications for consultation with a spine specialist. In these situations, surgery may be considered.

Return to play may be considered when the athlete is asymptomatic, neck range of motion is full and painless, and neurologic exam is normal.

Table 17-5   When to Refer Athlete with Acute Cervical Disk Herniation

- Progressive neurological deficits
- Fracture
- Instability
- Muscle atrophy
- Myelopathy

Serious Neck Injury

Cervical spine fractures, subluxations, and dislocation can be devastating because they can damage the spinal cord, which is housed within the vertebral column. Sporting events are the fourth leading cause of spinal cord injury (behind motor vehicle accidents, violence, and falls). Sports typically associated with cord injury are football, wrestling, diving, and gymnastics. More recently, cord injuries have been seen from skiing, surfing, ice hockey (10), and trampoline.

The most common mechanism of injury is axial loading to the spine with a slightly flexed neck. This occurs when the athlete lowers his or her head and strikes an object with the crown of the head. The object could be another player or a stationary object, such as a wall, a goalpost, or the ground. Normally, maintaining a slight lordosis (concavity), which allows the neck muscles to absorb axial forces, protects the neck. However, in slight neck flexion of 30 degrees, the lordosis is lost (Figure 17-7). In this

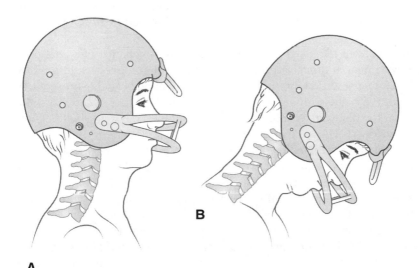

B

A

Figure 17-7   (A) When the neck is in the normal upright position, the cervical spine is slightly extended because of its natural lordosis. (B) When the neck is flexed slightly (to about 30 degrees), the cervical spine is straightened and converted into a segmented column.

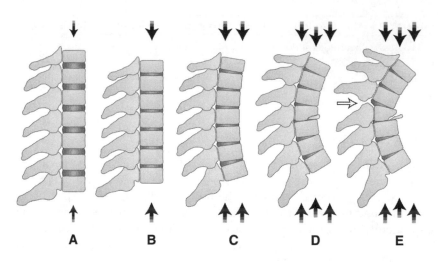

Figure 17-8   Biomechanically, the straight cervical spine responds to axial load force like a segmented column. Axial loading of the cervical spine first results in compressive deformation of the intervetebral disks (A & B). As energy input continues and maximum compressive deformation is reached, angular deformation and buckling occur. The spine fails in flexion mode (C) with resulting fracture, subluxation, or dislocation (D & E). Compressive deformation to failure with resulting fracture, dislocation, or subluxation occurs in as little as 8.4 msec.

straightened position, the spine is vulnerable to fracture and/or dislocation because axial loads cannot be dissipated (Figure 17-8). Less common mechanisms for serious neck injury are maximal forced flexion, extension, rotation, or side-bending of the neck.

The narrower the spinal canal, the greater is the chance of spinal cord injury with neck trauma. Furthermore, neurologic recovery is less likely after fracture-dislocation injuries if a narrow or stenotic canal is present (7).

In the 1960s and early 1970s, an increase in the number of cervical spine injuries in football were noted. This was around the time hard-shell helmets were developed. These helmets reduced head injuries but increased neck injuries. The improved helmets allowed tacklers to strike an opponent leading with the head, using the crown of the head as a battering ram. This "spearing" technique produces a significant axial load on the spine, leading to increase spinal injury. In the late 1970s and 1980s, rules were implemented to prohibit spearing and head-butting, resulting in a significant drop in the number of neck injuries and quadriplegia (11).

On-the-field evaluation and management are described below. As with cervical strains and sprains, the mechanism of injury causing fracture and/or dislocation includes excessive flexion, extension, bending, rotation, and compression, either alone or in some combination. Most injuries occur at the C4, C5, or C6 level, which can result in quadriplegia. Injuries at C1, C2, or C3 may result in death due to paralysis of the diaphragm. Athletes with documented spinal cord injury should receive high-dose methylpred-nisolone. A dose of 30 mg/kg within 8 hours of injury has been shown to have a positive effect on neurologic recovery (12). Some fractures have high association with cord injury and others do not. Some fractures are stable and only need immobilization with a neck collar; others are unstable and need surgical stabilization (13). The author suggests that a primary care physician refer all C-spine fractures, except the "clay shoveler's" fracture, to a spine specialist for appropriate treatment. Return to play decisions after serious neck injury are best made by the spine specialist.

Serious neck injury may be prevented in several ways. It is important to have properly trained clinicians covering athletic events. Instruction on proper tackling techniques and rules against checking and spearing can also reduce the incidence of injury. Strengthening of the neck muscle and use of neck collars may also provide protection. Before diving, water depth should be checked to be at least 10-12 feet.

On-the-Field Evaluation and Management

Physicians covering sporting events should prepare for handling a neck injury before the season begins. The necessary equipment should be readily available and fully functional, and the physician, certified athletic trainers, and other designated personnel should be proficient in its use. The sports medicine team should rehearse the protocols for head- or neck-injured athletes. The team physician usually is designated the leader of the team.

The usual scenario involves a player lying on the ground, unwilling or unable to get up. Any athlete suspected of having a head or spinal injury should not initially be moved, unless it is necessary to maintain airway, breathing, and circulation. Movement of the spine could injure or further injure the cord if a fracture or instability is present. When initially approaching the athlete, the physician must assess the "ABCs" (airway, breathing, and circulation). The most immediate threat to patients with spinal cord injuries at C3 or above is hypoxemia from apnea (14). In this instance, an airway must be established and breathing maintained. Emergency services are activated as soon as there is any suspicion of serious neck injury. If the athlete is lying on his or her back, a jaw thrust can also be used to clear the airway, allowing mouth-to-mouth resuscitation if a mask is not available. If not lying on the back, the athlete should be log-rolled onto the back, keeping the spine immobilized and moving the head and truck as a unit (Figure 17-9). If a helmet is on, it should be left in place and the faceguard should be removed with a bolt cutter or screwdriver, allowing access for respirations. The importance of not removing the helmet cannot be overemphasized, as the removal of a helmet from a football player with full pads will cause the head to fall into hyperextension, which may actually worsen the insult. Chest compressions must be performed if

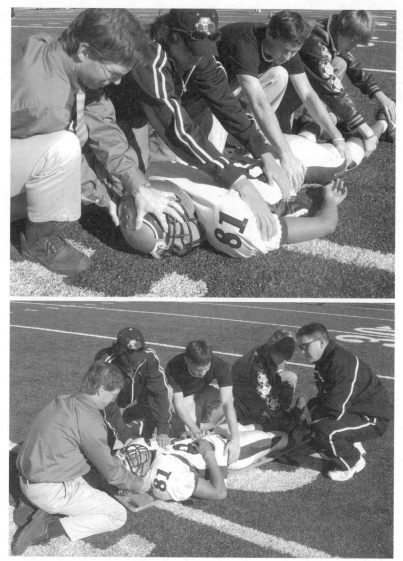

Figure 17-9   Handling the athlete with on-field neck injury utilizing the log-roll technique

there is no pulse. The fronts of the shoulder pads may be opened to allow access for chest compressions and defibrillation.

The vast majority of neck injuries are less serious, and the athlete is conscious and able to move. The physician must tell the athlete to lie still, however, to avoid further potential neck injury until the condition is assessed completely. Initial evaluation is directed to the possibility of a spinal cord injury. In addition to posterior neck pain, the player is asked about the ability to feel and move the extremities. Numbness, tingling, burning or weakness in the extremities may indicate cord injury. Next, a thorough neurologic exam is performed, including testing of reflexes and strength, tests of sensation to light touch and pinprick, and assessment of proprioception. The neck is examined for midline tenderness, swelling, and ecchymosis. Focal midline tenderness over the spinous processes may be from a neck strain/sprain, but one must assume it represents a vertebral fracture, subluxation, or dislocation, until proven otherwise.

If there is a possibility of cervical fracture or dislocation, the neck must be immobilized and the athlete transferred to a medical facility for radiographs. A rigid cervical collar is placed on the athlete and then he or she is placed on a backboard, keeping the spine in a neutral position. Lifting the injured athlete onto the board is best accomplished with at least four people working as a team. The head/helmet is additionally secured with bolsters or sandbags on each side and then taped or strapped to the board. Helmeted athletes should be immobilized with the helmet and shoulder pads left on to maintain neutral spine position (14). While these measures may seem extreme in some cases, missing the occasional cervical fracture or instability can be catastrophic.

Indications for radiographs for acute neck injury have been discussed earlier. The initial x-ray obtained in the emergency department is the cross-table lateral view of the cervical spine to include the C7-T1 junction. If no fracture or dislocation is present, anteroposterior and open-mouth odontoid views may be ordered. Flexion/extension and oblique views may be performed in certain circumstances. Advanced imaging (MRI and/or CT scanning) can be ordered.

Minor neck injuries with no extremity symptoms, no midline tenderness, and normal motor exam can be treated as a neck strain/sprain. Only athletes with full, painless cervical ROM and strength can be considered for return to play that day.

Case Study 17-2

A 20-year-old soccer player was tripped while running full speed and hit the goal post hard with the top of his head. He lay face down, complaining of severe neck pain. He was conscious, breathing and circulation were not compromised, and he was able to move his arms and legs. He was instructed to lie still. A neurological exam revealed no abnormalities. There was moderate midline tenderness in the posterior neck. He was placed into a rigid cervical collar and log-rolled onto his back by the medical personal, maintaining neutral position of the neck. He was then secured on a backboard and transferred to the local hospital via ambulance. X-rays revealed a displaced fracture of C4. The neurosurgical service took over his care at that point. He underwent surgical stabilization and had full recovery without neurological sequelae. A decision on return to play was made by the neurosurgeon.

REFERENCES

1. **Stiell IG, Wells GA, Vandemheen KL, et al.** The Canadian C-spine Rule for radiography in alert and stable trauma patients. JAMA. 2001;286:1841-8.

2. **Torg JS, Sennett B, Vegso JJ.** Axial loading injuries to the middle cervical spine segment: an analysis and classification of twenty-five cases. Am J Sports Med. 1991;19:6-20.

3. **Cantu RC, Micheli IJ.** Criteria for return to competition after head or cervical spine injury. In: Cantu RC, Micheli LJ, eds. ACSM's Guidelines for the Team Physician. Philadelphia: Lea & Febiger; 1991:205-8.

4. **Torg JS, Naranja RJ, Pavlov H.** The relationship of developmental narrowing of the cervical spinal canal to reversible and irreversible injury of the cervical spinal cord in football players: an epidemiological study. J Bone Joint Surg Am. 1996; 78:1308-14.

5. **Cantu RC.** The cervical spinal stenosis controversy. Clin Sports Med. 1998;17:122-6.

6. **Torg JS, Ramsey-Emrhein JA.** Suggested management guidelines for participation in collision activities with congenital, developmental or postinjury lesions involving the cervical spine. Med Sci Sports Exerc. 1997;29:S256-72.

7. **Miller MD.** Clinics in Sports Medicine: Head and Neck Injuries in Sports Medicine. Philadelphia: WB Saunders; 2003:22.

8. **Cantu RC, Bailes JE, Wilberger JE.** Guidelines for return to contact or collision sport after a cervical spine injury. Clin Sports Med. 1998;17:137-46.

9. **DeLee JC, Drez D.** Orthopaedic Sports Medicine: Principles and Practice. Philadelphia: WB Saunders; 1994:429-30.

10. **Davis PM, McKelvey MK.** Medicolegal aspects of athletic cervical spine injury. Clin Sports Med. 1998;17:147-54.

11. **Torg JS, Vegso JJ, Sennett B.** The national football head and neck injury registry: 14-year report on cervical quadriplegia (1971-1984). Clin Sports Med. 1987;6:61-72.

12. **Steinberg GG, Akins CM, Baran DT.** Orthopaedics in Primary Care, 2nd ed. Baltimore: Williams & Wilkins; 1992:24.

13. **Arendt EA.** Orthopaedic Knowledge Update: Sports Medicine 2. Rosement, IL: American Academy of Orthopaedic Surgeons; 1999:400.

14. **Chiles BW, Cooper PR.** Acute spinal injury: current concepts. N Engl J Med. 1996;334:514-20.

18

■ ■ ■

Shoulder Disorders

Michael J. Milne, MD

houlder symptoms are some of the most common in sports medicine. The number of active patients with shoulder injuries may range from 4%-8%. Primary care physicians can use historical clues that may help in diagnosis. For example, an athlete who performs repetitive overhead activities such as pitching or overhead serving in volleyball or tennis may be at risk for impingement syndrome. Simple physical exam maneuvers explained in this chapter can further delineate the chief complaint. Once the problem is identified, a structured rehabilitation program can be developed that allows the patient expedient return to his or her sport. Orthopedic referral may be necessary in some situations to restore normal anatomy and function.

Anatomy

The shoulder is composed of four distinct articulations: the glenohumeral joint, the acromioclavicular joint, the sternoclavicular joint, and the scapulothoracic articulation (Figure 18-1). Three bones interface in these joints: the scapula, clavicle, and humerus.

The glenohumeral joint has the greatest degree of freedom of motion of any joint in the human body. Although the glenohumeral joint is often regarded as a ball-and-socket joint, it more resembles a ball-and-saucer joint, because only approximately one-third of the humeral head is covered by the glenoid.

The glenohumeral joint derives its stability from static and dynamic constraints. Static constraints include bony architecture, glenoid labrum (which increases the concavity and surface area of the glenoid), negative intraarticular pressure, ligamentous structures (superior, middle, and inferior glenohumeral ligaments), and capsule. Dynamic constraints include

Shoulder

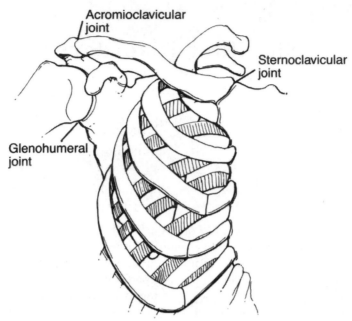

Figure 18-1 Articulations of the shoulder joint. (From Delee's Orthopedic Sports Medicine. Philadelphia: WB Saunders; 1994; Chapter 15; with permission.)

rotator cuff musculature (supraspinatus, infraspinatus, teres minor, and subscapularis), scapular musculature, and long head of the biceps (intraarticular attachment to the superior glenoid labrum) (Figures 18-2 and 18-3).

The acromioclavicular joint consists of the acromioclavicular ligaments and capsule (which cross the joint), the coracoclavicular ligaments, and an intraarticular disc. The acromioclavicular ligaments primarily constraint anteroposterior translation. The coracoclavicular ligaments constrain inferior displacement of the acromion relative to the clavicle.

The sternoclavicular joint has a similar intraarticular disc to the AC joint. Dislocations and fractures of this joint are uncommon. The scapulothoracic articulation is the articulation of the undersurface of the scapula and the chest wall. Several bursa and muscular attachments become important in shoulder movement and physical diagnosis.

History

Like most diagnoses in medicine, a careful history and physical examination can diagnose most shoulder complaints. In the shoulder, the most important initial facts are chief complaint and patient age.

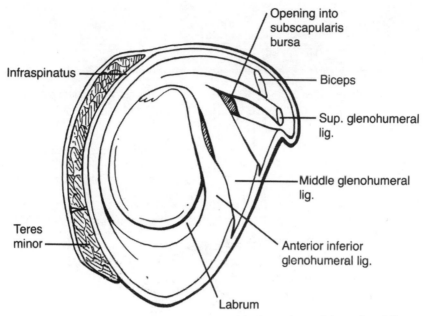

Figure 18-2 Static stabilizers of the ligamentous labral complex and dynamic stabilizers of the rotator cuff. (From Delee's Orthopedic Sports Medicine. Philadelphia: WB Saunders; 1994; Chapter 15; with permission.)

It is crucial to identify the patient's chief complaint: pain, stiffness, instability, weakness, swelling, deformity, paresthesias, or functional disability. Identifying the chief complaint usually is fairly straightforward, yet the patient may report combinations of the above, making diagnosis more difficult.

Pain as a chief complaint is common in both acute and chronic injuries. A description of pain must be elucidated to determine quality of pain (sharp, aching, radiating, and so forth), and degree of pain by using the visual analogue scale (i.e., a grading scale used to objectively quantify the level of pain). Pain at night or chronic pain with overhead activity can be consistent with rotator cuff pathology. This condition is often seen in the dominant shoulder of middle-aged to older individuals. Rotator cuff pathology is often seen in overhead athletes (for example, baseball pitchers). In the presence of night pain and/or constitutional symptoms, neoplasm and infection must be ruled out.

Stiffness as a chief complaint can be the result of true mechanical blocks or pain-related inhibition. Physical examination and specific testing (including impingement testing and selective injections) can help differentiate mechanical symptoms and pain-related inhibition. These tests are described later in this chapter.

Instability is a common complaint in the shoulder. Patients will report that the shoulder "slides in and out" or that they are afraid to throw a

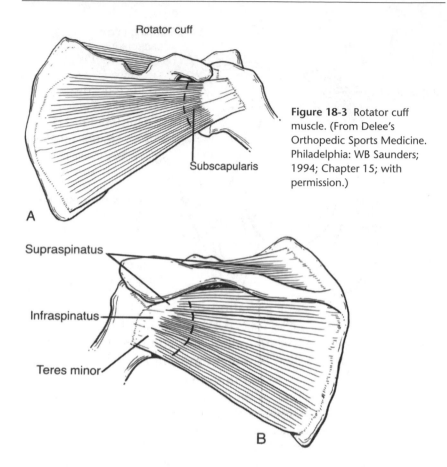

Rotator cuff

Subscapularis

Figure 18-3 Rotator cuff muscle. (From Delee's Orthopedic Sports Medicine. Philadelphia: WB Saunders; 1994; Chapter 15; with permission.)

A

Supraspinatus

Infraspinatus

Teres minor

B

ball for fear of dislocation or subluxation. Important considerations in evaluating shoulder instability include degree (frank dislocation versus subluxation), onset (traumatic versus atraumatic), chronicity (multiple dislocations, length of symptoms), direction (anterior, posterior, inferior, or multidirectional), and disability (how much the problem affects the patient's life). Instability as a chief complaint is often seen in football or hockey players or in the general population who slip and fall on an outstretched or abducted arm. Chronic instability is a common complaint seen in swimmers.

Weakness in the shoulder is a common complaint. Weakness is caused by true musculotendinous deficiency or neurologic deficiency. By far, the most common cause of weakness in the shoulder in the older population is rotator cuff tears. There is often prodromal tendinitis or a history of trauma in this presentation. Neurological weakness can be caused peripherally (by cervical root impingement or peripheral nerve impingement) or centrally (by upper motor neuron deficiency; for example, stroke or multiple sclerosis).

Swelling around the shoulder can be associated with acute injury or with infection or inflammation. The chronicity, location, and degree can help in the diagnosis. Spontaneous, painless swelling can be associated with neoplasm or systemic inflammatory disease. *Deformity* is a less common presenting complaint. It can be the result of congenital causes or related to previous trauma, metabolic disorder, infection, neoplasm, or degenerative joint disease. *Paresthesias* may be noted in patients with cervical root compression syndromes or in the multidirectional instability patient with no root compression.

Functional disabilities may be noted in the athlete or laborer. Factory workers may state that they cannot do their job all day without breaks like they used to or pitchers may report lost velocity. The degree of the disability must therefore be expressed as it may affect therapeutic options.

Physical Examination

A thorough physical examination is required and is correlated with the patient's history. It is important to complete a thorough examination of the cervical spine first as several C-spine problems can produce shoulder symptoms.

Observation alone can yield important diagnostic clues, including muscle atrophy, deformity, and position. The shoulder should be adequately exposed for a complete examination. The patient should be asked to point to the location of pain with one finger. The examiner can then distinguish the anatomic origin (i.e., acromioclavicular joint, lateral insertion of the rotator cuff, or impingement syndrome).

Palpation can yield tenderness (acromioclavicular joint and rotator cuff footprint) and deformity (AC separations, clavicle fractures and glenohumeral dislocation). Range-of-motion and translational testing is performed and compared with the contralateral shoulder. Normal range of motion is 160 degrees of forward flexion, 45-70 degrees of external rotation (elbow at side), and internal rotation to the T6 vertebra (thumb).

Translational testing is also compared to the contralateral side. This is performed with the patient seated with the examiner standing behind the patient. With the arm in a resting position and the elbow flexed, the examiner stabilizes the scapula with one hand and inferiorly translates the humerus with downward traction on the upper arm.

Anterior and posterior translational testing is performed again by stabilizing the scapula and applying anterior and posterior forces to the humeral head. The patient should be instructed to report sensations similar to instability symptoms, pain, or apprehension during translational testing.

Muscle strength testing is important to elucidate deltoid, biceps, and rotator cuff muscle problems. The examiner should test the strength of both the affected and contralateral side for comparison.

Deltoid Testing

Abduction of the arm in three planes can delineate anterior, middle, or posterior one-third deltoid weakness. This is performed by asking the patient to abduct his or her arms at 30 degrees forward of neutral, at neutral, and 10 degrees posterior of neutral.

Biceps Testing

Biceps testing includes Speed's test and supination strength. Speed's test is performed with resisted elevation of the arm with the palm up (full supination). Pain in the shoulder is a positive test. Yergason's test is resisted supination with the elbow at 90 degrees and the arm at the side. Again, shoulder pain is a positive result. One can also palpate over the long head of the biceps to appreciate subluxation during resisted supination. It is important to remember that the biceps is the most powerful supination muscle in the arm.

Rotator Cuff Testing

The physician may begin with testing for range of motion. Decreased motion with forward flexion, abduction, or internal or external rotation may indicate adhesive capuslitis, apprehension secondary to pain (for example, rotator cuff or subacromial inflammation) or weakness such as that seen in rotator cuff tears. Strength testing may be useful in assessing rotator cuff pathology. External rotation tests the infraspinatous and teres minor muscle groups. Internal rotation tests the subscapularis muscle. Testing the supraspinatous against resistance is performed by having the patient place both arms at 90 degrees of abduction and 30 degrees of forward flexion. The patient should turn his or her thumbs down (as if emptying a can) and resist a downward force by the physician. Weakness is a positive *empty-can test* and can symbolize rotator cuff tendinitis or a frank tear.

Provocative tests may help further delineate rotator cuff pathology (Table 18-1). The *drop-arm test* is performed by asking the patient to fully abduct the arm to 180 degrees and slowly lower it to his or her side. A positive test occurs if the patient "drops" the arm the last 60 degrees of the arc. This may signify a rotator cuff tear. The *impingement sign* is defined as pain that occurs when the arm is passively forward flexed greater than 90 degrees (Figure 18-4). A positive test may signify subacromial inflammation such as that seen with rotator cuff tears or subacromial bursitis (that is, impingement syndrome). Another well-accepted test for impingement syndrome is the *Hawkins test*. In this test, the arm is passively flexed to 90 degrees and internally rotated (Figure 18-5). Pain is interpreted as a positive test and results from the greater tuberosity of the humerus and the rotator cuff tendons impinging on the undersurface of the acromion. The

Table 18-1   Rotator Cuff Testing

Test	Designed to Test	Comments
Impingement sign	Subacromial space inflammation (rotator cuff tear or bursitis)	Hawkins test also used to test for impingement syndrome
Impingement test	Subacromial space inflammation after an injection	Relief of pain without restoration in strength is considered positive and may indicate rotator cuff tear
Drop-arm test	Rotator cuff muscle strength	Positive test may indicate major rotator cuff tear
Empty-can test	Supraspinatus muscle strength	Weakness may indicate tendinitis or frank tear

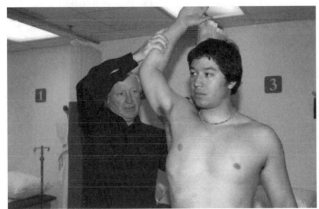

Figure 18-4
Impingement sign test.

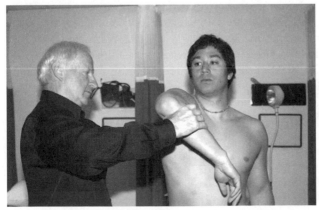

Figure 18-5 Hawkins test.

Impingement test is a diagnostic maneuver used to help distinguish rotator cuff tear from subacromial bursitis. The technique for diagnositic/therapeutic injection in the subacromial space is described later in this chapter. A positive impingement test is defined as pain that disappears partially or fully when the impingement sign is repeated after the anesthetic injection. If strength testing is performed and pain does not return after the injection, this may also be considered a positive test. Longstanding tendinitis may produce a false-positive. No pain relief is a negative impingement test. A positive test may signify a rotator cuff tear, which generally requires orthopedic consultation.

Other Tests

Like the impingement test and impingement sign, the apprehension and relocation tests are related. These tests are designed to test instability in the glenohumeral joint. The apprehension test is performed with the patient supine on the exam table with the affected shoulder near the edge of the table. The arm is passively flexed to 90 degrees and externally rotated to 90 degrees (throwing position) plus/minus anterior force on the proximal humerus (Figure 18-6, *A*). Visible apprehension on the patient's face or the report of "fear of dislocation" defines a positive result (Figure 18-6, *B*). With the relocation test, the arm is passively flexed and externally rotated to the same position as in the apprehension test but with a posterior force placed on the proximal humerus (Figure 18-7). Relief of apprehension defines a positive result and correlates with anterior instability.

The posterior apprehension test is performed again with the patient in a supine position on the examination table. The arm is passively flexed to 90 degrees and internally rotated. A posterior force is then placed through the flexed elbow. Again, visible or verbal apprehension of posterior subluxation or dislocation is a positive result and correlates with posterior instability.

Two tests have been accepted to correlate with subscapularis rupture or insufficiency. They are the lift-off test and the belly-press test. The lift-off test is easily performed during examination of range of motion. When testing internal rotation, the patient slides the dorsum of the hand up the spine and touches the highest spinous process possible. Afterward, it is easy to have the patient slide his or her hand down to the belt line. By stabilizing the elbow with one hand and asking the patient to lift his or her hand posteriorly off the back against the examiner's hand, the examiner can test competency and strength of the subscapularis muscle/tendon (Figure 18-8). Similarly, the belly-press test is performed with the patient seated or standing. The examiner asks the patient to place both hands just below the chest, palms down with the fingers interlaced. The examiner then asks the patient to bring both elbows forward. Asymmetric movement can point to a subscapularis insufficiency (Figure 18-9). The belly-press test is sometimes done with one hand.

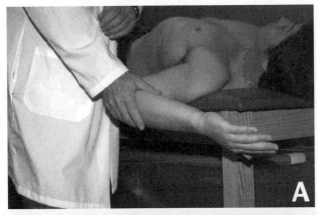

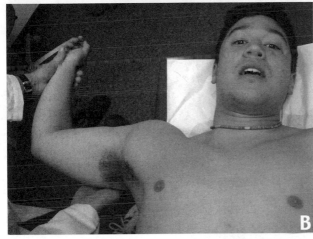

Figure 18-6
Apprehension test.

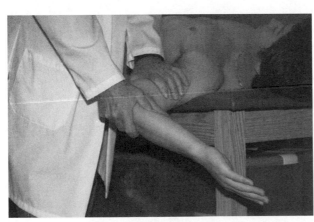

Figure 18-7 Relocation test.

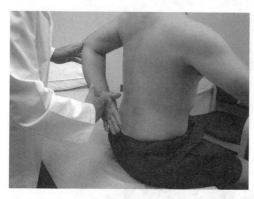

Figure 18-8 Lift-off test.

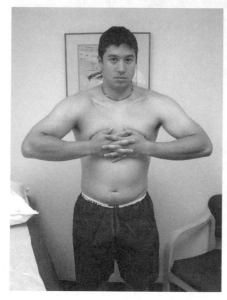

Figure 18-9 Belly-press test.

Acromioclavicular and/or arthritis pain can be elicited on physical examination by performing the crossed-arm adduction test. This is performed with the patient seated and the arm passively flexed to 90 degrees and adducted fully across the chest. This test loads the AC joint and is positive with pain. An AC joint injection with lidocaine (discussed later in this chapter) can be performed and the crossed-arm adduction test repeated to further confirm the AC joint as a source of the patient's pain.

Biceps tendinitis is also a significant cause of shoulder pain. Tenderness to palpation at or proximal to the biceps groove on the proximal humerus can direct an examiner to biceps tendinitis as a contributing factor to a patient's shoulder pain. Two tests, Speed's test and Yergason's test (discussed earlier in this chapter), have been accepted to correlate well with this diagnosis.

Imaging Studies

Radiographic evaluation of the shoulder begins with plain radiographs. The basic trauma series includes anteroposterior of the glenohumeral joint and axillary lateral view. Most fractures around the shoulder, glenohumeral dislocations, and glenohumeral arthritis may be visualized with these two views.

Other, special radiographic views can help delineate subacromial spurring, Bankart lesions on the glenoid (depression fracture of the glenoid or separation of the labrum from the glenoid), Hill-Sachs lesions (impression fractures) of the humeral head, sternoclavicular injuries, and AC arthritis/osteolysis.

CT scanning is helpful in fracture classification and in detecting bony changes as in Bankart lesions and Hill-Sachs lesions. Most of its use is seen in the acute injury phase. These imaging exams are helpful in decision-making regarding operative intervention versus rehabilitation. CT scans are an excellent means of detecting bony injury and should be ordered in the face of a grossly unstable glenohumeral joint (for example, a joint that dislocates easily or during sleep).

MR imaging has become a common test when rotator cuff or intracapsular abnormalities (SLAP [superior labrum anterior posterior] lesion, labral pathology, biceps tendonopathy) are suspected. Image quality, MRI techniques, and radiologist interpretation have become more refined over the last several years, making subtle findings more frequent. The use of arthrography has declined over the last 5-10 years, but MR arthrography has become more useful.

Case Study 18-1

A 26-year-old football player presented with left shoulder pain. He stated that 2 weeks ago he was tackling an opponent while his left arm was outstretched and abducted. His arm bent backwards as he missed the tackle, and his shoulder "came out of its socket" but then went back in. Since that time, he has had pain when raising his arm, and he is worried that his shoulder will come out again.

On physical examination, the patient had near full range of motion with pain at the extremes. Skin was intact. Impingement sign was negative. Apprehension test and relocation test results were positive. He was neurologically intact.

Radiographic evaluation revealed positive anterior/inferior Bankart lesion and Hill-Sachs lesion on the humerus.

Advanced imaging was considered given his x-ray findings. Because Bankart lesions are commonly associated with labral pathology, MRI was chosen to evaluate the labrum. This athlete likely suffered a dislocation with spontaneous reduction. The insult of the dislocation resulted in glenohumeral labral injury. The patient was referred to an orthopedist who performed labral repair surgery.

Specific Disorders

Instability

Instability presents as a chief complaint in one of two ways. First, the patient reports a history of trauma (that is, falling during a football game or off of a ladder) and a frank dislocation. The patient has sought medical treatment, including reduction of the dislocated shoulder. Second, the patient may give a history of pain, especially with certain movements. A typical history may include feeling the shoulder slide in and out while lifting boxes or when the arm is placed in certain positions. This sliding is more commonly referred to as subluxation.

One of the most common complaints about the shoulder, instability can severely limit the strength and function of the affected extremity. The glenohumeral joint, because of its architecture, has the least static constraints in the body. Much of the stability of the shoulder is derived from the rotator cuff muscles and the glenohumeral ligaments. The glenohumeral joint is also the most commonly dislocated joint.

Instability can be divided into frank dislocations and subluxations. A good way to determine which is the cause of the patient's complaint is to ask the patient if they have ever had to go to the hospital or have someone "put their shoulder in." A majority of true dislocations are anterior. These are most common in sports injuries (for example, contact sports like football and hockey) and falls. The mechanism of injury is usually collision or fall on an abducted or extended arm. Posterior dislocations can also be seen in acute injuries (rare) but are most commonly associated with seizures. Acutely, axillary lateral radiographs must be performed to define anterior and posterior dislocation before relocation is attempted. The pneumonic TUBS can help one remember the typical dislocation pattern seen in younger patients: Traumatic, Unilateral (usually anterior), Bankart lesion, Surgery. A redislocation rate between 65%-90% has been reported in younger patients with nonoperative management. Similarly, a pneumonic for chronic shoulder instability is AMBRI: Atraumatic, Multidirectional, Bilateral shoulder involvement, Rehabilitation, and Inferior capsular shift (if necessary).

Important associated injuries with dislocations include axillary nerve injuries, rotator cuff tears, and tuberosity fractures.

Shoulder instability may be treated with rotator cuff strengthening programs. If conservative therapies fail or if dislocations recur, orthopedic referral may be useful.

Impingement Syndrome

Impingement typically presents in patients over 50 years old (or manual laborers) as pain in the dominant shoulder with overhead movements or while sleeping. By age 65, most people will have rotator cuff tears identifiable by MRI. Rotator cuff tears causing impingement syndrome may present as shoulder weakness and pain. However, most of these tears are asymptomatic. Rotator cuff pathology has been associated with acromial spurring, decreased subacromial space, older populations, throwing athletes, and repetitive overhead activity.

Bigliani has categorized acromion morphology into three types. Type I are flat, type II have a downward slope, and type III are hooked. Type II and III acromions have been associated with impingement syndrome.

The supraspinatus tendon is the most commonly torn rotator cuff tendon. Larger tears can extend into the infraspinatus or subscapularis. Physical examination findings include a positive drop arm test and weakness in the "thumbs down" position (empty can test).

Small or partial thickness rotator cuff tears can be treated nonoperatively. Common treatment modalities include physical therapy for rotator cuff strengthening, activity modification, anti-inflammatory medications, and subacromial corticosteroid injections. Arthroscopic decompression and rotator cuff repair may be performed for larger tears or when nonoperative measures have failed. Impingement syndrome without a rotator cuff tear may be treated conservatively with NSAIDs and structured physical therapy. Occasionally, a therapeutic injection may help relieve pain and allow therapy to begin earlier.

Case Study 18-2

A 56-year-old right-hand-dominant male who works as a heavy machinery mechanic complained of right shoulder pain. He stated that the pain had increased over the last 3 months. He complained of pain with overhead activity. NSAIDs seemed to make the pain better. On physical examination, the skin was intact bilaterally. Forward flexion was painful beyond 140 degrees. Impingement sign and Hawkins tests were positive. He had a negative drop arm test and no weakness with other rotator cuff muscle strength testing. On x-ray, type II acromion was identified. No glemohumeral arthrosis was found.

A diagnosis of impingement syndrome was made. The patient underwent 2 weeks of limited overhead activity at work and therapy with over-the-counter NSAIDs. At his return visit, his symptoms had improved somewhat but had not resolved. He then had a therapeutic injection of corticosteroids in the subacromial space and was enrolled in a structured physical therapy program with gradual return to full duty at work.

Labral Tears at the Biceps Anchor

The long head of the biceps is intracapsular in the glenohumeral joint. It attaches to the superior glenoid labrum at the 12 o'clock position. In the early 1990s, the superior labrum and biceps tendon were identified as a source of pain in the shoulder, primarily in throwing athletes. The SLAP lesion was identified by Snyder and colleagues to be a source of shoulder pain. It is suspected in the overhead athlete or laborer who describes vague shoulder pain that increases with activity. With this lesion, there is tearing and separation at superior labrum at the biceps attachment (biceps anchor). Six types of SLAP lesions have been identified, and their treatment ranges from rest, physical therapy, NSAIDs, and icing to arthroscopic stabilization.

Acromioclavicular Joint

The two most common disorders of the acromioclavicular (AC) joint are separations ("shoulder separation") and arthritis. AC separations are the result of trauma and usually occur with a fall or direct blow to the superior aspect of the shoulder. Patients will have pain over the AC joint and often palpable dislocation of the distal clavicle. AC arthritis is a repetitive-load type injury often seen in heavy weight lifters and laborers.

AC separations have been classified into six types based on displacement and injured structures. Type I consists of AC sprain with no displacement seen on radiographs. Type II AC separation consists of tearing of the AC ligaments and capsule with intact coracoclavicular ligaments (conoid and trapezoid). On radiographs, the acromion is displaced 50%-100% downward from the distal clavicle. Treatment for types I and II consists of protection, analgesics, and physical therapy. The type III AC separation requires disruption of both the AC and CC ligaments. Currently, surgical versus nonsurgical treatment for the type III separation is debated. Most surgeons are opting for nonoperative treatment, at least in the acute phase. Types IV, V, and VI are more severe injuries and usually require early operative intervention.

AC arthritis is common in the face of previous trauma and in older patients, laborers, and athletes. Diagnosis can be made by a positive crossed-arm adduction test, joint space narrowing on plain radiographs, and tenderness to palpation of the joint. Treatment options include corticosteroid injections and arthroscopic or open distal clavicle excision, often in conjunction with subacromial decompression. Distal clavicle osteolysis (that is, a disappearing bone at the distal end of the clavicle on a plain radiograph) can be seen primarily in weight lifters. Treatment includes activity modification and/or distal clavicle excision.

Disorders of the Biceps Tendon

Biceps tendinitis is common. Anterior shoulder pain and pain with lifting are often chief complaints. Physical examination findings include tenderness at or above the bicipital groove and positive Speed's and Yergason's tests. NSAIDs and activity modification are the mainstay of nonoperative treatment. Arthroscopic debridement, release, or tenodesis lead to complete relief in a majority of patients who fail nonoperative treatment options.

Biceps subluxation refers to subluxation from the bicipital groove, which is often associated with subscapularis rupture. The tendon usually is released or tenodesed, often in conjunction with supscapularis repair.

Adhesive Capsulitis

Often referred to as "frozen shoulder," adhesive capsulitis is common in diabetics and after shoulder injury or surgery (that is, immobilization). It may also be associated with rotator cuff tears, neoplasms, systemic diseases, and/or autoimmune disorders. The findings are pain and restricted range of motion. The condition is usually self-limited with three phases. The first phase is characterized by diffuse pain about the shoulder. Second phase findings include continued pain and decreased range of motion. The third phase is sometimes referred to as "thawing." In this phase, there is gradual return of function and range of motion. This process can last as long as 14 months. Adjunctive therapeutic aids can include NSAIDs, physical therapy, modalities such as ultrasound, iontophoresis (administered by a physical therapist), and occasionally manipulation under anesthetic, and/or arthroscopic releases.

Injection Treatments

Subacromial Injection

After obtaining informed consent, including risks of infection, neurovascular damage, hypopigmentation of the skin, allergic reaction, and fatty necrosis of the skin, position the patient seated on the examination table to allow access to the entire shoulder region. The first step in subacromial injection is to palpate and identify the clavicle, AC joint, and acromion. Perform a sterile prep with betadyne or an equivalent sterile scrub. Prepare one 3 ml syringe with 1% lidocaine. Palpate the anterior corner of the acromion and drop anterolateral to this landmark 1-2 cm. Using a 25-27-gauge syringe, instill the lidocaine into this area. After allowing time for the analgesic to set up, prepare a second syringe (10 ml) with 3 ml 1% li-docaine, 3 ml 0.25% marcaine, and 3 ml triamcinolone acetonide (corticos-teroid). Using a $1^1/_2$-inch, 22-gauge needle, instill this solution under the acromion into the subacromial space. It is important to bathe the rotator cuff insertion with the injection but *not* inject the tendon itself. Finish by cleaning the area and placing a small bandage on it. Many favor a posterior or anterior approach, but the present author finds this approach the most direct and reproducible in ensuring proper placement of the injection.

After the injection is completed, perform the impingement test by asking the patient to move the shoulder around and describe his or her im-provement. A helpful way to quantify this is to ask: "Is it 25%, 50%, 75%, or 90% better, or is there no change?" This information is then documented in the record. Because of the combination of local analgesics and corticos-teroids, this injection has both diagnostic and therapeutic value.

Acromioclavicular Joint Injection

After obtaining informed consent, as above, position the patient again to allow access to the entire shoulder. The first step in acromioclavicular joint injection is to palpate the clavicle, acromion, and spine of the scapula. The AC joint will lie directly anterior to the point where the spine of the scapula and the distal clavicle meet. After a sterile betadyne prep, as with the sub-acromial injection, prepare one 3 ml syringe with 1.5 ml 1% lidocaine and 1.5 ml triamcinolone acetonide (corticosteroid). Standing directly in front of the patient, use a 22-gauge syringe to enter the capsule of the AC joint di-rectly from above. The joint has an even smaller volume when arthritic, and 3 ml total is the maximal amount to be injected. Clean the area and place a small bandage on it.

Test the relief that this injection provides by repeating the crossed-arm adduction test after a few minutes. Ask the patient to classify the relief as zero, 25%, 50%, 75%, or 90% improvement, and document the result.

SELECTED READING

Caborn DM, Fu FH. Arthoscopic approach and anatomy of the shoulder. Op Tech Orthop. 1991;1:126-33.

Cooper DE, O'Brien SJ, Warren RF. Supporting layers of the glenohumeral joint: an Anatomic Study. Clin. Orthop. 1993;289:144-55.

Gartsman GM. Arthrscopic management of rotator cuff disease. J Am Acad Orthop Surg. 1998;6:259-66.

Iannotti JP, Gabriel JP, Schneck SL, et al. The normal glenohumeral relationships: an anatomic study of 140 shoulders. J Bone Joint Surg Am. 1992;74:491-500.

Neer CS, Welch RP. The shoulder in sports. Orthop Clin North Am. 1977;8:583-91.

Rockwood CA, Lyons FR. Shoulder impingement syndrome: diagnosis, radiographic evaluation, and treatment with a modified Neer acromioplasty. J Bone Joint Surg Am. 1993;75:409-24.

Snyder SJ, Karzel RP, Del Pizzo W, et al. SLAP lesions of the shoulder. Arthroscopy. 1990;6:274-9.

Warner JJP, Greis PE. Frozen shoulder: diagnosis and management. J Am Acad Orthop Surg. 1997;5:183-91.

Zebas CJ, Loudon K, Chapman M, et al. Musculoskeletal injuries in a college-age population during a one-semester term. J Am Coll Health. 1995;44:32-4.

19

■ ■ ■

Elbow Injuries

John P. Jamison, MD

njuries to the elbow in the athlete can be divided into traumatic and atraumatic (or overuse) types. Traumatic injuries, such as fracture, dislocation, and tendon rupture, are common in the nonathletic population as well. Overuse injuries, including medial tension overload, lateral compression injuries, and epicondylitis, most frequently are seen in the athletic population, and it is this latter group of injuries that has received the most attention in recent years. Advances in the diagnosis and treatment of overuse injuries, particularly in the overhead-throwing athlete, have extended the careers of these players significantly.

Anatomy

The bony anatomy of the elbow consists of the distal humerus, which articulates with the radial head, and the proximal ulna (Figure 19-1). The medial compartment consists of the articulation between the humerus and the ulna, and the lateral compartment consists of the articulation between the humerus and the radial head. The ulnohumeral joint is one of the most congruous joints in the body. The olecranon locks into the olecranon fossa in extension, and the radial head and coronoid process lock into their fossae in full flexion. This makes the elbow quite intolerant to abnormal motions (1). Medial stability is provided by the medial collateral ligament (MCL) complex, which consists of the anterior bundle, the posterior bundle, and the transverse ligaments (Figure 19-2, C). This is also sometimes referred to as the ulnar collateral ligament complex (UCL). The anterior bundle is the primary restraint to valgus instability (2). The lateral collateral ligament (LCL) complex, which consists of the lateral ulnar collateral ligament, radial collateral ligament, and annular ligament, provides lateral stability (Figure 19-2, *B*). These structures blend into a complex of interdependent fibers.

Muscles attaching to the lateral epicondyle of the elbow include the extensor carpi radialis brevis (ECRB), the extensor carpi radialis longus, extensor digitorum communis, and extensor carpi ulnaris. The ECRB is most

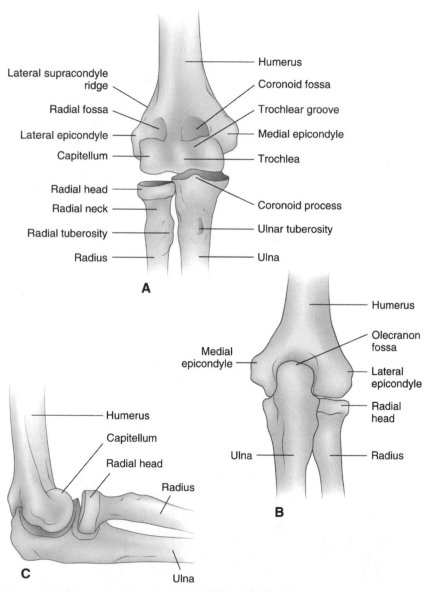

Figure 19-1   Anatomy of the elbow. (A) Anterior view. (B) Posterior view. (C) Lateral view.

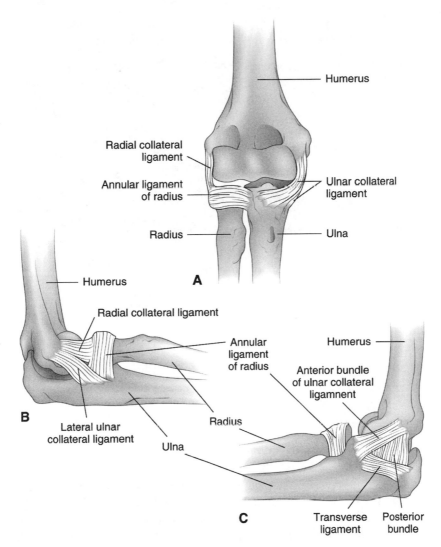

Figure 19-2 Ligaments of the elbow. (A) Anterior view. (B) Lateral collateral ligament (LCL) complex. (C) Medial collateral ligament (MCL) complex.

commonly implicated in "tennis elbow." The medial epicondyle serves as the origin of the flexor-pronator mass, consisting of the pronator teres, the flexor carpi radialis, and the flexor carpi ulnaris. The ulnar nerve passes posterior to the medial epicondyle in the ulnar groove (Figure 19-3).

Biomechanics of Throwing

The motion used in pitching in baseball has been thoroughly evaluated and has been broken down into several phases to facilitate understanding of

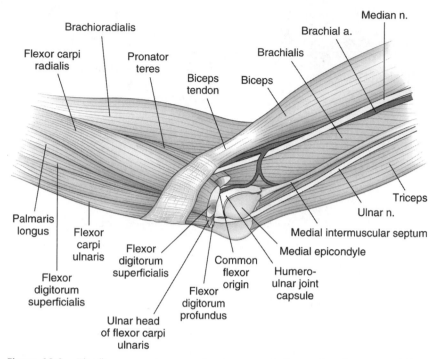

Figure 19-3 The flexor-pronator group has been resected, revealing the course of the ulnar nerve as it runs around the medial epicondyle, passing distally before entering the plane between the flexor carpi ulnaris and the flexor digitorum profundus.

the motion. These phases include windup, early cocking, late cocking, arm acceleration, arm deceleration, and follow-through. Video and EMG analyses have shown that the elbow is maintained at about 85 degrees of flexion during windup and cocking. It then extends at a rate of approximately 2300 degrees per second during early acceleration to a position of 20 degrees of flexion at the time of ball release. Elite pitchers can generate forces as high as 100 to 120 N•m between late cocking and acceleration. The primary restraint to these forces is the anterior band of the MCL. EMG studies have shown very limited capacity for the surrounding muscles to provide stability in the absence of an intact MCL (3-6). The same motion that puts tension on the medial structures of the elbow also places the lateral structures such as the capitellum and radial head under high compressive forces (Figure 19-4). High forces are also generated in the posterior elbow during the acceleration and deceleration phases of throwing. Analogous forces are generated during other sports activities such as serving a tennis ball, golf, or volleyball.

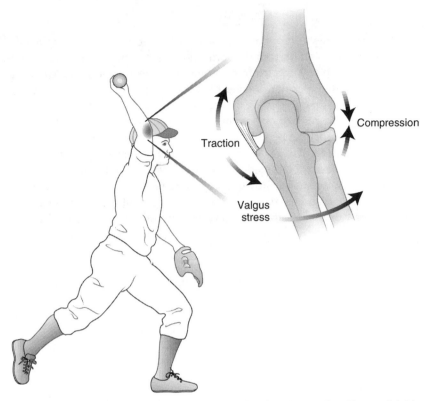

Figure 19-4   The forces about the elbow during the throwing motion. The medial side of the elbow experiences tensile forces and the lateral side experiences compressive forces.

Medial Collateral Ligament Injuries

Loss of MCL function is a debilitating injury for the throwing athlete. The vast majority of these injuries are caused by repetitive overload rather than by a sudden event. The athlete usually is involved in a sport requiring repetitive overhead activities. Onset of pain typically is insidious, and the development of pain with even moderate throwing effort is highly suggestive of attenuation of the MCL. The patient may report a feeling of instability during throwing that prevents maximum effort. Chronic cases may be associated with symptoms of locking or catching associated with loose body formation. Rarely, acute rupture may occur that is characterized by a "pop" and a sudden sharp pain at the medial side of the elbow. MCL injuries are sometimes associated with stretching of the ulnar nerve, resulting in paresthesias in the ulnar two digits (6,7).

Case Study 19-1

A 15-year-old high school quarterback developed pain on the medial side of his elbow on his throwing arm three games into the season. He did not reveal his symptoms to his trainer or coach, because he feared losing his starting position. He did not have symptoms of numbness or tingling in his arm or hand. He was able to play through the pain.

During a midweek practice session, he attempted to throw a long pass and felt a painful pop on the medial side of his elbow. He rapidly developed swelling and was unable to continue throwing. X-rays revealed an avulsion of the medial epicondyle of the distal humerus with moderate displacement. Growth plates were not yet closed. He underwent reduction and fixation of the avulsed fragment with a screw approximately one week after the injury. His fracture healed uneventfully, and he was able to return to throwing activities 3 months post-op.

Physical examination begins with range-of-motion testing. Loss of extension may be present due to anterior capsular contracture or posterior compartment impingement. Osteophytes may form at the tip of the olecranon due to abnormal posterior compartment mechanics secondary to an incompetent MCL. A proximal injury to the MCL may be manifested by tenderness over the medial epicondyle. The valgus stress test, performed at 30 degrees of flexion, can be used to evaluate an injury to the MCL (Figure 19-5). In full extension, the bony anatomy may disguise instability. In more than 30 degrees of flexion, it becomes very difficult to stabilize the distal humerus sufficiently to get an accurate exam. Valgus stability can also be tested using the moving valgus stress test (Figure 19-6) and the milking maneuver. The milking maneuver is performed by placing the elbow in supination and 90 degrees or more of flexion and pulling on the thumb with the other hand by reaching around behind the forearm of the involved

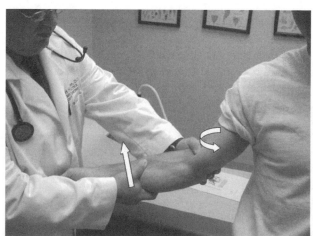

Figure 19-5   Valgus stress test.

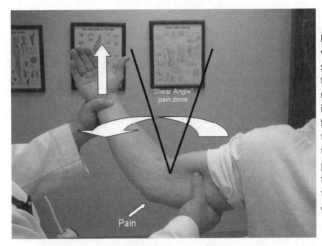

Figure 19-6 Moving valgus stress test for symptomatic partial tears of the MCL. A moderate valgus torque is applied to the fully flexed elbow, which is then extended. A positive test is noted by reproduction of pain as the elbow passes between 120 and 90 degrees.

limb (6). A thorough neurological exam of the extremity is important, since ulnar neuropathy is commonly associated with MCL injury.

AP and lateral radiographs are obtained to look for degenerative changes and loose bodies. Calcifications may be present in the MCL in chronic injuries. MRI is currently the imaging modality of choice and allows visualization of the anterior bundle of the MCL, as well as cartilage surfaces, surrounding muscles, and nerves. The anterior bundle of the MCL is the primary medial stabilizer of the elbow (see Figure 19-2, C). CT arthrography may demonstrate subtle undersurface tears of the MCL not apparent on MRI (8).

Treatment of MCL injuries is dependent on the severity of the injury and the functional demands of the athlete. Generally speaking, mild strains of the MCL can be successfully treated with rest, ice, NSAIDs, and physical therapy. Even with severe MCL injuries, nonthrowing athletes are usually asymptomatic after conservative management, and are frequently able to return to high-level competition. However, athletes who participate in sports that require high-demand upper extremity motions, such as pitching, volleyball, or tennis, usually fare poorly with nonsurgical treatment. Attempts at simple repair of the MCL have yielded disappointing results in the past, and reconstruction of the ligament with a graft is now the treatment of choice (6). The ipsilateral palmaris longus tendon is the most commonly used graft. Throwing athletes in whom a MCL tear is suspected should be referred for orthopedic evaluation and possible surgical treatment. For nonthrowing athletes, a trial of conservative treatment is reasonable.

Lateral Compression Injuries

Compressive forces are produced on the lateral side of the elbow during the late cocking and acceleration phases of throwing. Repetitive microtrauma to the area can produce a variety of lesions that tend to be age-dependent. In adolescents and young adults, osteochondritis dissecans (OCD) may occur. Older individuals may present with chondral injury to the capitellum, resulting in chronic pain.

The exact cause of OCD is not well understood. OCD involves loss of the blood supply to a segment of bone, which may result in that portion of the bone becoming unstable or loose within the joint. Subchondral fracture and osteonecrosis are assumed to play a role. OCD lesions in the lateral compartment of the elbow are quite debilitating to a throwing athlete or gymnast and usually end the player's competitive career before adulthood. The typical patient presents in the second decade of life with symptoms of insidious onset of pain, restriction of motion, swelling, and catching. Diagnosis can usually be made on routine anterior and lateral radiographs, although tomograms or MRI may further delineate the lesion. Radiographs will frequently show a vague lucency in the capitellum, sometimes accompanied by one or more loose bodies.

The prognosis of OCD of the elbow is age-related. Group 1 (age < 13, asymptomatic) typically has good results without surgical intervention; group 2 (adolescent or adult with loose bodies and acute pain) has fair results and often requires surgical removal of loose fragments; group 3 (adults with joint incongruity and chronic pain) has a poor prognosis. Surgical options include fragment removal or reattachment, drilling, or debridement. Thus far, however, it appears that surgical intervention has little hope of returning the athlete to competitive sports or preventing long-term symptoms (6,9,10).

Valgus Extension Overload

The posterior compartment of the elbow experiences high forces during the acceleration and deceleration phases of throwing and during gymnastic activities. This can result in a spectrum of chronic injuries resulting in flexor-pronator tendinopathies, valgus instability, posteromedial impingement, ulnar neuritis, and, ultimately, lateral compression syndromes. This syndrome has been termed valgus extension overload (6). Diagnosis can usually be made by a careful history and physical exam. The history usually consists of pain with throwing activities and is associated with an inability to fully extend the elbow. Examination includes application of a hyperextension stress in terminal extension to elicit posterior symptoms and valgus stress at 30 degrees of flexion to test for instability. Treatment generally consists of arthroscopy, removal of loose bodies and spurs, and olecranon fenestration. Studies have shown significant improvement in pain, motion, strength, and function after arthroscopic treatment. Stress fractures of the olecranon are occasionally seen in pitchers and gymnasts. Diagnosis can be made with plain radiographs, bone scan, or MRI. Patients are treated with activity restriction and usually can return to sport activities within 3 to 6 months. Refractory cases may require internal fixation (6,9).

Epicondylitis

Epicondylitis is one of the most frequently encountered problems in the elbow. It typically occurs in young to middle-aged adults who participate in sports or occupations that require repetitive upper extremity motions (Table 19-1). Histological studies have demonstrated that epicondylitis is a degenerative process rather than an inflammatory process as the name would imply.

Lateral Epicondylitis (Tennis Elbow)

Although the cause of lateral epicondylitis is poorly understood, the injury generally is attributed to repetitive microtrauma resulting in a microscopic tear at the origin of the ECRB (11). It accounts for 80% 90% of all cases of elbow epicondylitis and is the most common reason that patients seek medical help for elbow pain. The extensor digitorum communis, extensor carpi radialis longus, and extensor carpi ulnaris may also be involved (9). Diagnosis is made by a history of lateral elbow pain accompanied by an exam revealing tenderness over the lateral epicondyle associated with pain on resisted extension of the wrist and with grasping activities. Radiographs are usually negative but will occasionally reveal calcification over the lateral epicondyle. MRI is not necessary to confirm the diagnosis but may help with surgical planning in recalcitrant cases.

Nonsurgical treatment involves a coordinated rehabilitation protocol aimed at increasing strength and stamina in the wrist extensors. It should

Table 19-1   Common Activities Leading to Epicondylitis

	Lateral	*Medial*
Recreational	Tennis (ground strokes)	Golf
	Racquetball	Rowing
	Squash	Baseball (pitching)
	Fencing	Javelin throwing
		Tennis (serving)
Occupational	Meat cutting	Bricklaying
	Plumbing	Hammering
	Painting	Typing
	Raking	Textile production
	Weaving	

Republished with permission from Jobe FW, Ciccoti MG. Lateral and medial epicondylitis of the elbow. J Am Acad Orthop Surg. 1994;2:1-8.

begin with activity modification, as well as active and passive range-of-motion routines three to five times a day. Strengthening should then begin with wrist exercises performed with and without resistance, progressing to a forearm supination and pronation program. Finally, the use of light weights is permitted to regain strength. Rotator cuff strengthening also is performed to maintain balance in the upper extremity. Ice and NSAIDs are used in conjunction with the exercise program (6,9,12). A limited number of corticosteroid injections (a maximum of 3) may be considered, although recent studies have shown only short-term improvement with injections. Counterforce braces also are commonly used. In patients who fail to respond to a well-designed conservative program over 2 to 4 months, surgery should be considered. Current surgical treatment most often involves removing the degenerated portion of the tendon and repairing the resulting defect. Surgical treatment is effective in 85%-90% of patients. It is estimated that only 20% of patients with lateral epicondylitis will ever require surgical treatment (9).

Case Study 19-2

A 37-year-old female right-handed recreational tennis player developed pain on the lateral side of her right elbow midway through her tennis league season. At first, she had pain only when playing tennis. Backhand shots were particularly uncomfortable. Eventually, she started having pain with daily activities, such as lifting grocery sacks and milk cartons or even brushing her hair. A diagnosis of lateral epicondylitis, or "tennis elbow," was made. She was treated with a counterforce brace and NSAIDs, and her symptoms decreased but did not resolve. Because her symptoms were tolerable, she continued to play tennis.

After 4 months, she continued to experience lateral elbow symptoms. She was given a steroid injection at the lateral epicondyle and was started on a physical therapy program. Her symptoms resolved completely for 3 weeks, and she continued to play tennis. After 3 weeks, her pain gradually returned to its previous level and remained there despite continued rest, NSAIDs, and physical therapy exercises.

Eight months after the onset of symptoms, the patient underwent debridement of the extensor carpi radialis brevis origin. She was in a sling for 2 weeks post-op. She was then able to gradually resume activities of daily living. She was able to start hitting tennis balls 3 months after surgery and was completely pain-free 6 months after the procedure.

Medial Epicondylitis (Golfer's Elbow)

Medial epicondylitis represents only 10%-20% of epicondylitis cases. This condition is an overuse syndrome usually involving the flexor-pronator muscle mass of the dominant extremity. Patients typically report insidious onset of chronic elbow pain exacerbated by wrist flexion and pronation activities. Athletes with medial epicondylitis most commonly participate in golf, racquet sports, and swimming. Grip weakness and radiating forearm pain also may be present. Physical exam reveals pain to palpation over the medial epicondyle. Pain can also be elicited through provocative maneuvers, such as resisted wrist flexion and forearm pronation.

The standard nonsurgical treatment protocol for medial epicondylitis is similar to that for lateral epicondylitis. It consists of activity modification, counterforce bracing, physical therapy, and oral NSAIDs. Steroid injections provide temporary relief but do not affect the natural history of the condition. Surgery consisting of debridement and repair of the involved tendon is indicated for patients who fail conservative treatment (6,9,12).

Nerve Injuries

Overhand sports can frequently lead to ulnar neuropathy caused by traction, friction (subluxation), or compression of the nerve at the elbow. During the throwing motion, fibers of the ulnar nerve may be subjected to injury in four locations: 1) the medial cord of the brachial plexus at the coracoid, 2) the ulnar nerve at the elbow, 3) the ulnar nerve at the flexor-pronator insertion, and 4) the ulnar nerve at the wrist. Symptoms may include vague medial elbow and forearm pain, clumsiness, and decreased performance. EMGs may help in making the diagnosis. Treatment consists of rest, NSAIDs, and avoidance of direct pressure over the ulnar nerve. Surgery is indicated for patients who have had symptoms for more than 6 weeks, have motor denervation, or who have associated MCL incompetence (9).

Elbow Injuries in Skeletally Immature Athletes

Skeletally immature athletes present a unique set of problems due to the presence of open growth plates. One of the most commonly affected areas is the medial epicondyle. Medial epicondylar stress lesions also are referred to as "Little League" elbow. This condition results from repetitive valgus stress combined with pull from the flexor muscle mass. Symptoms include progressive pain and decreased throwing effectiveness. Physical findings are confined to point tenderness over the medial epicondyle. X-rays reveal subtle widening or fragmentation of the epiphyseal line when compared with the asymptomatic elbow (Figure 19-7) (13). Treatment involves simple rest from throwing activities. Pain will usually resolve in 2 to 3 weeks, and throwing can be resumed in 6 weeks (14). In an adolescent, one occasionally will see an avulsion of the medial epicondyle caused by the simple act of throwing a ball (Figure 19-8). Direct trauma can also cause fracture through the physis. Although fractures that are displaced < 1 cm will heal

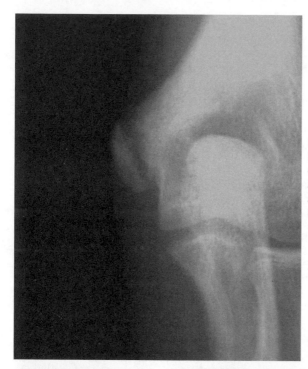

Figure 19-7   "Little League" elbow (medial epicondyle apophysitis). The apophyseal line is widened and slightly irregular (cf. Figure 19-8, *B*).

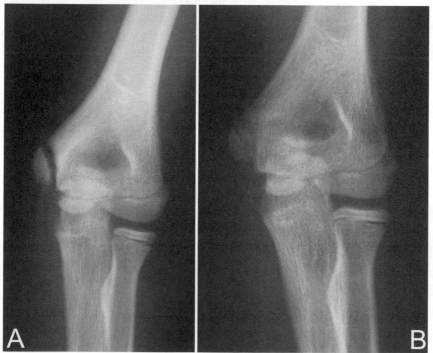

A

B

Figure 19-8   (A) Avulsion of the medial epicondyle. (B) Normal elbow.

without surgery, they may cause disability for athletes who require elbow stability, such as throwers and gymnasts. These patients frequently require surgical fixation of the fractured medial epicondyle.

Traumatic Injuries of the Elbow

Fractures and dislocations about the elbow are far more common in the general population than in athletes. These injuries include distal humerus fractures, radial head fractures, olecranon fractures, coronoid fractures, and elbow dislocations (with or without associated fracture). Elbow fractures are fraught with complications and require considerable judgment and experience to manage appropriately. Even with the best possible treatment, a fracture about the elbow may end the athlete's career.

Other rare traumatic injuries of the elbow include rupture of the distal biceps tendon and rupture of the triceps tendon. Distal biceps tears typically occur in middle-aged males and result from powerful eccentric contraction of the biceps against a fixed elbow. Findings include ecchymosis in the antecubital fossa and weakness on supination of the forearm. There may be a visible or palpable defect in the distal biceps tendon. Triceps ruptures occur with either a direct blow to the elbow or forced elbow flexion with a strong eccentric contraction of the triceps. Patients have inability to extend the arm against gravity, usually with a palpable defect just above the olecranon. MRI is useful in confirming both of these conditions. Both conditions are best treated with prompt surgical repair (15).

REFERENCES

1. **Andrews JR, Meister K.** Overuse injuries of the athlete's elbow. In: Griffin I, ed. Orthopedic Knowledge Update Sports Medicine. Rosemont, IL: American Academy of Orthopedic Surgeons; 1994:1179-90.

2. **Smith J, O'Driscoll SW.** Elbow functional anatomy and Biomechanics. In: Arendt EA, ed. Orthopedic Knowledge Update: Sports Medicine 2. Chicago: American Academy of Orthopedic Surgeons; 1999:207-16.

3. **DiGiovine NM, Jobe FW, Pink M, et al.** An electromyographic analysis of the upper extremity on pitching, J Shoulder Elbow Surg. 1992;1:15-25.

4. **Callaway GH, Field LD, Deng XH, et al.** Biomechanical evaluation of the medial collateral ligament complex of the elbow. Am J Sports Med. 1995;23:396-400.

5. **Hamilton CD, Glousman RE, Jobe FW, et al.** Dynamic stability of the elbow: Electromyographic analysis of the flexor pronator group and the extensor group in pitchers with valgus instability. J Shoulder Elbow Surg. 1996;5:347-54.

6. **Williams RJ III, Altchek DW.** Atraumatic injuries of the elbow in athletes. In: Arendt EA, ed. Orthopedic Knowledge Update: Sports Medicine 2. Chicago: American Academy of Orthopedic Surgeons; 1999:229-36.

7. **Fealy S, Rohrbough JT, Allen AA, et al.** Athletic Injuries and the Throwing Athlete: Elbow. In: Norris TR, ed. Orthopedic Knowledge Update: Shoulder and Elbow 2. Chicago: American Academy of Orthopedic Surgeons; 2002:297-312.

8. **Timmerman LA, Schwartz MI, Andrews JR.** Preoperative evaluation of the ulnar collateral ligament by magnetic resonance imaging and computed tonography arthrography: evaluation in 25 baseball players with surgical confirmation. Am J Sports Med. 1994;22:26-31.

9. **O'Driscoll SW.** Acute, Recurrent, and Chronic Elbow Instabilities. In: Norris TR, ed. Orthopedic Knowledge Update: Shoulder and Elbow 2. Chicago: American Academy of Orthopedic Surgeons; 2002:313-24.

10. **Bianco AJ.** Osteochondritis dissecans. In: Morrey BF, ed. The Elbow and Its Disorders. Philadelphia: WB Saunders; 1993:254-9.

11. **Boyer MI, Hastings H II.** Lateral tennis elbow: "Is there any science out there?" J Shoulder Elbow Surg. 1999;8:481-91.

12. **Field LD, Savoie FH.** Common elbow injuries in sport. Sports Med. 1998;26:193-205.

13. **Bennett JB, Tullos HS.** Ligamentous and articular injuries in the athlete. In: Morrey BF, ed. The Elbow and its Disorders. Philadelphia: WB Saunders; 1993:502-22.

14. **Wilkins KE.** Fractures and dislocations of the elbow region. In: Rockwood CD Jr, Wilkins KE, King RE, eds. Fractures in Children. Philadelphia: JB Lippincott; 1991:689-705.

15. **Hamilton CD.** Traumatic elbow injuries in the athlete. In: Arendt EA, ed. Orthopedic Knowledge Update: Sports Medicine 2. Chicago: American Academy of Orthopedic Surgeons; 1999:217-28.

20

■ ■ ■

Wrist Injuries

S. Craig Veatch, MD
David M. Harsha, MD

W rist injuries frequently occur in relation to sporting activities. Up to 10% of all athletic injuries are attributable to the wrist (1,2). When wrist pain is diagnosed as a "sprain," a more serious injury may be overlooked, such as a fracture or ligamentous instability. Generally, wrist pain and its assessment can be grouped into two categories: acute traumatic injury and chronic overuse injury (3,4). This chapter reviews the essential anatomy, history, and physical examination of wrist pain, as well as the evaluation and management of common wrist injuries.

Anatomy

An understanding of the surface and bony anatomy of the wrist is essential in assessing wrist pain. Eight carpal bones functioning as an intercalated segment form a proximal row (lunate, triquetrum, pisiform) with the scaphoid serving as a bridge to the distal row (trapezium, trapezoid, capitate, hamate) (Figure 20-1). The anatomic position of the scaphoid provides stability to the carpal bones (5). This critical function underscores the importance of recognizing scaphoid injuries in a timely fashion. Scaphoid fracture is the most common of the wrist fractures. The anatomical snuffbox is found just distal and dorsal to the radial styloid, bordered on the radial side by the abductor pollicis longus (APL) and extensor pollicis brevis (EPB) and on the ulnar side by the extensor pollicis longus (EPL). The snuffbox serves as the site for palpation of the scaphoid (navicular) bone (Figure 20-2). The tubercle of the radius (Lister's tubercle) lays one-third of the way across the dorsum of the wrist from the radial styloid process. It is a small bony prominence or nodule. Just distal to Lister's tubercle is the lunate. The lunate is

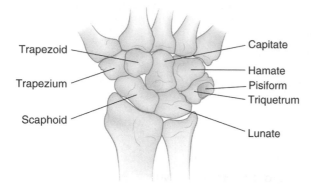

Figure 20-1 Carpal bone anatomy of the wrist (dorsal view). Note that the space between the distal ulna and triquetrum is where the triangular fibrocartilage complex (TFCC) lives.

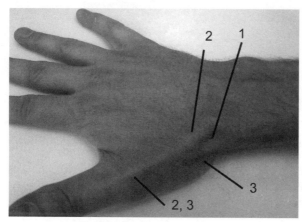

Figure 20-2 Dorsal surface anatomy of the hand and wrist demonstrating the anatomic snuffbox (1). The extensor pollicis longus (2) forms the ulnar border. The abductor pollicis longus and extensor pollicis brevis (3) form the radial border, with the scaphoid forming the floor of the triangle.

the most frequently dislocated and second most often fractured bone in the wrist. It articulates proximally with the radius and distally with the capitate. On the palmar ulnar side of the wrist, the pisiform and the hook of the hamate can be palpated, and the depression between these bones is the tunnel of Guyon (Figure 20-3). This tunnel contains the ulnar nerve and artery and is a site for compression injuries (6).

Physical Examination

A detailed physical exam of the wrist can help localize symptoms to the correct anatomic region and aid in the correct diagnosis.

Inspection

Observe the uninjured side to serve as a baseline; look for swelling (diffuse or localized) on the dorsal and palmar surfaces. Look for atrophy of

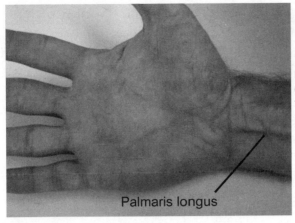

Figure 20-3   Palmar (volar) surface anatomy of the wrist demonstrating prominent palmaris longus.

Palmaris longus

the thenar muscles (median nerve innervated) and hypothenar muscles (ulnar nerve innervated) suggesting possible nerve injury or entrapment. Look for asymmetric deformities suggesting possible fracture or dislocation. Look for discrete soft tissue prominences that may represent ganglion cysts on the dorsal or palmar surface of the wrist (7).

Palpation

1. Palpate for bony tenderness over the anatomical snuffbox for a scaphoid injury (ulnar deviation facilitates scaphoid palpation).
2. Palpate the distal radius and ulna for deformity and tenderness suggesting fracture.
3. Palpate the distal radioulnar joint.
4. Palpate Lister's tubercle on the dorsum of the radius and just distal to that the lunate.
5. Move radially to palpate the scapholunate joint.
6. Palpate the base of the thumb carpometacarpal (CMC) joint for tenderness; this is a common place for osteoarthritis between the trapezium and first metacarpal.
7. Palpate over the radial styloid for crepitus and tenderness in the first dorsal compartment containing the APL and EPB, where tenosynovitis is common.
8. Palpate the pisiform and hook of hamate on palmar ulnar surface for bony tenderness.
9. Palpate the distal ulnar styloid for tenderness (palpable tenderness over dorsal ulnar aspect of wrist between ulnar styloid and carpus may indicate triangular fibrocartilage complex [TFCC] injury) (see Figure 20-1).

Table 20-1   Wrist Range of Motion and Neuromuscular Function

	Range of Motion	Nerve Responsible	Muscle Innervated
Flexion	75-80 degrees	Median, C7 Ulnar, C8	Flexor carpi radialis Flexor carpi ulnaris
Extension	65-70 degrees	Radial, C6 Radial, C6 Radial, C7	Extensor carpi radialis longus Extensor carpi radialis brevis Extensor carpi ulnaris
Radial deviation	20-25 degrees		
Ulnar deviation	30-35 degrees		
Supination	90 degrees	Musculocutaneous, C5, C6 Radial, C6	Biceps Supinator
Pronation	90 degrees	Median, C6 Anterior interosseous branch, C8, T1	Pronator teres Pronator quadratus

Range of motion: Assess active range of motion first using bilateral comparison; if unable to complete due to pain or difficulty, then passive range-of-motion tests may be considered if fracture has been ruled out. Measure active wrist motion from a neutral or straight wrist position (Table 20-1). Special tests for physical diagnosis are mentioned under specific injuries later in the chapter.

Specific Injuries

Acute Wrist Injuries (Trauma)

History

Falling on an outstretched hand with the wrist in dorsiflexion is the most common mechanism of injury to the wrist (8). Pain and swelling are often immediate. This type of mechanism can produce a scaphoid fracture or distal radius fracture, or it may injure the intercarpal ligaments or the triangular fibrocartilage complex. Less commonly, carpal dislocations can occur, most often involving the lunate. Pain that follows swinging a racquet, club, or bat that strikes a hard object may produce a fracture to the hook of the hamate. Forced ulnar deviation and rotational stress may injure the TFCC on the ulnar side of the wrist (9).

Physical Examination

It is helpful to localize the site of injury, specifically to distinguish between volar and dorsal wrist pain (Table 20-2). Swelling is often diffuse, but on occasion, localized pain and swelling can identify the area of concern.

Range of motion is usually limited by pain and swelling. Neurovascular assessment should always be included in the exam. An understanding of the muscles responsible for wrist motion and the nerves that control those movements is important (see Table 20-1).

Imaging
Standard radiographs to rule out bony injury after acute trauma include posterior-anterior (PA), neutral, lateral, and oblique views. The lateral view assesses alignment of the distal radius with the lunate, capitate and third metacarpal (Figure 20-4). Additional views can include clenched-fist PA to evaluate for scapholunate instability by looking for widening of the gap between the scaphoid and lunate of 3 mm or more (Figure 20-5). For suspected scaphoid injuries, obtain PA ulnar deviation and PA 45 degrees pronation views (see Figure 20-4). A carpal tunnel view with the wrist in dorsiflexion should be obtained to look for injury to the hook of the hamate, pisiform, or trapezium ridge. Comparison films of the uninjured wrist are often helpful.

Fluoroscopy allows for dynamic examination to evaluate possible instability.

Bone scan is useful to further evaluate suspected fractures or subtle fractures not seen on plain radiographs.

CT scanning helps to further define bony injuries and to evaluate the distal radial ulnar joint and fractures of the hook of the hamate or

Table 20-2   Causes and Location of Acute and Chronic Wrist Pain

	Radial	*Ulnar*	*Volar*	*Dorsal*
Acute wrist pain	Scaphoid injury, distal radius fracture, scapholunate dissociation	Triangular fibrocartilage complex tear (TFCC), distal ulnar fracture, hamate fractures, traumatic ulnar artery thrombosis	Hook of hamate fracture, Kienböck's disease (acute)	Scaphoid fracture, scapholunate dissociation, lunate fracture, distal radius fracture, distal radioulnar joint injury
Chronic wrist pain	De Quervain's tenosynovitis, missed scaphoid fracture, intersection syndrome	Ulnar nerve compression (Guyon's tunnel syndrome), TFCC tear, distal radioulnar joint instability, extensor carpi ulnaris tendinopathies, flexor carpi ulnaris tendinopathies	Kienböck's disease, carpal tunnel syndrome, flexor carpi tendinopathies, ulnar tunnel syndrome, ganglion cyst	Kienböck's disease, ganglion cyst, extensor tendinopathies, intersection syndrome, osteoarthritis

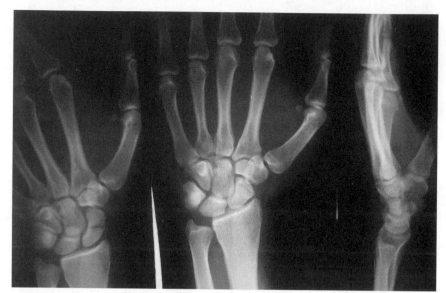

Figure 20-4   Three views of the wrist (*left to right:* PA ulnar deviation, PA, lateral) demonstrating the importance of specific scaphoid views to identify fractures. Wrist fracture of the middle one third of the scaphoid is best seen in the PA ulnar deviation view.

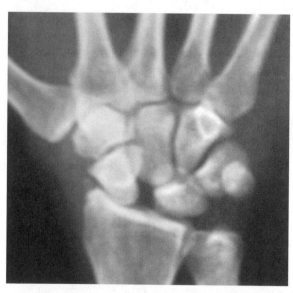

Figure 20-5   Clenched-fist PA view of wrist demonstrating scapholunate dissociation with > 3 mm separation between the scaphoid and lunate bones.

trapezium (Figure 20-6). CT scanning is not helpful in assessing ligament injury.

Arthrography can be useful in defining ligamentous injuries and TFCC tears. Arthography has questionable sensitivity and specificity. It is used in conjunction with MRI on occasion (10).

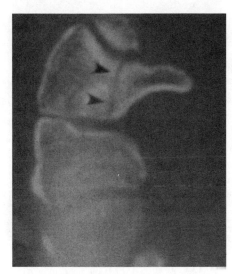

Figure 20-6   CT scan demonstrating hook of the hamate fracture.

MRI is being used more often to assess wrist pain. It is useful for evaluation of ligaments, TFCC, soft tissues about the wrist, as well as bony injury. Musculoskeletal-trained radiologists and appropriate equipment are essential when using this modality to assess wrist pain (11).

Arthroscopy is being used more frequently as both a diagnostic and therapeutic procedure. It is useful in assessing ligament disruptions and chronic ulnar-sided wrist pain (12,13).

Treatment

Treatment depends on the specific injury. In general, if no obvious fracture or abnormality is discovered on initial evaluation, but the wrist is painful and swollen, immobilization in a splint or cast is appropriate. The patient should be reevaluated in 2 weeks. Specific wrist injuries and their treatment are discussed in the sections that follow.

Scaphoid Fractures

Scaphoid fracture is the most common and problematic fracture in the wrist, accounting for 70% of all carpal bone injuries in adults. It is the most common sports-related bony injury to the wrist. As mentioned, the scaphoid serves as the bridge between the two rows of carpal bones and is the principal bony block to hyperextension at the wrist; thus it is susceptible to fracture (14).

The scaphoid most commonly fractures in the middle third or "waist" (70% of scaphoid fractures), followed by fractures of the proximal third (20%), and fractures of the distal third, including the distal tubercle (10%).

These fractures are notoriously problematic due to the tenuous blood supply to the scaphoid that arises distally from branches of the radial artery. The proximal pole of the scaphoid is completely dependent on the distal blood supply. Due to the vascular anatomy entering distally and running proximally, middle and proximal fractures are more prone to delayed healing, avascular necrosis (AVN), and nonunion (3,4).

The majority of scaphoid fractures result from a fall on an outstretched hand with the wrist hyperextended and in ulnar deviation. Alternatively, they occur via a blow to the palm from contact with another person. Patients will present with pain and or swelling in the anatomical snuffbox on the dorsal radial aspect of the wrist. Scaphoid fractures are often diagnosed late due to the patient's delay in seeking treatment or being misdiagnosed as a "wrist sprain."

X-rays should include PA, lateral, and special scaphoid views with ulnar deviation (see Figure 20-4). The radiographs are often normal, or the fracture is extremely subtle. If suspicious for scaphoid injury and plain radiographs are normal, place the patient in a short-arm thumb spica cast or splint (if there is moderate swelling) and reevaluate with x-rays in 2 weeks (Table 20-3). If the patient is still symptomatic and x-rays are negative, continue immobilization for 2 more weeks. Four weeks post-injury, if the patient is still symptomatic and x-rays are negative, proceed to bone scan or MRI for diagnosis. If a diagnosis needs to be made more promptly in an

Table 20-3   Treatment Guidelines for Suspected and Nondisplaced Scaphoid Fractures

	Suspected	Distal 1/3	Middle 1/3	Proximal 1/3
Cast type	Short-arm thumb spica splint or cast (thumb IP joint free)	Long-arm thumb spica cast × 6 weeks, then short-arm thumb spica cast until clinical and radiographic union	Long-arm thumb spica cast × 6 weeks, then short-arm thumb spica cast until clinical and radiographic union	Long-arm thumb spica cast, followed by short-arm thumb spica cast versus ORIF
Length of immobilization	Until diagnosis confirmed	10-12 weeks	12-14 weeks	12-20 weeks
Healing time	—	12-14 weeks	14-16 weeks	18-24 weeks
Follow-up	Every 2 weeks until diagnosis confirmed, bone scan or MRI at 4 weeks from injury if plain films still negative	Every 2-3 weeks until radiographic union	Every 2-3 weeks until radiographic union	Consider referral due to high risk for poor healing, need for prolonged immobilization and possible ORIF

athletic setting, a bone scan no sooner than 72 hours post-injury is extremely sensitive and very specific for scaphoid fracture; conversely, an MRI can be obtained but is a few hundred dollars more expensive.

Risk factors for delayed union, nonunion, and AVN include displaced fractures (> 1 mm separation), involvement of both bone cortices on either side of the fracture, proximal one-third pole fractures, and delayed presentation of injury greater than 2 weeks (5,15). Strong consideration for referral to an orthopedic surgeon for further management is warranted in these cases. Nonunion occurs in up to 20%-30% of proximal third fractures and 10%-20% of middle third fractures, rarely in distal pole fractures. AVN occurs in up to 5% of middle third waist fractures and in up to 10% of proximal pole fractures. Nonunion can lead to significant chronic pain and arthritis (14).

Definitive treatment of nondisplaced middle and proximal third fractures includes 6 weeks in a long-arm thumb spica cast, followed by a short-arm thumb spica cast with repeated out-of-cast x-rays every 2-3 weeks until the fracture is healed (radiographic union). Average total time in cast is 8-12 weeks for distal third and middle third nondisplaced fractures and 12-20 weeks for proximal third nondisplaced fractures. CT scanning or MRI can be used to confirm union (see Table 20-3).

Displaced fractures of the scaphoid typically undergo open reduction and internal fixation (ORIF). A symptomatic delayed union or nonunion is an indication for surgery with bone grafting. Treatment of an asymptomatic delayed union or nonunion of a scaphoid fracture is controversial. In the young athlete, bone grafting with internal fixation is suggested based on natural history studies. Careful review of the options with the patient and family is warranted (5,16).

Return to play in short-arm thumb spica orthosis is reasonable for certain sports a week after cast removal, as long as risks are understood. In general, impact loading of the wrist is to be avoided for 2-3 months after immobilization. Referral to a surgeon for consideration of Herbert screw fixation is reasonable for the athlete who cannot accept the prolonged immobilization time for healing. The screw fixation technique has demonstrated earlier return to play with middle-third fractures and good union rates (15).

Case Study 20-1

A 35-year-old bicyclist presented to the office complaining of right wrist pain after a fall from her bicycle onto an outstretched arm 2 days earlier. She had no previous injury to the wrist.

Physical exam revealed limited wrist extension secondary to pain and tenderness at the anatomical snuffbox. There was no pain with palpation over the ulnar styloid or proximally up the forearm. Neurovascular exam was unremarkable.

Initial radiographs did not reveal any fractures or dislocations; however, a scaphoid injury was suspected. The patient was placed in a thumb spica splint and told to return for a follow-up visit in 10 days. Examination at that time revealed pain with wrist dorsiflexion and palpation of the snuffbox. Pain was not appreciated over the distal radius or ulna. Popping or clicking was not appreciated with range-of-motion assessment.

Repeat films revealed a fracture of the distal third of the scaphoid with no other abnormalities. After discussion with the patient, it was decided to place her in a long arm thumb spica cast for 6 weeks followed by a short arm cast for 6 more weeks.

Fractures of the scaphoid occur most frequently at the wrist followed by the distal then proximal pole. Because most fractures are nondisplaced, radiographs may be unremarkable at initial presentation. Special views or advanced imaging may be helpful, however. For recreational athletes who are suspected of having a scaphoid fracture, conservative measures as described above are appropriate. Obtaining radiographs 10 to 14 days after the acute insult will allow bony reaction; therefore repeat radiographs will likely confirm the diagnosis.

Distal Radius Fractures

Distal radial fractures make up 10%-12% of all bone injuries and are seen in the athletic population frequently. The most common mechanism of injury is a fall on the outstretched hand causing dorsal displacement of the distal fragment. These fractures of the distal radius are often termed *Colles' fractures*. The extensor pollicis longus tendon and the median nerve run in close proximity to the distal radius and may be injured in association with a distal radius fracture. There is typically pain and swelling at the distal radius, primarily on the dorsal side. A deformity referred to as a "silver fork" is due to the dorsal displacement of the distal fragment from a Colles' fracture. There is point tenderness and pain that limits range of motion. Radiographs to evaluate the distal radius should include an anteroposterior, lateral, and oblique view. The Colles' fracture is an extraarticular fracture that usually occurs within 2 cm of the distal radial articular surface (3).

Stable distal radial fractures can be treated by cast immobilization. Most fractures that are displaced, angulated, intraarticular, or comminuted are unstable and should be referred to an orthopedic surgeon. Displaced intraarticular fractures usually require operative fixation to achieve and maintain anatomic reduction. Nondisplaced extraarticular fractures are treated initially with a sugar tong splint (splinting along the dorsal aspect of the wrist and forearm down to and around the elbow, which is flexed at 90 degrees, and up the volar side of the forearm back to the wrist creating a "sugar tong" that is then wrapped with an ace bandage). This is followed by a short-arm cast to total 4-6 weeks. It is advised to repeat radiographs through the cast weekly for 2 weeks and then every 2 weeks to assure alignment is maintained. Fractures requiring reduction are unstable and are treated in a long-arm cast followed by a short-arm cast to total 6-8 weeks. Weekly radiographs for 3 weeks, followed by every 2 weeks, are advised to assure stability (14). The goal of treatment is to restore normal anatomy, particularly in the young athlete, to minimize radial shortening.

Hamate Fractures

Fractures to the body of the hamate are caused by a direct blow to the hypothenar region and are uncommon. Fractures to the hook of the hamate commonly are seen in baseball, tennis, and golf. They are due to repetitive stresses of a racquet handle, golf club, or baseball bat impinging and impacting the hypothenar eminence (5). Hook fractures are commonly missed and should be suspected with ulnar-sided wrist pain (see Table 20-2). There is typically tenderness to deep palpation of the hook of the hamate in the base of the palm and along the dorsoulnar side of the hamate. Radiographs should include PA, lateral, carpal tunnel, and supinated oblique views to best assess the hamate. Often plain films are negative, and a CT scan is needed for definitive diagnosis (see Figure 20-6).

Nondisplaced body fractures are treated in a short arm cast for 4-6 weeks. Displaced body fractures should be referred for open reduction and internal fixation. Hook of the hamate fractures, if untreated, result in chronic ulnar palmar pain and the possibility of flexor tendon rupture or ulnar nerve injury. Cast immobilization for 6-12 weeks to achieve union is an option. Most authors recommend excision of the fracture fragment, because it allows an earlier return to play (about 7-10 weeks postsurgery) for athletes. Patients with delayed presentation of hook fractures (> 2 weeks from initial injury) should undergo excision (14,15).

Scapholunate Dissociation

Scapholunate dissociation is due to a tear of the volar-sided scapholunate ligament from a fall on the outstretched hand or from a scaphoid nonunion. Examination will reveal tenderness distal to Lister's tubercle along the radial side of the lunate and involve the volar and dorsal aspects of the scapholunate joint (17). Watson's test will be positive, revealing scapholunate dissociation. To perform Watson's test, the examiner places the thumb on the scaphoid tuberosity (palmar) with the wrist in ulnar deviation and places the four fingers of the same hand on the dorsal aspect of the distal radius. The wrist is deviated radially while pressure is placed on the scaphoid with the thumb. If the scapholunate ligaments are ruptured, the thumb will prevent the scaphoid from palmar flexing and force it to move dorsally, causing the patient pain dorsally with a painful click (7).

PA radiographs may show the scapholunate space to be greater than 3 mm. Bilateral clenched-fist PA views will likely highlight a gap greater than

3 mm between the scaphoid and lunate on the injured side (see Figure 20 5). This gap is often referred to as the Terry-Thomas sign (named after the gapped-tooth English entertainer). These injuries should be referred to the orthopedic surgeon.

Acute treatment of scapholunate dissociation involves open reduction and repair of the ligaments with internal fixation versus closed reduction and percutaneous pinning. Chronic instability often requires capsulodesis with scapho-trapezio-trapezoidal fusion (17).

Triangular Fibrocartilage Complex Injury (TFCC Tears)

The TFCC houses the triangular fibrocartilage, the meniscus homologue, articular disk, ulnar collateral ligament, dorsal and volar radioulnar ligaments, and the extensor carpi ulnaris sheath. It functions as the stabilizer of the distal radioulnar joint, serves as a cushion for axial loads to the ulnar side of the wrist, and acts as a sling for the carpal bones from the radius (18). The TFCC is a common site of ulnar wrist pain. A positive ulnar variance (in which the ulna is longer than or more distal than the radius) predisposes to tearing of the TFC secondary to impingement of the distal ulna on the TFC. TFCC injuries can be traumatic or degenerative. Mechanisms of injury include wrist extension and hyperpronation of the forearm with axial loading and ulnar deviation. This can tear the cartilage. Racquet sports players, gymnasts, and divers are prone to these injuries (9).

The physical exam reveals swelling and tenderness distal to the ulnar styloid on the dorsal side of the wrist. Dorsiflexion of the wrist with ulnar deviation and rotation causes pain and clicking in TFCC tears. The press test involves a seated patient grasping the arms of the chair and pressing down on the chair to lift up to a standing position. This invariably creates pain on the ulnar side of the wrist in someone with a TFCC injury.

Special radiographs can be obtained to evaluate for ulnar fracture or subluxation. In addition, CT scanning, MRI, or arthrography can be helpful in identifying TFCC tears. CT imaging can evaluate subtle distal radio-ulnar joint subluxation, and arthroscopy can be used as a diagnostic and therapeutic tool (11,13).

Treatment for acute injuries begins with immobilization with a long-arm cast for 4-6 weeks, followed by splinting and therapy for strengthening and range of motion. For refractory cases, consider referral for potential debridement. Degenerative tears secondary to impingement from positive ulnar variance are amenable to ulnar shortening procedures (18).

Overuse Wrist Injuries

Overuse wrist injuries result from repetitive microtrauma involving overload and breakdown of the involved musculoskeletal structure. This typically involves inflammation of the tendon (tendinitis) or tendon sheath (tenosynovitis). When overuse persists, tissue breakdown without adequate healing occurs (19). As a result, chronic pain develops from disordered healing with fibrosis and scar tissue deposition (tendinosis).

History

A detailed history, including circumstances surrounding the onset of wrist pain, will help in determining whether the pain is from overuse versus a prior trauma or injury that went untreated or undiagnosed. Activities that worsen the pain provide insight into the location of the involved tendon, muscle, nerve, or ligament. The timing of the pain (worse at night, stiff after rest, worse with activity) also provides clues at to the cause of the pain. Finally, location of the wrist pain aids in narrowing the differential diagnosis (see Table 20-2).

Physical Examination

Swelling, tenderness to palpation, crepitus, pain with passive range of motion, or passive stretching and pain with active resistance are all indicators of inflammation involving tendons or tendon sheaths. Tinel's testing (tapping over a nerve to reproduce the pain or an altered sensation in the distribution of the nerve) or noting muscle atrophy can indicate compression neuropathies. Volar or dorsal soft tissue masses seen on inspection could represent ganglion cysts.

Treatment

Treatment is similar for most overuse injuries of the wrist. The general principles of relative rest, ice, and nonsteroidal anti-inflammatory medications apply. Correction of the underlying problem and rehabilitation exercises are important. Modalities of physical therapy including ultrasound, phonophoresis, iontophoresis, contrast baths, and augmented soft-tissue mobilization can be beneficial. Corticosteroid injections for tenosynovitis and certain chronic tendinopathies are helpful. Splinting or bracing to allow pain-free activity often plays a role in recovery. Once pain is absent with rest, progressive strengthening exercises can be implemented. The goal is to return to activity pain-free, with full range of motion and normal strength.

De Quervain's Tenosynovitis

The first dorsal compartment of the wrist houses the abductor pollicis longus and extensor pollicis brevis tendons in a synovial sheath on the dorsal radial side of the wrist, near the radial styloid (Figure 20-7). De Quervain's tenosynovitis is swelling or stenosis of that sheath. Localized pain and swelling develops as inflamed tendons move through the sheath. Patients often complain of a triggering or locking sensation and creaking as they move their thumb. This condition arises from repetitive motion of the

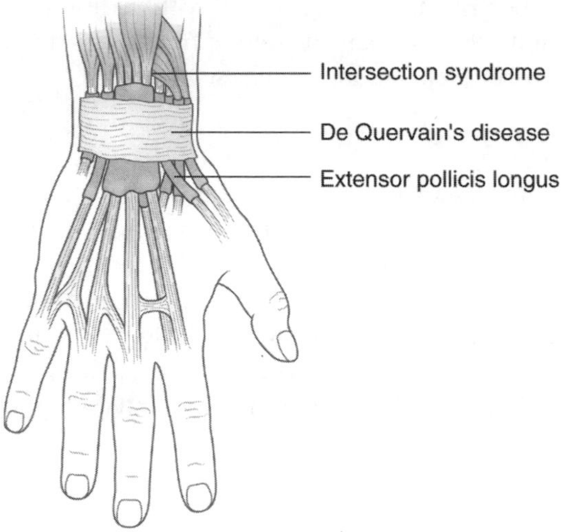

Intersection syndrome

De Quervain's disease

Extensor pollicis longus

Figure 20-7   De Quervain's tenosynovitis location in the first dorsal compartment of the wrist (housing the abductor pollicis longus and extensor pollicis brevis). Also, note the more proximal location of the intersection syndrome where the first dorsal compartment intersects with the extensor carpi radialis tendons.

wrist and thumb and is exacerbated by forceful grasping or ulnar deviation of the wrist. It is commonly seen in racquet sports players, golfers, rowers, and fishermen. The differential diagnoses of de Quervain's tenosynovitis are shown in Table 20-4.

Physical exam reveals swelling and tenderness of the tendons passing over the radial styloid. Crepitus may often be felt with thumb motion. Finkelstein's test is diagnostic for de Quervain's tenosynovitis. This test is performed by having the patient flex the affected thumb into the palm, flex the fingers over the thumb making a clenched fist, and ulnarly deviate the wrist. This maneuver will elicit pain in patients with de Quervain's tenosynovitis.

Treatment includes thumb spica splinting, NSAIDs, icing, and corticosteroid injections. A typical course of treatment is to immobilize the thumb and wrist in a thumb spica splint for 10-14 days, along with NSAIDs and icing. If this fails to resolve the pain, a steroid injection into the tendon sheath is often very effective. In rare cases, surgical release is needed for patients who fail conservative treatment (19).

Table 20-4   Differential Diagnoses for de Quervain's Tenosynovitis

- Scaphoid fracture
- CMC arthritis of thumb
- Dorsal ganglion
- Flexor carpi radialis tendinitis
- Wrist arthritis

Case Study 20-2

A 40-year-old white female daycare worker and bicyclist presents with bilateral wrist pain. She is right-handed dominant and notes symptoms are worse in that hand. The pain has been noticeable for the last 2 months; more recently, however, it has been less tolerable and she notes a sticking sensation with particular motions of the wrist. She denies any wrist trauma. There is no significant past medical history.

Physical exam revealed no erythema or swelling over the wrists. Range of motion is symmetrical bilaterally. Pain is reproduced with palpation just distal to the radial styloid over the extensor pollicus brevis and abductor pollicus longus tendon. Finkelstein's test revealed pain over the first dorsal compartment. These symptoms were present in the left wrist but not as noticeable.

The patient is diagnosed with de Quervain's tenosynovitis, an overuse injury likely the result of her frequent lifting of children at work. The etiology is a friction tendinitis with repetitive motion of the extensor pollicus brevis and abductor pollicus longus as they run under the extensor retinaculum near the radial styloid. A thickening over the first dorsal compartment can be appreciated on occasion. An acute version can occur with direct trauma to the area.

Treatment options are discussed, and the patient decides to have the right wrist injected with a corticosteroid. An injection into the tendon sheath of the first dorsal compartment is performed. She is asked to use bilateral thumb spica splints, placed on a course of NSAIDs, given a handout for home and physical therapy, and referred to occupational therapy to educate her on proper lifting techniques to prevent recurrence.

The patient returns 2 weeks later for a follow-up visit. She notes significant improvement. She is told to keep wearing her splints, especially during work, to continue home physical therapy, and to use NSAIDs as needed. Her condition continues to improve, and over the next 4 weeks she discontinues use of the wrist splints. She has no further incidents of wrist pain.

Intersection Syndrome

Intersection syndrome is a tenosynovitis or bursitis at the site where the first dorsal compartment tendons (APL, EPB) cross over the extensor carpi radialis tendons. This occurs proximal to de Quervain's disease on the dorsal radial side of the wrist (see Figure 20-7). The condition is seen in weight lifters, canoeists, and rowers, in whom repetitive wrist extension and radial deviation is common. This syndrome is thought to be due to inflammation and bursitis at the intersection point of the first dorsal compartment and the extensor tendons of the wrist or due to a tenosynovitis of the extensor carpi radialis tendons themselves (4).

Physical exam reveals tenderness, swelling, and crepitus about 3 inches proximal to Lister's tubercle at the dorsal radial aspect of the forearm.

Treatment is similar to de Quervain's tenosynovitis that occurs distal to intersection syndrome. Relative rest, thumb spica splinting, NSAIDs, and corticosteroid injections are effective in most cases (3). Surgical decompression and debridement is rarely necessary.

Carpal Tunnel Syndrome

Entrapment of the median nerve at the wrist is the most common compression neuropathy in the upper extremity and with sporting activities. Cyclists, throwers, and tennis players have been found to have a higher incidence of carpal tunnel syndrome (CTS). The syndrome is also associated with pregnancy, thyroid dysfunction, and diabetes (20). The median nerve can be compressed as it travels through the carpal tunnel on the volar side of the wrist along with the flexor tendons beneath the transverse carpal ligament. Repetitive wrist activities or activities requiring the wrist to be held in a fixed flexed or extended position for prolonged times predispose to carpal tunnel syndrome. The differential diagnoses of carpal tunnel syndrome are shown in Table 20-5.

Typical symptoms include an aching pain with numbness or paresthesia along the distribution of the median nerve. This includes the thumb, the index and middle fingers, and the radial side of the ring finger. The pain is often worse at night and causes nocturnal awakenings with signs of numbness. The pain can radiate to the forearm and up into the shoulder. More chronic symptoms involve weakness of pinch and grip.

Clinical findings include a positive Phalen's test that involves placing the wrists in a hyperflexed position. Aching and numbness in the median nerve distribution within 60 seconds is considered a positive Phalen's test for carpal tunnel syndrome. Tinel's sign is positive in a little less than half of patients with CTS. This test involves tapping over the median nerve along the volar aspect of the wrist. This will produce a tingling or shooting sensation in some or all of the digits the median nerve innervates. The median nerve compression test is now considered one of the best exam findings to correlate with CTS. Applying thumb pressure over the median nerve at the wrist for 30 seconds will elicit pain or numbness in the median distribution. Other exam findings include decreased vibratory sensation and diminished two-point discrimination (< 5 mm) in the sensory distribution of the median

---

Table 20-5   Differential Diagnoses for Carpal Tunnel Syndrome

• C6 cervical radiculopathy	• Proximal arm median nerve compression
• CMC arthritis of thumb	• Ulnar neuropathy
• Volar ganglion	• Wrist arthritis
• Underlying diabetes	• Flexor carpi radialis tendinitis
• Underlying hypothyroidism	

nerve (7). Thenar atrophy is seen in more advanced cases. Electro-myograms (EMG) and nerve conduction studies (NCS) are helpful objective diagnostic tests. These studies may be of benefit in predicting prognosis of surgical intervention and information on chronicity, severity, and regenera-tion (4); they are typically obtained before any surgical intervention. However, in 10%-20% of patients with carpal tunnel syndrome, EMG and NCS testing are normal.

Treatment for mild cases includes splinting the wrist in slight dorsiflex-ion (cock-up splint) in an attempt to relieve pressure on the median nerve. This should be worn at night at a minimum and during the day if not pro-hibitive for work activities. Work-place ergonomic modifications, such as keyboard or forearm supports, adjusting chair or computer table height, and avoiding chronic wrist flexion positions, are important. Avoidance of activities that precipitate symptoms and short courses of NSAIDs or oral corticosteroids can be tried. If symptoms persist, corticosteroid injection into the carpal canal can be beneficial. Acute carpal tunnel syndrome often responds well to injected corticosteroids. This is performed with a 25-gauge needle inserted at a 30-45 degree angle 1 cm proximal to the distal palmar wrist flexion crease, ulnar to the palmaris longus in alignment with the ring finger. If the patient reports paresthesias, redirect the needle. Inject 1 ml of steroid with 1-2 ml of local anesthetic into the carpal canal (7). Surgical re-lease of the transverse carpal ligament through open procedure or arthroscopy is indicated when conservative measures fail or in more ad-vanced cases diagnosed clinically or by nerve conduction studies.

Ulnar Nerve Compression at the Wrist (Guyon's Tunnel Syndrome)

Also known as *cyclist's palsy*, ulnar nerve compression occurs as the nerve traverses Guyon's canal between the pisiform and hamate bones on the ulnar side of the wrist. The nerve is divided into the deep motor branch and the superficial sensory branch. Symptoms can vary depending on where the compression occurs. Symptoms include paresthesias and pain in the distribution of the ulnar nerve (specifically the ulnar side of the palm), the fifth digit, and the ulnar side of the fourth digit. This syndrome is common among competitive cyclists with direct compression of the ulnar nerve against the handlebars (Table 20-6). It is also seen in weightlifters, karate athletes, and baseball catchers, in whom chronic repetitive motion in the hypothenar region predisposes to ulnar nerve injury (19).

Table 20-6   Conditions Causing Ulnar Nerve Compression at the Wrist (Guyon's Tunnel Syndrome)

• Hook of hamate fracture	• Tumor
• Ulnar artery aneurysm	• Synovial cyst
• Extrinsic compression (handlebars)	• Lipoma
• Ulnar nerve compression more proximal	

Physical exam findings depend on where the compression occurs but can include decreased sensation and two-point discrimination in the ulnar nerve distribution, hypothenar muscle weakness or atrophy, and weakness of the adductor and flexor pollicis brevi muscles. Radiographs with carpal tunnel views are sometimes warranted to rule out associated fractures of the hook of the hamate.

Conservative treatment involves protective padding or splinting over the hypothenar area and NSAIDs. Changing the cyclist's grip on the handlebars is helpful. In resistant cases, EMG and NCS are beneficial to isolate the site of compression and aid in planning surgical intervention. Referral to an orthopedic surgeon is warranted in resistant cases and those cases involving obvious muscle weakness and motor loss.

Ganglion Cysts

Ganglion cysts arise from degeneration or tearing of the capsule of a joint or a tendon synovial sheath. They contain a gelatinous, clear fluid similar to joint fluid. Ganglia, the most common soft tissue tumors of the hand and wrist, are benign (7). They can vary in size and are most commonly found on the dorsum of the wrist or the volar radial side of the wrist. These cysts are often asymptomatic masses. Their size can "wax and wane," often depending on activity. Ganglion cysts become painful due to mass effect on surrounding structures.

Dorsal wrist ganglia usually arise from the scapholunate junction and become more prominent with wrist flexion. Volar-sided ganglia are less well defined and typically found on the radial side between the flexor carpi radialis tendon and the radial styloid. The cysts are mildly tender with palpation and if large enough will transilluminate with a penlight.

PA and lateral radiographs are recommended to rule out bony pathology. Most ganglion cysts are associated with normal x-rays. Treatment involves reassuring the patient that this is a benign entity. Relative rest and splinting to immobilize are helpful for acute severe symptoms. Aspiration of the cyst using an 18- or 20-gauge needle with or without injection of a corticosteroid can be performed on larger, symptomatic ganglia. If the ganglion cyst becomes recurrent, surgical excision is warranted.

Kienböck's Disease

Kienböck's disease is an idiopathic avascular necrosis of the lunate. Generally described as atraumatic in origin, it is believed that chronic repetitive trauma precipitates the lunate injury (15,20). It can present with chronic volar- or dorsal-sided wrist pain, swelling over the dorsum of the lunate, and wrist stiffness. Tenderness is usually on the dorsal side, and grip strength is diminished. Diagnosis is made by imaging. Plain radiographs often show a negative ulnar variance in association with AVN of the lunate. In the early stages, radiographs are normal but eventually the patient develops sclerosis, compression fracture, and carpal collapse. A bone scan or

MRI is essential if there is clinical suspicion for Kienböck's disease. Referral to an orthopedic specialist in a timely fashion is suggested. In the acute stages, immobilization can lessen symptoms, but in more advanced and chronic cases, complex surgical intervention is often necessary (15).

REFERENCES

1. **Mastey R, Weiss A, Akelman E.** Primary care of hand and wrist athletic injuries. Clin Sports Med. 1997;16:707-24.

2. **Rettig AC.** Epidemiology of hand and wrist injuries in sports. Clin Sports Med. 1998;17:401-6.

3. **Lillegard WA, Butcher JD, Rucker KS.** Handbook of Sports Medicine: A Symptom Oriented Approach. Boston: Butterworth-Heinemann; 1999:159-80.

4. **Brukner P, Khan, K.** Clinical Sports Medicine. Sydney: McGraw-Hill; 2001:292-306.

5. **Zemel N, Stark H.** Fractures and dislocation of the carpal bones. Clin Sports Med. 1986;5:710-24.

6. **Hoppenfeld S.** Physical Examination of the Spine and Extremities. Norwalk: Appleton & Lange; 1976:59-104.

7. **Greene WB.** Essentials of Musculoskeletal Care. Illinois: American Academy of Orthopaedic Surgeons; 2001:199-265.

8. **Wood MB, Dobyns JH.** Sports-related extraarticular wrist syndromes. Clin Ortho. 1986;202:93-103.

9. **Mooney JF III, Siegel DB, Koman LA.** Ligamentous injuries of the wrist in athletes. Clin Sports Med. 1992;11:129-39.

10. **Weissman B, Sledge CB.** Orthopedic Radiology. Philadelphia: WB Saunders; 1986:111-67.

11. **Fritz R, Brody G.** MR imaging of the wrist and elbow. Clin Sports Med. 1995; 14:315-50.

12. **Savoie F, Whipple T.** The role of arthroscopy in athletic injuries of the wrist. Clin Sports Med. 1996;15:220-33.

13. **Ekman EF, Poehling GC.** Arthroscopy of the wrist in athletes. Clin Sports Med. 1996;15:753-60.

14. **Eiff MP, Hatch RL, Calmbach WL.** Fracture Management for Primary Care. Philadelphia: WB Saunders; 1998:65-83.

15. **Griggs S, Weiss A.** Bony injuries of the wrist, forearm, and elbow. Clin Sports Med. 1996;15:373-400.

16. **Rettig AC, Weidenbener EJ, Gloieske R.** Alternative management of mid-third scaphoid fractures in the athlete. Am J Sports Med. 1994;22:711-4.

17. **Cohen MS.** Ligamentous injuries of the hand and wrist in the athlete. Clin Sports Med. 1998;17:533-50.

18. **Palmer AK.** Triangular fibrocartilage complex lesions: a classification. J Hand Surg. 1989;14A:14-28.

19. **Plancher K, Peterson R, Steichen J.** Compressive neuropathies and tendinopathies in the athletic elbow and wrist. Clin Sports Med. 1996;15:331-71.

20. **Schreibman KL, Freeman A, Gilula LA, et al.** Imaging of the hand and wrist. Orthop Clin North Am. 1997;28:537-79.

21

■ ■ ■

Spine Injuries

Melvin R. Manning, MD
Phil Page, PT

Spine pain is a common diagnostic challenge for the primary care physician covering sports related injuries. Fortunately, most spine pain is self-limited and without permanent impairment. However, if timely recovery is expected, accurate diagnosis followed by appropriate management is crucial. Unless impaired motion and disrupted functional anatomy is appreciated, no meaningful corrective therapeutic measures may be applied. Although it is difficult to accept, always remember that timely recovery is independent of what the athlete, coach, or other team members expect or hope for.

Anatomy

An appreciation of normal spinal anatomy is necessary before considering a differential diagnosis during an injury survey. The brief review of functional anatomy discussed below is focused toward spine regional anatomy of common injuries. Conventional anatomy lists 7 cervical, 12 thoracic, and 5 lumbar vertebra from superior to inferior in location. Each intervertebral disc consists of two basic components: a central nucleus pulposis surrounded by a peripheral annulus fibrosis (Figure 21-1). The last component of the intervetebral disc is the vertebral end-plate, which is composed of two layers of cartilage that cover the top and bottom aspects of each disc. The intervetebral discs' principal function is to allow movement between vertebral bodies and to transmit loads from one body to the next. Zygapophyseal joints, also known as "facet joints," are formed by the articulation of the inferior articular processes of one vertebra with the superior articular processes of the next vertebra. The joints exhibit features typical

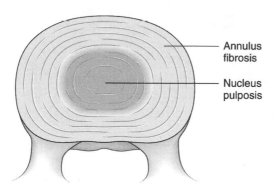

Figure 21-1   Each intervetebral disc consists of two basic components: a central nucleus pulposis surrounded by a peripheral annulus fibrosis.

of synovial joints. The par interarticularis runs obliquely between the superior and inferior articular processes and is responsible for dissipating considerably high forces during movement (particularly extension and rotation). The spinal cord is protected within the vertebral canal, just posterior to the vertebral body. The spinous process is the most posterior portion of the spine and many times is appreciated during examination (palpation). There are a series of ligaments and muscles that span the spine and interconnect vertebral bodies and surrounding soft tissue/fascia. There is a superficial and deep layer of spinal muscles. The deep muscle group within the cervical region includes the semispinalis cervicis, which arises on the transverse process of the thoracic and lower cervical vertebrae and inserts on the spinous processes of the upper cervical vertebrae. The deep cervical portion of the erector spinae consists of the iliocostalis, the spinalis, and the longissimus cervicis. The lumbar region has short intersegmental muscles known as the interspinales and intertransversarii medialis. The deep lumbar region has polysegmented attachments known as the multifidus. Compared with the cervical and lumbar regions, the height of the discs in the thoracic spine is decreased. However, the annulus fibrosis is thicker. Thoracic discs seem to be effective in limiting rotation. Ligaments and other soft tissue structures are not significantly different from cervical and lumbar segments.

Mechanical Low Back Pain

Mechanical low back pain (LBP) in athletes is often long-standing and recurrent, with no specific onset. Usually, diagnostic testing is unremarkable. Mechanical LBP can be differentiated from a lumbar sprain/strain by the former pain being chronic and recurring. As the diagnosis states, mechanical LBP is often a result of some biomechanical dysfunction involving the musculoskeletal structures. While the cause of the pain is often vague, it often involves malignment of bony structures or imbalance of muscular forces on joint surfaces.

Athletes with mechanical LBP often have a leg length discrepancy or rotation of the sacroiliac joint. These are usually noted by a bony asymmetry of the pelvis. Heel lifts are indicated in leg length discrepancy, whereas mobilization may be indicated for a sacroiliac rotation. Hip musculature plays a significant role in transferring forces from the lower extremity toward the spine during upright activities. Consequently, proximal lower-extremity muscle imbalance may play a major role in the development of low back pain (1,2). The most notable muscle imbalance appears to be within the hip extensors. Overall hip extension strength is typically weaker after episodes of low back pain. Additionally, significant side to side differences of hip extension have been used as a predictor of low back pain in female college athletes (3). Another important consideration of mechanical low back pain is dynamic regulation of spine motion. Under normal circumstances, spinal motion is initiated by the cerebral cortex and moderated by the spinal cord. As dysfunctional movements occur, there is abnormal control of the lumbar paraspinal musculature, causing erratic control of spine motion. As a result, rehabilitation is often focused toward restoring normal functional spinal motion, core body muscle strength and proximal lower extremity muscle balance, followed by an exercise maintenance program.

The muscular imbalances associated with mechanical LBP are determined and addressed with therapeutic exercise (4). Muscles found to be tight (usually the hip flexors, hamstrings, and thoraco-lumbar extensors), should be stretched using a contract-relax technique. Next, muscles found to be weak should be strengthened (abdominals, gluteus maximus, multifidus, and quadriceps).

Once muscle balance is restored, dynamic stabilization exercises are performed. Exercises that emphasize stabilization of the lumbo-pelvic region while incorporating movement of the extremities help teach the athlete how to control and protect their spine. Progressing patients from stable surfaces to more unstable surfaces, such as exercise balls, foam stability trainers, or wobble boards, may improve dynamic stabilization of the lumbo-pelvic region. Athletes gradually may be progressed to sport-specific activities to increase power and endurance while protecting the spine.

Sprains and Strains

Sprains occur as a result of injury to the ligamentous cervical and lumbar structures. Typically, injury occurs during lateral flexion or combined flexion-rotation injuries of the trunk. Although primary injury occurs within the ligament, studies reveal that primary failure occurs at the myotendinous junction (5,6). There is tenderness surrounding the myotendinous junction of the deep and superficial muscles. The most common result of this type of injury is decreased spinal motion without neurologic sequelae. Clinically, palpable myotendinous junctions lie short of the ribs near the insertions of the iliocostalis lumborum. More severe spine injuries involve subluxation or frank dislocation with catastrophic neurologic sequelae. Strains occur when paraspinal muscles are overloaded eccentrically. High-intensity forceful eccentric contraction increases risk of injury.

Important diagnostic tests include lateral radiographs with flexion and extension views to rule out subluxation/dislocation (Figure 21-2). Because of the excellent preinjury condition of these athletes, these injuries are usually self-limiting and resolve in 2-4 weeks with conservative management. Regular activity should be encouraged within pain tolerance; however, athletes should not participate in activities that increase their symptoms. Strains respond to occasional short-term immobilization, NSAIDs, and concurrent rehabilitation directed toward range of motion, flexibility, and strengthening exercises. Modalities are often helpful in managing acute sprains and strains. Cold modalities (ice packs, cold packs, ice massage) should be used within the first few days of injury and are often beneficial to apply after exercise or physical activity. Heat treatments (hot packs, heating pads, warm baths) can be used once the acute inflammatory stage is over, usually 2-3 days after injury. Electrical modalities, such as ultrasound or electrical stimulation, may be beneficial in the first 4 weeks after injury to assist in tissue healing but are of limited benefit after 4 weeks of back pain.

Exercises should also be prescribed to strengthen muscles that may have become damaged or that support damaged structures. Strengthening exercises involving the spine and extremities can help with tissue healing and prevent further injury. Athletes with recurrent spinal strains and sprains should emphasize a dynamic stabilization program to protect the spine.

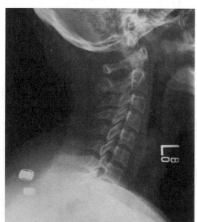

Figure 21-2   Normal lateral view of cervical spine.

Athletes should be taught how to voluntarily recruit their abdominal musculature while performing progressively more challenging exercises involving the extremities. Education on proper posture and body mechanics can be included to protect healing tissues. Sport-specific activities should be introduced and progressed to increase endurance. Although sprains are more likely to require short-term immobilization, the importance of rehabilitation can never be overemphasized. Poor rehabilitation may lead to recurrence of injury.

Spondylosis

The process of generalized degenerative changes in the cervical and lumbar spine is known as spondylosis and is the most common cause of upper and lower extremity pain in middle and older age athletes. Spondylosis is often asymmetric; however, when the symptoms occur, they are often localized to the center of the spine. Progression of spondylosis may include radicular symptoms such as hypertrophic changes and spurs that compress nerve roots. Common symptoms include morning stiffness in addition to stiffness after having been in one position for an extended period of time. Range of motion is often limited and rest often relieves pain. Radiographs are often diagnostic. Typical radiographic findings of spondylosis include extensive disc space narrowing and end-plate spurring (Figure 21-3).

Management is geared toward pain relief followed by improvement and provision of proper static and dynamic spine posture. Exercises include abdominal and spine isometric strengthening. When rehabilitation

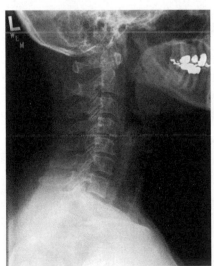

Figure 21-3 Extensive disc space narrowing and end-plate spurring can be seen throughout the cervical spine. These findings are consistent with spondylosis.

is difficult or initial muscle support is poor, consider application of an elastic spine support while attempts are made to improve strength of supporting muscle groups.

Facet Syndrome

Lumbar facet syndrome typically involves the L4/5 and L5/S1 joints. The syndrome includes back pain, which is exacerbated with hyperextension or rotation. There is usually pain with palpation over the involved facet joints. Occasionally, the pain refers to the buttock, hip, or thigh (after hyperextension or rotation). However, lumbar facet joints are rarely an isolated source of back pain. There is usually an associated degenerative component or segmental instability (7).

Management includes pain control through local measures. If cryotherapy and/or manual treatment is unsuccessful, a facet cortisone injection may be helpful. Once pain has been controlled and normal movement patterns begin, rehabilitation strategies should progress toward strengthening. Athletes should return to sport only after demonstration of full motion with excellent strength.

Disc Herniation

Disc herniation is relatively uncommon in athletes and usually is associated with a nonathletic event. The North American Spine Society has agreed to the following nomenclature for disc herniation:

1. The nonspecific term *herniation* should be used when a specific diagnosis cannot be made. This situation should only exist when attempts by CT, CT myelography, or suboptimal MRI are indeterminate and a definitive diagnosis cannot be made.
2. A concentric extension of the disc margins circumferentially beyond the vertebral margins should be termed an *annular bulge.*
3. If there is a focal and/or extension of nucleus beyond the ventral margin but remains beneath the outer annular wall, posterior longitudinal ligament complex, it should be termed a *protrusion.*
4. The extension of nuclear material completely beyond the outer annulus into the epidural space is termed an *extrusion.* Sequestration occurs as an extruded disc fragment separates from the parent body and becomes a free fragment of disc.

The diagnostic test of preference for herniations is MRI (Figure 21-4). Classic presentation includes pain or numbness in a dermatomal distribution often associated with weakness of the associated muscle group. Athletes with disc herination typically present with unilateral radicular leg

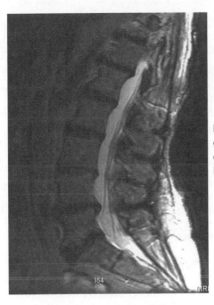

Figure 21-4   Lumbar lateral MRI T$_2$ view demonstrates disc space narrowing, nuclear dehydration, and herniation involving the L3/L4/L5 segment.

pain; myotomal leg weakness may not be present. Conservative care is the mainstay of treatment. Most patients with lateral disc herniation recover within 1 month, and the majority recover within 6 months. Conservative care includes NSAIDs, short-term analgesics, and muscle relaxants combined with physical therapy.

Rehabilitation should be directed toward core body muscle strengthening when there is a lumbar disc herniation and cervical isometrics when the cervical disc is involved.

With lumbar disc herniation, depending on the extent of the herniation, most athletes respond well to "McKenzie" extension exercises, popularized by Robin McKenzie. These exercises emphasize lumbar extension (such as a "press-up" or "lean back") rather than flexion in order to reduce a posterior bulge or herniation. Without the presence of myotomal weakness, the radicular pain may be self-limiting. It is very important to avoid any exercise or activity that increases leg pain, numbness, or weakness. These activities usually involve flexion of the spine; therefore, these athletes should be instructed to avoid the traditional "Williams' flexion" exercises ("knee to chest"), vigorous hamstring stretching, or slumped-sitting postures.

Dynamic lumbar stabilization, including exercises to improve reflexive activation of the deep abdominal and lumbar musculature, should be prescribed once the acute radicular symptoms have subsided. These dynamic exercises, including stabilization with an exercise ball, have been shown to decrease radicular symptoms by 96% in patients with herniated discs (8). Modalities may be beneficial acutely to decrease the symptoms of a herniated disc; however, they should be secondary to education to avoid increasing leg pain and specific exercises to reduce the herniation. Advanced conservative care options include epidural steroid or selective nerve root injections. If the athlete's condition is recalcitrant to conservative care, consider surgical intervention. It is important to restrict an athlete's activity during recovery from a herniation. Moreover, athletes should be advised against participation in high-impact and contact sports such as tennis, basketball, and football. Athletes should remain out of sports until pain has subsided and normal movement and strength patterns have returned. However, because the recovery after disc herniation usually requires a significant decrease in athletic participation, it is important that athletes continue to perform cardiovascular conditioning exercises to maintain their aerobic and anaerobic capacity. Swimming or deep water running, upper body ergometry, or treadmill walking can be used. Bicycling, jogging, or stair-climbing often aggravates radicular symptoms.

Scoliosis and Kyphosis

The cause of adolescent scoliosis is multifactorial. Typically, this problem is detected shortly after onset of puberty and is more common in females than males (9). Consequently, the incidence is higher in sports such as gymnastics, tennis, and volleyball. Traditional evaluation uses standing posterioanterior radiographs of the spine to assess lateral curvature with the Cobb angle. The most tilted vertebral bodies above and below the apex of the spinal curve are used to create intersecting lines that give degree of curvature (Figure 21-5). The forward bend test is universally accepted as the most useful physical exam tool.

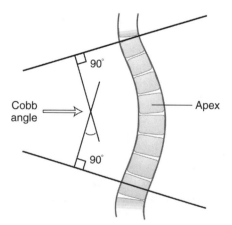

Figure 21-5 The most tilted vertebral bodies above and below the apex of the spinal curve are used to create intersecting lines that give degree of curvature. The Cobb method of determining the degree of scoliosis is shown here.

There is a general consensus that curves < 25 degrees require no active treatment and may be monitored. However, most authors believe that, in patients with immature skeletons and curves between 30 and 40 degrees, bracing may effectively halt progression of the curve. Correcting curves larger than 50% in rapidly growing athletes involves posterior spinal fusion, usually with instrumentation (10). The primary risk factors for curve progression are a large curve magnitude, skeletal immaturity, and female gender. Severe pain, a left thoracic curve, or an abnormal neurologic examination are Red Flags and should prompt the examiner to look for a secondary cause of spinal deformity.

Scheuermann's disease represents moderate-to-severe kyphosis in adolescents nearing growth spurt. The cause is unknown. Scheuermann's may present with acute back pain without history of trauma. Wedging of the vertebral bodies is associated with end-plate irregularities, Schmorl's nodes, and disc space narrowing. However, symptoms may spontaneously resolve after completion of the growth spurt. Fisk and colleagues (11) found that prolonged sitting was the important factor in pathogenesis of Scheuermann's disease compared with athletes lifting weights, undergoing compressive stresses, or doing heavy lifting and part-time work; the implications of this finding are important when considering sports such as rowing or kayaking. Initial management should consist of bracing. Severe kyphosis or persistent pain symptoms may require surgical fixation.

Spondylolysis and Spondylolisthesis

"Spondylo-" injuries are common in athletes involved in repetitive hyperextension, particularly gymnasts, and are the most common cause of back pain in adolescent athletes. Patients may present with lumbar spine pain that worsens with extension and, at times, rotation. The pain may refer to the buttocks or posterior thigh but rarely below the knee. Hamstring tightness is also commonly noted (12).

Spondylolysis occurs as a result of a defect within the pars interarticularis. This region connects the lamina to the superior articular facet. The progression from spondylolysis to spondylolisthesis indicates an increase in the hypermobility of the damaged vertebral segment. Spondylolisthesis occurs after loss of posterior stabilization, at which point the vertebral body may "slip" or sublux forward.

Initial presentation of spondylolysis is often during prepubescent years. However, spondylolisthesis most often occurs during puberty and/or a growth spurt. Spondylolysis and spondylolisthesis occur in more than 20% of female gymnasts and disproportionately affects adolescents who participate in diving, weight lifting, football, wrestling, high jumping, and rowing (13).

Initial diagnostic testing should include anteroposterior, lateral, and oblique films. Oblique films show the defect of the pars interarticularis (Figure 21-6), whereas the lateral view will reveal any forward slippage/subluxation that may present. If radiographs are negative, consider bone scan for acute injury or CT scan/MRI for subacute or chronic discomfort. Serial follow-up radiographs are helpful in monitoring the progression of listhesis (Figure 21-7). Also consider follow-up CT scan after 8-12 wks of conservative care (discussed below) for assessment of healing.

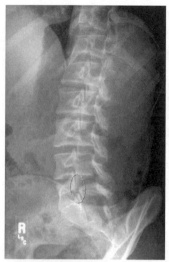

Figure 21-6   Lumbar oblique (also known as "Scottie dog view") film showing defect of pars interarticularis.

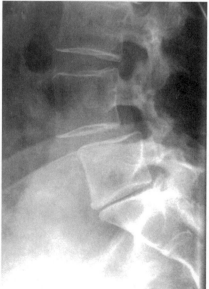

Figure 21-7   Spondylolisthesis occurs after loss of posterior stabilization at which point the L4 vertebral body "slips" or subluxes forward relative to the L5 vertebral body.

Conservative treatment includes relative rest and removal from sports. A lumbar support brace is often used concurrent with rehabilitation focused toward hamstring stretching and core body strengthening exercises. A thoracolumbar brace may also be used for minor spondylolisthesis. The lumbar instability seen with the progression of spondylolysis to spondylolisthesis must be controlled by the dynamic secondary stabilizers of the spine: the musculature. Sinaki and colleagues suggest that conservative rehabilitation emphasize flexion movements, isometric back strengthening, and avoidance of extension movements (14). Therefore, the main emphasis of rehabilitation is to first avoid hyperextension and promote dynamic stabilization exercises in functional positions. The goal of rehabilitation is to teach the athlete to perform functional activities in a neutral spine position to avoid anterior translation of the hypermobile segment during extension.

Additional emphasis should be placed on strengthening the neuromuscular control of the lumbar extensors, particularly the multifidus. Care must be taken to avoid hyperextension and to maintain abdominal bracing with these exercises. Nonoperative treatment of mild spondylolisthesis relieves pain in two-thirds of patients (15). Once symptoms have resolved and the athlete is able to demonstrate full motion with adequate lower extremity strength, sport participation may resume. Surgical intervention should only be considered for major listhesis or persistent symptoms, despite conservative care that includes oral medication and rehabilitation efforts.

Case Study 21-1

A 15-year-old male golfer presents with low back pain of 6 weeks duration. He states that he has been practicing extensively over this period in an effort to improve his game and make the varsity squad later in the year. If he does not hit any balls for a day or two, the pain improves, but it is exacerbated when he resumes practice. He denies any radiation of the pain into his legs or any lower extremity weakness.

Pain on exam is reproduced by having the patient stand on one leg and hyperextending the spine. Plain films, including a "Scottie dog" view of the lumbar spine, are normal. A bone scan is ordered because of the duration of symptoms and physical exam that is suggestive of pars interarticularis injury. Increased uptake is appreciated in the lumbar vertebrae, and a diagnosis of spondylolysis is made.

The patient is advised to refrain from golf and any twisting/hyperextension activity indefinitely. It is recommended that he continue putting practice and begin restricted cardiovascular activities (e.g., stationary cycling). Rehabilitation is ordered to begin 4 weeks following the initial assessment with a focus on strengthening trunk musculature.

The patient returns after 6 weeks rehabilitation, noting resolution of his pain. He is allowed to slowly resume his complete golf game and advised to continue basic core strengthening exercises to help prevent recurrence.

Fractures

Unfortunately, there is no consistent or universally excepted classification system of cervical fractures. Cervical fractures that are isolated to the lamina or spinous process are typically stable. Flexion-extension x-rays reveal no evidence of instability. Cervical vertebral body compression fractures occur as the result of axial loading. Simple wedge or end-plate compression fractures and isolated anterior-inferior vertebral body fracture or "teardrop" fractures are also considered stable. These fractures should respond to conservative management and rarely, if ever, are associated with neurologic sequelae. These injuries require no active treatment other than immobilization within a cervical collar. Once radiographs show sufficient healing and the athlete is able to demonstrate pain-free motion with normal strength, contact sport participation may resume. There are no experimental or clinical data to help the physician predict the stability of healed spinal fractures or fusions when placed under extreme degrees of mechanical load.

As mentioned previously, the thoracic spine has limited rotational movement. Consequently, considerable violence is necessary to produce fractures or fracture-dislocations with the thoracic spine. Most of the bony injuries occur in flexion and axial loading (secondary to limited rotation). Additionally, the spinal cord is frequently injured as a result of the violent forces created.

The most common lumbar spine fracture in contact sports involves the posterior column. Fractures of the transverse or posterior spinous process are usually stable and are rarely associated with neurologic injury. Management includes local measures in an attempt to control pain. Oral medications and cold therapy are appropriate during initial treatment. As pain decreases, rehabilitation should begin.

Compression fractures represent anterior column injury. Axial loading of the anterior column in flexion until it fails produces disruption of the anterior vertebral body with likelihood of associated ligamentous injury, segmental instability, and chronic deformity (16,17). Compression fractures of less than 50% are treated conservatively with a thoracolumbar spinal orthosis. Compression fractures of more than 50% are considered unstable and often require surgical intervention.

Direct axial loading causes burst fractures. Additionally, these fractures may be caused by a combination of flexion and axial loading to the point of anterior and middle column failure. Burst fractures are unstable because of the involvement of at least two spinal columns. Management of burst fractures includes spinal fixation in an effort to remove pelvic bony/soft tissue fragments and restore height of vertebral body. Absolute contraindication to contact sports includes > 3.5 mm of herniation displacement or > 11 degrees of rotation between two adjacent vertebrae.

Acute Spine Injury

Sports medicine physicians who are involved in event coverage should be very comfortable with appropriate management of acute spine injuries. Sports physicians who are not involved in event coverage should have a working knowledge of the guidelines that direct appropriate care of spine-injured athletes. All sports physicians should practice and review the skills identified below before they are needed in an emergency situation.

Football will be the sport examined for the purpose of this discussion. In May 1998, the Inter-Association Task Force for Acute Care of the Spine Injured Athlete issued its guidelines (18). The Task Force encourages the development of a local emergency care plan regarding the prehospital care of an athlete with a suspected spinal injury. This plan should include communication with the institution's administration and those directly involved with the assessment and transportation of the injured athlete. Key points of the guidelines are as follows:

1. Any athlete suspected of having a spinal injury should not be moved and should be managed as though a spinal injury exists.
2. The athlete's airway, breathing, circulation, neurologic status, and level of consciousness should be assessed.
3. The athlete should not be moved unless absolutely essential to maintain airway, breathing, and circulation.
4. If the athlete must be moved to maintain airway, breathing, and circulation, he or she should be placed in a supine position while maintaining spinal immobilization.
5. When moving a suspected spine-injured athlete, the head and trunk should be moved as a unit. One accepted technique is to manually splint the head to the trunk.
6. The emergency medical services system should be activated.
7. The face mask should be removed before transportation, regardless of the current respiratory status.
8. Those involved in the prehospital care of injured football players should have the tools for face mask removal readily available.
9. Spinal immobilization must be maintained while removing the helmet. In many cases it may be helpful to remove cheek padding and/or deflate air padding before helmet removal.
10. The front of the shoulder pads may be opened to allow access for CPR and defibrillation.

In a second meeting, the Task Force made several recommendations to helmet manufacturers about safety information (19). The safety information includes literature about proper emergency removal of helmet and face guard. Additional recommendations were made toward equipment manufacturing. Football helmet face guards should be attached by loop straps—not bolted on—to facilitate appropriate emergency management by medical personnel. The loop straps should be made of material that is easily cut, and necessary tools for removal should be supplied. In review, the face mask should be removed immediately to allow airway access. The helmet and pads should remain in place until adequate assessment of cervical spine stabilization can be performed in the hospital.

Spear tackler's spine was given its name in 1993 after careful evaluation of data from the National Football Head and Neck Registry (20). Permanent neurologic injury occurred in four athletes who were identified as having the following characteristic combination of abnormalities on plain cervical films: 1) developmental cervical canal stenosis, 2) persistent straightening or reversal of the normal cervical spine lordotic curve, 3) evidence of preexisting posttraumatic radiographic abnormalities of the cervical spine, and 4) documentation of having previously used spear tackling techniques.

Other Considerations

Discitis is recognized to be a form of infectious spondylitis in children. It involves a pyogenic infection of the vertebra-disc unit, and treatment requires antibiotic therapy (21). Athletes with infection of the spinal column present with back pain with and without fever. Similarly, osteomyelitis may present with varying degrees of lower back pain. *Staphylococcus aureus* and *Mycobacterium tuberculosis* are the two common pathogens that cause bacterial and tubercular osteomyelitis, respectively. Bone scanning is sensitive but provides less-than-optimal specificity. MRI is the test of choice for early diagnosis. CT-guided needle biopsy is helpful if a specific pathogen needs to be isolated for treatment. The treatment of choice is intravenous antibiotics. Spinal cord tumors and primary bone tumors of the spinal column (osteoid osteoma/osteoblastoma) may be a cause of painful scoliosis.

Osteoarthritis

Cervical and lumbar osteoarthritis (OA) are common among older athletic individuals. Increased age is the primary risk factor. Symptoms such as pain and stiffness are common, and OA presence is confirmed by x-ray findings of degenerative changes and/or spurring. Unfortunately, conservative treatment will not reverse the bony changes associated with OA. The goal of rehabilitation is to minimize inflammation, strengthen associated musculature, and prevent further damage to the joint(s) affected. Heat modalities are often beneficial to promote activity, and ice may be more beneficial in an acute flare-up. It is best to recommend the athlete use heat before and ice after physical activity if it helps decrease pain or soreness.

Osteoarthritis typically responds well to active movement. Athletes should be encouraged to perform gentle, repetitive movements with minimal weight bearing. Walking, biking, and swimming are ideal activities that can be incorporated into rehabilitation or daily activity. Athletes participating in higher-impact or spinal-demand sports should be encouraged to modify their activities, depending on the extent of the OA.

Strengthening of the musculature surrounding the neck or back should be encouraged, including the arms and legs, respectively. Dynamic stabilization exercises may also be of benefit to teach the athlete to use deep stabilizer muscles to protect osteoarthritic segments. Aquatic rehabilitation is an excellent option, particularly for athletes with lumbar osteoarthritis.

REFERENCES

1. **Torg JS, Sennett B, Pavlov H, et al.** Spear tackling spine: an entity precluding participation in tackle footbal and collision activities that expose the cervical spine to axial injury inputs. Am J Sports Med. 1993;21:640-9.

2. **Nadler SF, Malanga GA, Feinberg JH, et al.** Relationship between hip muscle imbalance and occurrence of low back pain in collegiate athletes: a prospective study. Am J Phys Med Rehabil. 2001;80:572-7.

3. **Ville Leinonen BM, Markku K, Olavi A, Osmo H.** Back and hip extensor activities during trunk flexion/extension: effects of low back pain and rehabilitation. Arch Phs Med Rehabil. 2000;81:32-7.

4. **Janda V.** Muscles and motor control in low back pain: assessment and management. In: Twomey LT, ed. Physical Therapy of the Low Back. New York: Churchill Livingstone; 1987:253-78.

5. **Garrett WE, Nikoloau PK, Ribbeck BM, et al.** The effect of muscle architecture on the biomechanical failure properties of skeletal muscle under passive tension. Am J Sports Med. 1988;16:7-12.

6. **Garrett WE, Saffrean MR, Seaber AV, et al.** Biomechanical comparison of stimulated and nonstimulated skeletal muscle pulled to failure. Am J Sports Med. 1987; 15:448-54.

7. **Esses SI, Moro JK.** The value of the facet joint blocks in patient selection for lumbar fusion. Spine. 1993;18:185-90.

8. **Saal JA, Saal JS.** Nonperative treatment of herniated lumbar intervertebral disc with radiculopathy. Spine. 1989;14(4):431-7.

9. **Morrisy RT, Weinstein SL, eds.** Lovell and Winter's Pediatric Orthopedics, 4th ed. Philadelphia: Lippincott-Raven; 1996.

10. **Beaty JH, ed.** Orthopedic Knowledge Update. Rosemont, IL: Academy of Orthopedic Surgeons; 1999.

11. **Fisk JW, Baigent ML, Hill PD.** Scheuermann's disease: clinical and radiological survey of 17 and 18 year olds. Am J Sports Med. 1984;63:18-30.

12. **Weltse LL, Jackson DO.** Treatment of spondylolisthesis and spondylolysis in children. Clin Orthop. 1976;117:92.

13. **Jackson DW, Wiltse LL, Cirincione RJ.** Spondylolysis in the female gymnast. Clin Orthop. 1976;117:6.

14. **Sinaki M, Lutness MP, Ilstrup DM, et al.** Lumbar spondylolistheses: retrospective comparison and three-year follow-up of two conservative treatment programs. Arch Phys Med Rehabil. 1989;70:594-8.

15. **Pizzutillo PD, Hummer CD.** Nonoperative treatment for painful adolescent spondylolysis and spondylolisthesis. J Pediatr Orthop. 1989;9:538-40.

16. **White AA, Panjabi MM.** Clinical Biomechanics of the Spine. Philadelphia: JB Lippincott; 1978.

17. **White AA, Johnson RM, Panjabi MM.** Biomechanical analysis of clinical stability in the cervical spine. Clinical Orthop. 1975;109:85-93.

18. Guidelines from Inter-Association Task Force for Appropriate Care of the Spine-Injured Athlete. First meeting. May 1998; Indianapolis.

19. Guidelines from Inter-Association Task Force for Appropriate Care of the Spine-Injured Athlete. Second meeting. January 1999; Dallas.

20. **Torg JS, Wiesel SW, Rothman RH.** Diagnosis and management of cervical spine injuries. In: Athletic Injuries to the Head, Neck and Face. Philadelphia: Lea & Febiger; 1982.

21. **Ring D, Wenger DR.** Magnetic resonance imaging scans in discitis: sequential studies in a child who needed operative drainage: a case report. J Bone Joint Surgery [Am]. 1994;76A:596.

22

■ ■ ■

Hip and Pelvic Injuries

Luis Palacios, MD

ip and pelvic injuries may occur as a result of trauma or overuse. Injuries to the hip and pelvis are less common than injuries of the other extremities, in part because the greater mass of the muscles of the hip and pelvis provide greater protection as well as decreased exposure to trauma or overuse. When they do occur, however, these injuries can present a diagnostic dilemma for the primary care physician given the additional nonmuscular structures in the area. Both the gastrointestinal and genitourinary structures may be the actual source of pain or discomfort in patients presenting with pelvic pain. The location of the pain may also be misleading, because hip problems may present as pain in other areas (for example, the knee), while hip pain may actually indicate a problem with the spine. In addition, injury cause may be age-specific (for example, overuse traction injuries are more common in skeletally immature adolescents). For these reasons, proper attention to the history and a focused physical examination are crucial.

Anatomy

The hip and pelvis are surrounded by multiple large, powerful muscles, which provide support and are a major basis for locomotion. Many of these muscles originate and insert within the pelvic borders, whereas others traverse the area. There are four functional muscle groups: 1) hip flexors, 2) hip adductors, 3) hip abductors, and 4) hip extensors. In addition, these four groups collaborate to produce the movements of external and internal rotation of the hip (Table 22-1). The cluneal nerves cross the posterior aspect of the iliac crest and supply sensation over the iliac crest, between the posterior superior iliac spine and the iliac tubercle, and over the buttocks. The posterior cutaneous nerve supplies sensation to the posterior

Table 22-1   Muscles of the Hip and Pelvis

Flexors	Adductors	Abductors	Extensors	External Rotators	Internal Rotators
Iliopsoas	Gracilis	Gluteus medius	Gluteus maximus	Gluteus minimus	Gluteus medius
Sartorius	Pectinius	Gluteus minimus	Hamstrings	Piriformis	Adductor magnus
Rectus femoris	Adductor longus, adductor brevis, adductor magnus	Tensor fascia lata		Obturator internus, quadratus femoris	Semimembranosus and semitendinosis, gracilis

thigh from the gluteal crease to just below the popliteal fossa. The anterior femoral cutaneous nerve serves the anterior thigh. The lateral femoral cutaneous nerve is located superficially in the anterior pelvis and runs over the anterior superior iliac spine (ASIS), innervating the anterolateral thigh.

History

Adequate attention to history, review of systems, and a physical examination will enable the clinician to identify most problems. The history should take into account the age of the patient, daily activity level, other medical problems, and current medications.

Developmental and acquired problems, including congenital dislocation of the hip and coxa vara (a deformity of the proximal femur associated with a decrease of the normal neck/shaft angle), may manifest in adulthood as hip and pelvic pain. Some hip and pelvis disorders may be age-specific. Degenerative arthritis and neuropathic joints are more common after the age of 40, whereas apophyseal avulsion fractures occur in the skeletally immature patient. In children, toxic synovitis, Legg-Calvé-Perthes disease (epiphyseal aseptic necrosis of the proximal femur), and slipped capital femoral epiphysis (SCFE) would be of consideration.

It is important to understand factors that may precipitate the patient's pain. If the patient has sustained a high-impact injury, then immediate attention to possible pelvic organ or vascular injury is of prime importance. If the patient is involved in sports and the injury is subacute in nature, then overuse injuries or stress fractures should be considered in the differential diagnoses.

If there is no history of direct trauma, but there is a history of overuse, several historical factors may be helpful. In runners with hip pain, the clinician should ask about changes in terrain or running on uneven surfaces, type and condition of shoes, changes in training schedule and/or increased mileage, and the character and quality of the pain during the activity. Hip problems do not always present with pain; the patient may present with symptoms of decreased motion at the hip, muscle weakness, or gait disturbances. Older patients may report difficulty with gait, dressing, putting on shoes, or getting up from a chair. The clinician must inquire about factors that aggravate or relieve the pain, including whether ambulation or direct pressure on the hip increases the pain.

The location of hip or pelvic pain may not be very helpful in determining the cause of the pain. Hip problems may present as knee pain, whereas problems in the spine or pelvis may present as hip pain. Lower lumbar disease often causes pain radiation to the gluteal region, whereas upper lumbar lesions cause pain radiation to the anterior thigh. Back pain is often aggravated by stooping or lifting and improves with walking, but true hip pain is made worse by walking.

Physical Examination

The physical examination should be focused and tailored according to the information obtained in the history, particularly the time frame of the symptoms and the mechanism of injury. The practitioner should develop his or her own style and procedure with a goal of performing a thorough examination that includes the elements of inspection, palpation, range of motion, strength testing, and sensation. Practitioners should also familiarize themselves with special testing of the hip and pelvis, which will add to their diagnostic capabilities.

Inspection

The examiner should observe the patient for gait disturbances, body habitus, and signs of obvious pain, as well as how the patient transfers onto the exam table if able to walk unassisted. The hip and pelvic area should be inspected for any obvious deformities, wounds, contusions, swelling, or erythema. With the patient standing, the ASIS should be level and symmetrical. Posteriorly, the gluteal folds and dimples over the posterior superior iliac spines should be symmetric. The curvature of the spine should also be assessed. Absence of the normal lumbar lordosis should be noted, as this suggests paravertebral muscle spasm or weak abdominal musculature. The presence of scoliosis is determined by having the standing patient flex forward at the waist. With the patient supine, the position and orientation of the leg and calf should be observed. Shortening or rotation of the lower extremities may indicate a hip fracture, a leg length discrepancy, or tilted pelvis.

Palpation

The hip and pelvic area should be checked for warmth or point tenderness. With the patient standing, the ASIS should be level. The greater trochanter should be palpated and the presence of point tenderness assessed. As the patient flexes the hip, the examiner may feel a "snap" or "pop" as the tensor fascia lata glides over the greater trochanter. Anteriorly, the symphysis pubis may also be tender, possibly due to osteitis pubis, a condition caused by the shearing forces of running, biking, or playing soccer. Posteriorly, the examiner should palpate the sacroiliac joint, posterior superior iliac spines, the sciatic nerve and piriformis area, and ischial tuberosities.

With the patient supine, the examiner should palpate the femoral triangle for the femoral pulse and abnormal lymph nodes. Tenderness of the origin of the sartorius and adductor longus muscles should be assessed at the anterior superior iliac spine and the pubic symphysis, respectively. Other muscles that can be palpated include the adductor longus, gluteus medius, gluteus maximus, rectus femoris, quadriceps, and hamstrings. Localized tenderness is consistent with a possible strain or tear of these muscles.

Range of Motion

Both active and passive range of motion (ROM) of the hip should be assessed with the patient in the supine position. Normal active range of motion is abduction 45 degrees, adduction 20 degrees, extension 30 degrees and flexion 135 degrees. Passive internal rotation should be about 35 degrees, and external rotation about 45 degrees. Internal rotation and external rotation of the hip should be tested with the hip in both flexion (while sitting on the exam table) and extension (lying prone on the exam table).

Femoral neck anteversion or retroversion can cause excessive internal or external hip rotation. Femoral anteversion is due to an increase in the anterior angulation of the neck of the femur in relationship to the long axis of the shaft of the femur and the femoral condyles. Femoral anteversion causes greater internal rotation of the hip and is commonly manifested clinically as in-toeing ("pigeon-toed"). In-toeing is thought to be caused by positioning while in utero, and in most cases, it is benign and tends to resolve by the ages of 8-10. Rarely is a femoral osteotomy required for correction. It does not predispose individuals to degenerative arthritis. A decreased anterior angulation (retroversion) results in greater external rotation. This is much less common and presents itself in childhood with an out-toeing gait. As with femoral anteversion, this usually resolves in childhood.

Muscle Testing and Sensation

Manual muscle testing should be done on the four functional muscle groups (abduction, adduction, flexion, and extension). Sensory testing may detect lesions involving the lower thoracic and lumbosacral spine or peripheral nerve lesions.

Special Tests

Trendelenburg Test
The Trendelenburg test (Figure 22-1) assesses the function of the gluteus medius muscle. To perform the Trendelenburg test, the patient should stand and bear weight evenly on both legs. The dimples over the posterior superior iliac spines should be even. As the patient stands on one leg, the gluteus medius muscle on the supported side (the leg the patient is standing on) should contract and elevate the pelvis on the unsupported side. If the pelvis on the unsupported side drops, the Trendelenburg test is positive, which indicates abnormal function of the gluteus medius muscle on the supported side. The patient may also demonstrate a Trendelenburg gait, a lurching gait that counteracts the imbalance caused by the descending hip.

Ober Test
The Ober test (Figure 22-2) is used to test for contraction of the iliotibial band. To perform the test, the patient should be in the decubitus position, with the affected leg in the superior position. The patient's leg should be abducted slightly and the knee flexed to 90 degrees, while keeping the hip in neutral position. The abducted thigh is then released while the examiner

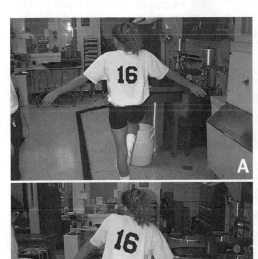

Figure 22-1 Trendelenberg test. With the patient standing and viewed from behind, he or she is asked to stand on one foot. Tilting or "falling" of the hip of the unsupported side signifies weak gluteus medius strength and tone on the supported side. (A) Normal test. (B) Positive test.

holds the patient's foot. If the iliotibial band is tight, the thigh will not return to the adducted position. Iliotibial band contracture can cause pain over the greater trochanter due to traction on the trochanteric bursa.

Patrick (FABER) Test

The Patrick test, or FABER (Flexion, Abduction, and External Rotation) test (Figure 22-3), is used to assess function in the hip or sacroiliac joint. With the patient supine, the examiner asks the patient to abduct the thigh and flex the knee while externally rotating the leg and placing the foot on the opposite knee. To stress the sacroiliac joints, the examiner stabilizes the pelvis with one hand at the anterior aspect of the opposite iliac

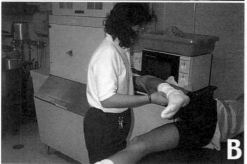

Figure 22-2 Ober test. With the patient lying on his or her side, the leg being tested is abducted with the knee flexed to 90 degrees. Holding on to the patient's knee and ankle in the neutral position (or slightly extended), the examiner releases the knee. The knee on the leg being tested should touch the knee not being tested. (A) Negative exam: tested knee falls to opposite leg. (B) Positive exam: patient unable to "adduct" tested leg due to pain.

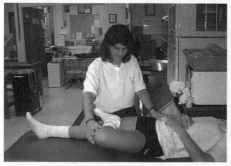

Figure 22-3 FABER test. With the patient supine, the leg on the side being tested is flexed, then internally rotated with the ankle of the test leg resting on the opposite knee, then externally rotated with augmentation by pushing down on the externally rotated leg at the knee. Pain with this maneuver may point to sacroiliac joint problems.

crest while pressing down on the medial aspect of the flexed, externally rotated knee. Pain in the lower back with this maneuver indicates sacroiliac pathology.

Thomas Test

The Thomas test (Figure 22-4) is used to detect hip flexion contractures and to evaluate the range of hip flexion. The patient is supine on the examining table with the pelvis level and square to the trunk. The examiner stabilizes the pelvis by placing one hand under the lumbar spine while flexing the patient's hip with the other hand. The examiner should note the point at which the patient's back touches the hand as the hip is flexed; further flexion originates only in the hip joint. Normal flexion allows the anterior thigh to rest on the abdomen. As the patient fully flexes one hip, the patient's other leg (which is extended) should be observed. If the contralateral leg does not extend fully, the patient has a flexion contracture of that hip. Most flexion contractures are treated with stretching/physical therapy. Hip flexion contractures can also be detected by having the patient lie prone with the knees flexed to 90 degrees. The examiner stabilizes the pelvis with one hand on the lumbar spine or iliac crest, then lifts the patient's thigh with the other hand placed under the patient's knee. Normal hip extension is about 30 degrees. This maneuver also stretches the femoral nerve. A positive test may produce sciatic symptoms and indicate radiculopathy at the L5 level.

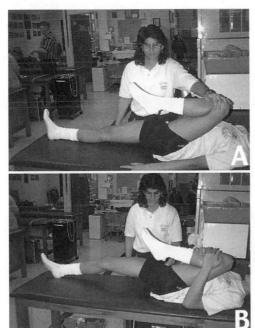

Figure 22-4 Thomas test. The patient is examined in the supine position. The patient is asked to grab one knee with both hands and to bring it to his or her chest. The test is for the opposite leg. The ability to keep the knee straight is examined on the opposite side. The test is positive when the opposite knee flexes and points to tight hip flexors. The physician may augment this test by applying pressure on the knee if it flexes in an attempt to keep it straight. (A) Negative exam. (B) Positive exam.

Test for Leg Length Discrepancy

Leg length discrepancy can be evaluated by several methods. One method is by measuring the distance between the anterior superior iliac spine and the medial malleolus on each leg. Another is by looking for pelvic tilt with the patient standing. A third method involves looking for differences with the patient lying prone, by visualizing the medial malleoli. It often requires about a 2 cm difference between leg length before a limp is obvious. A more accurate measurement would require radiographs (entire lower limbs of both sides and measurement of lengths of both limbs).

Ancillary Studies

Imaging Studies

Imaging studies may be necessary in the assessment of hip and pelvic pain when fracture is suspected. Routine plain films are often sufficient, but selected patients (for example, those with stress fractures) require additional diagnostic tests, such as scintigraphic bone scan, CT, or MRI.

Plain Radiographs. Routine plain radiographs in hip and pelvic disorders include an AP view of the hip and pelvis and a lateral view of the affected hip. The AP view of the pelvis is particularly important in cases of trauma to detect occult pelvic fractures. For most patients, a frog-leg lateral view is obtained, but in cases of trauma, a surgical lateral view is preferred to avoid displacement of potential fractures. In young patients involved in trauma or sports activities, an oblique view of the hip may provide better visualization of avulsion fractures. Radiographic changes may be subtle, and therefore diagnosis may be difficult. Stress fractures may not be visible on plain radiograph or can present as a radiolucent line on radiograph. In children with SCFE, the fracture may not be apparent, or the only sign may be a widened epiphysis. Abnormalities may be seen in patients with OA, sclerosis, osteophyte formation, and/or narrowing of the joint. A radiolucent line, the crescent sign, is seen before subchondral collapse of the femoral head with avascular necrosis of the skeletally immature patient.

Bone Scan. Technetium-99m pyrophosphate bone scan is particularly helpful in detecting stress fractures. Stress fracture should be considered in a patient who presents with hip pain and a history of repetitive weight-bearing exercise. If plain radiographs of the hip are normal, but clinical suspicion of a stress fracture of the femoral neck or shaft is high, the physician should instruct the patient not to bear weight and obtain a bone scan. A bone scan is less helpful in the evaluation of the older patient who falls and has negative plain radiographs but in whom clinical suspicion of a fracture persists. The bone scan may not be positive for up to 5 days due to osteoporosis and delayed remodeling of bone. An MRI may be more appropriate and cost effective in these older patients. Bone scans are also useful in detecting bony metastases in the patient with cancer.

CT/MRI. CT and MRI scans are very useful in the diagnosis of hip and pelvic problems. CT scan is most helpful when the plain radiographs are nondiagnostic. CT may help by providing a three-dimensional analysis of the femoral epiphysis as well as a detailed assessment and pattern of a known fracture or metastatic lesion. MRI is most helpful in the patient with poorly characterized injuries or symptoms and is particularly effective in showing bone bruises or avascular necrosis. MRI can be very useful for assessment of fluid or effusion (for example, in the work-up of an inflammatory arthritis or septic joint).

Laboratory Studies

In general, laboratory studies are not helpful in establishing the diagnosis for patients with hip and pelvic pain. Exceptions to this rule include the patient with fever or a possible septic joint and the patient with symptoms suggestive of arthritis. In these patients, a complete blood count (CBC), erythrocyte sedimentation rate (ESR), and RA latex and antinuclear antibody (ANA) may be helpful. The ESR is almost always elevated in cases of septic arthritis, whereas it is normal in OA. The erythrocyte count may not be significantly elevated, but there may be relative elevation of polymorphonuclear leukocytes. Joint aspiration and fluid analysis are essential for the timely diagnosis of the septic hip, but an orthopedic consultant usually is required for this procedure.

Differential Diagnosis

Hip and pelvic pain can be seen throughout the patient spectrum, from children to adults. There are problems that are specific to pediatric patients or to adults and the elderly. Some of these problems are similar in both adolescents and adults (for example, trauma). Some diseases causing hip and pelvic pain may lead to further problems at a later date (for example, osteoarthritis secondary to improperly treated Legg-Calvé-Perthes disease).

Hip and pelvic pain in adults may, in other cases, be related to stress and trauma placed on the hip joint and pelvis. Partially due to the large muscle mass, greater forces are applied to the joint and surrounding tissues. Causes of hip and pelvic pain include traumatic injuries such as muscle strain, bursitits, and fracture, compression/overuse syndromes, and degenerative joint disease.

Specific Disorders

Table 22-2 summarizes the hip and pelvic injuries discussed below.

Table 22-2   Hip and Pelvic Injuries

Injury	Adult or Child/Adolescent	Examples	Presenting Complaints/Symptoms	Diagnosis	Additional Studies	Treatment
Apophyseal injuries	Child/adolescent	AIIS, ASIS, ischial tuberosity, lesser trochanter, iliac crest	May have occurred acutely or chronically; pain, weakness, tenderness to palpation over affected site	Tenderness, ± swelling, weakness over affected site	Plain radiographs may reveal irregularity of apophysis or widening compared with unaffected side	NSAIDs, ice, compression, and pain control; protective padding for RTP
Muscle strain	All	Quadriceps, adductors, rectus abdominis, hamstring	Acute onset; tenderness with attempted activity	Tenderness with passive stretch and resisted contraction	Usually not necessary unless complete disruption suspected	NSAIDs, ice, compression, and pain control; protective padding for RTP
Compression	Adult, rarely adolescent	Meralgia, paresthetica	Numbness, burning over lateral aspect of thigh down to knee	Occasionally reproduced by tapping over ASIS	None	Loose clothing, avoidance of inciting postural positions, rarely injection; exercises, NSAIDs
		Piriformis	Pain, numbness in buttock down the posterior aspect of the leg in sciatic nerve distribution	Hyperextending leg while patient in prone position	None	
Friction	Adult and adolescent (but "snapping hip" more likely in late adolescent and adult)	Bursitis	Localized pain to bursae site but may be difficult to localize with deeper bursae	Pain over affected bursae but with deeper bursae may have pain with stretch of overlying muscle	X-ray not helpful; for deeper bursae, CT or MRI may be diagnostic	Ice, NSAIDs, exercises; for greater trochanter, aspiration and injection of steroid possible; radiological guidance for deeper bursae

		Clinical presentation	Examination	Diagnostic	Treatment
"Snapping hip"		Pain/discomfort with "popping", "snapping" sound which may be localized to affected side but difficult to localize if deeper structures affected.	Pain over affected muscle but difficult to localize/palpate with deeper structure involvement	CT or MRI may be helpful for localization and surgical referral	If symptoms are mild and do not affect function/performance, ice, stretching, and NSAIDs; severer cases require orthopedic referral for nodule excision
Osteitis pubis		Pain (burning, aching) in the suprapubic area; history of increased running or hurdling	Pain in suprapubic, inguinal, or abdominal areas to palpation and with resistive adduction	X-ray with sclerosis, irregularity, or widening of the symphysis pubis	Ice, relative rest, and NSAIDs; resistant cases may benefit from steroid injection into pubis
Avulsion fracture	Child and adolescent	Rectus femoris (AIIS), sartorius (ASIS), iliopsoas (lesser trochanter), tranversus abdominis (iliac crest), hip adductors (pubic symphysis), semitendinosis and biceps femoris (ischial tuberosity)	Pain/discomfort over affected muscle; difficulty with ambulation, swelling, weakness in affected muscle	Pain with palpation over affected muscle and with resistive action of affected muscle; palpable defect if muscle retracts	X-ray reveals bony avulsion over affected site	Treat similarly to strain, with ice, rest, NSAIDs, crutch walking; severity of symptoms dictates RTP; okay to RTP once symptoms resolve —up to 6 weeks; if displacement or avulsion > 2 cm, may need surgical repair

Cont'd.

Table 22-2   Hip and Pelvic Injuries (Cont'd)

Injury	Adult or Child/Adolescent	Examples	Presenting Complaints/Symptoms	Diagnosis	Additional Studies	Treatment
Stress fracture	Adolescent and adult	Femoral neck	Pain and discomfort in the inguinal, anterior thigh, or buttock area; limp or difficult gait	Pain with range of motion of hip; decreased internal rotation with hip flexed	X-ray reveals fracture; MRI or CT scan if increased suspicion but x-ray nondiagnostic	Refer to orthopedics; in compression side fractures, may treat with orthopedist with strict non-weight-bearing until pain-free
Fracture		Slipped capital femoral epiphysis	Pain in knee (referred) or hip; limping gait	Limited internal rotation; positive "log roll"	X-ray usually diagnostic	Refer to orthopedics
Genito-urinary	All	Cystitis	Pain in suprapubic area; dysuria	Normal exam; pain in suprapubic area	US if pyelonephritis or nephrolithiasis suspected; urinalysis test of choice	Treat with antibiotics; increase fluids
	Adolescent and adult	Pelvic inflammatory disease	Purulent vaginal discharge; fever, pelvic and/or flank pain	Pain with palpation in suprapubic area; purulent vaginal discharge, uterine tenderness	US, cultures	Treat with antibiotics; hospitalize if toxic
	Adult; occasionally late adolescent	Prostatitis	Deep suprapubic tenderness/burning, dysuria	Prostate tender on exam	X-ray not indicated	Treat with antibiotics

Adolescent and adult	Pregnancy	Vague discomfort, weight gain	Depending on gestation—enlarged uterus	Positive pregnancy test	Refer for pregnancy care; okay to continue with exercise if appropriate
Adolescent	Testicular torsion	Inguinal or scrotal pain	Scrotal swelling and pain with palpation; some relief with testicular elevation	Testicular US	Refer to urology
Late adolescent and adult	Sports hernia	Vague lower quadrant or inguinal pain	Nonspecific findings	MRI occasionally helpful	Refer to general surgery

RTP = return to play.
NSAID = nonsteroidal anti-inflammatory drug.
US = ultrasonography.

Trauma-Caused Disorders

Muscle Strain

As mentioned previously, the large muscles that surround and support the hip and pelvis are susceptible to contusion or strain with the powerful contractions they can produce. With trauma, patients will communicate a history of being struck in the affected muscle. In strains, the musculotendinous junction is the area most commonly involved. The patient may describe hearing a loud pop or snap with sudden onset of pain. In overuse injuries, the patient will describe a recent increase in frequency, intensity, and/or duration of a specific inciting activity.

Quadriceps Strain. The quadriceps is composed of three muscles: the rectus femoris, vastus lateralis, and vastus medius. Of these, the rectus femoris is the most commonly affected. Athletes involved in explosive running or hurdling activities are at risk for quadriceps strain. Treatment consists of relative rest, ice compression, and elevation (RICE), protected weight bearing, and range-of-motion exercises. NSAIDs may be used for a short course to control pain. Rehabilitation activities are progressed as tolerated to include restoration of full range of motion and strength. Once this is established, sports-specific skills are incorporated into the rehabilitative process before return to sport/activity. Time away from activity varies depending on the severity of the injury, but it can be up to 4-6 weeks, even with a proper rehabilitation program.

Quadriceps Contusions. Quadriceps contusions are common in contact sports such as football. One will appreciate significant swelling and pain over the quadriceps. Treatment should include keeping the knee flexed for 1 or 2 days (use of a body Ace wrap will facilitate this) and avoiding NSAID use during the first 24 hours after the injury. These treatment maneuvers are an attempt to avoid the development of myositis ossificans (heterotopic ossification) within the quadriceps, a disabling disorder.

Adductor Strains. Groin pain occurs acutely with adductor strains. Athletes who perform cutting maneuvers are most likely to have this injury. The physical exam will reveal tenderness to palpation in the groin area. The patient will be tender to passive abduction and resistive adduction. Treatment is similar to that for quadriceps strain.

Hamstring Strains. Patients with this injury will have pain in the posterior thigh or the bottom of the buttock. The three hamstring muscles are the biceps femoris (laterally) and the semitendinosis and semimembranosis (medially). Of the three, the biceps femoris is the most commonly injured, usually in the proximal musculotendinous junction. Treatment is with RICE, protected weight bearing, and NSAIDs. A progressive rehabilitative program is initiated until full range of motion and strength is obtained. Then sports-specific skills are begun. Only after the athlete has accomplished these skills may he or she return to full athletic activity or competition.

Bursitis

There are three major bursa in the hip joint: the trochanteric bursa, the iliopsoas bursa, and the ischial bursa (Figure 22-5). This is an inflammatory problem caused by repetitive or direct trauma. The patient may have had a recent change of activity (for example, increase in frequency, amount, duration, or change in walking/running surface).

The trochanteric bursa is located over the greater trochanter and underneath the tensor fascia lata; therefore it is somewhat superficial and susceptible to shear stresses and blunt trauma. An increase in activity is common historical information collected from patients with trochanteric bursitis, although trauma can cause the condition as well. If due to overuse, the precipitating cause of trochanteric bursitis is friction caused by the tensor fascia lata as it sweeps over the bursal sac. Pain may occur in the lateral aspect of the hip over the greater trochanter, with occasional radiation to the buttocks or down the lateral thigh along the tensor fascia lata. Initially, pain may be localized and occur only with activity, but eventually the symptoms progress and the patient experiences pain even at rest. On physical examination, the patient may demonstrate an antalgic gait. In females, an increased quadriceps angle or Q angle (that is, the angle formed by drawing a line from the ASIS to the patella, then a line transecting the patella; normal is < 15 degrees) may precipitate the bursitis. Leg length discrepancy has also been associated with an increased incidence of trochanteric bursitis.

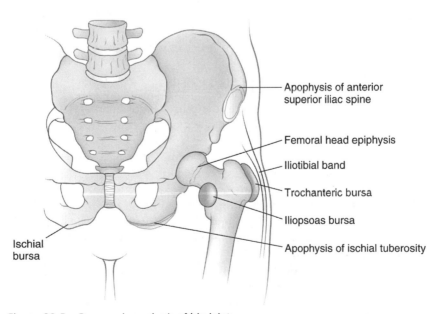

- Apophysis of anterior superior iliac spine
- Femoral head epiphysis
- Iliotibial band
- Trochanteric bursa
- Iliopsoas bursa
- Apophysis of ischial tuberosity

Ischial bursa

Figure 22-5   Bursa and apophysis of hip joint.

The iliopsoas bursa overlies the hip joint and is located between the iliofemoral and pubofemoral ligaments. It is the largest bursa in the body, with normal dimensions of 6 cm by 3 cm. The most common cause for inflammation of the iliopsoas bursa in a younger or more active population is overuse or trauma. It can also be associated as a complication of osteoarthritis, rheumatoid arthritis, or septic arthritis. The patient with iliopsoas bursitis presents with pain deep in the groin or inguinal area. Pain may be elicited by palpation of the lesser trochanter, performed with the hip flexed and externally rotated.

Ischial bursitis is fairly uncommon and usually due to trauma. The bursa lies over the ischial tuberosity and underneath the gluteus maximus. The patient reports a history of trauma to the ischial area with subsequent pain on sitting. Because of its location, it is sometimes confused with a hamstring strain. Physical examination may reveal a limping gait, plus tenderness to palpation of the ischial tuberosity.

Bursitis of the hip may be chronic because of the overuse nature of its cause. This chronicity can lead to changes in the tendinous unit overlying the bursae and lead to a distinct problem known as the "snapping hip" (discussed in more detail later in this chapter).

Treatment for bursitis usually includes relative rest, NSAIDs, and modalities including ice or heat, in addition to range of motion exercises. Once range of motion exercises have been successfully completed, the rehabilitative process should progress to resistive and then strengthening exercises. Additional treatment modalities may include aspiration of the bursa with or without injection of an anesthetic (lidocaine) steroid mixture. In practice, the trochanteric bursa may be the only bursa for which injection treatment is possible due to the easy accessibility of this bursa; the other bursa would require radiological guidance for access.

Case Study 22-1

A 36-year-old female presented to the office complaining of right hip pain. She stated that the pain began one month ago after changing her exercise routine in which she had started a step aerobics class. She had never experienced this problem before and noted an increase in symptoms during exercise. Symptoms were relieved with rest. The pain was localized over the lateral portion of her hip.

Physical exam revealed no gross swelling or defect over the hip. Gait was normal. Passive and active range of motion were normal. She had tenderness to palpation over the greater trochanter, and the Ober test was positive on the right side.

The patient was diagnosed with trochanteric bursitis with a secondary diagnosis of a tight illiotibial band. Treatment options were reviewed with the patient. She was instructed to modify her exercise routine by doing fewer step workouts. She was given an educational brochure on illiotibial band stretching and instructed to ice the area daily. Over-the-counter NSAIDs were advised. She was able to gradually return to her aerobics class in 4 weeks and continued her stretching program.

Hip Fractures

Patients may present with fractures of the hip or pelvis. Fractures of the hip are due to direct blunt trauma, in most cases. In the young, hip fracture is usually caused by severe trauma (for example, sudden deceleration such as occurs in a motor vehicle accident).

Pelvic Fractures

Pelvic fractures can be caused by avulsion of a muscle insertion site, blunt trauma causing compression forces that disrupt the pelvic ring, or direct force to the pelvis. Avulsion fractures caused by direct blows are stable, cause little or no displacement of the pelvic ring, and are classified as "minor" fractures. A minimally displaced fracture of the pubic rami is an example of a minor fracture that is stable and is treated conservatively. Other minor fractures include: 1) avulsion fracture of the pelvic brim, 2) undisplaced fracture of the coccyx, 3) undisplaced fracture of the sacrum, 4) fracture of the ischium, and 5) fracture of the ilium. Radiographs may reveal avulsion fractures due to traction by the attached muscle or direct trauma to the area. Treatment for these fractures is usually supportive and includes ice, compression, and pain control with analgesics. Patients may be able to continue to participate in athletic activities if the injured site is protected by taping or padding.

Major pelvic fractures are usually due to severe trauma from a fall from a height or a motor vehicle accident. They are unstable fractures and may be vertically and/or rotationally unstable or have associated life-threatening complications. They are usually seen in emergency room settings with patients presenting with multiple trauma. Large blood vessels cross the brim of the pelvic floor, so care must be taken to rule out vessel trauma. The basic principles of resuscitative care should be incorporated during initial evaluation (that is, attention must be paid to airway, breathing, circulation, disability, exposure, and so forth).

There are three common fracture patterns: 1) the straddle type, which involves all four pubic rami or in combination with symphysis pubis disruption, and which is associated with genitourinary and pelvic floor injury; 2) the double-vertical type, which involves one set of rami or pubis in addition to the sacroiliac joint; and 3) ilium disruption, which is associated with severe neurologic, GI, and genitourinary damage.

Radiographs are helpful to quickly identify area and type of fracture. Because serious complications are common with pelvic fractures, CT scan may be warranted to determine and localize soft-tissue trauma involving vascular, neurological, bowel, and bladder damage. Patients with these injuries must be referred promptly for definitive care.

Stress Fractures

Stress fractures are more common in a younger population. These injuries are due to repetitive trauma from overuse caused by excessive running or marching and may involve the femoral neck, the femoral shaft, and the pelvis. The repetitive trauma exceeds the body's ability to regenerate, which leads to bony failure at the site. The patient presents with a history of increased activity or an altered training regimen. Initially, pain symptoms occur only with activity, but as the disease process worsens, pain symptoms can occur with activities of daily living or even at rest.

Stress fractures of the femoral neck account for less than 2% of all stress fractures but are more commonly encountered among military recruits and female athletes. Amenorrheic female athletes are at risk for stress fractures due to osteopenia, and military recruits are at risk due to the continual stress on the femur from marching. The patient usually reports pain localized to the inguinal or groin area. On physical examination, the patient is tender in the inguinal or groin area and demonstrates limited hip rotation due to pain at the femoral neck. Plain radiographs of the hip area may demonstrate a stress fracture of the femoral neck. The earliest radiographic sign is a sclerotic line that indicates the site of the fracture. The fractures are classified by location, whether they occur on the superior aspect of the femoral neck (that is, the tension side) or at the inferior aspect of the femoral neck (that is, the compression side). Continued stress and/or weight bearing may cause a displaced fracture of the femoral neck, which is an orthopedic emergency due to the risk of avascular necrosis of the femoral head. Bone scan may aid diagnosis and is indicated if hip pain persists in the patient with a history of overuse and negative plain radiographs.

Treatment of compression side fractures consists of early recognition, non-weight-bearing crutch use, and follow-up x-rays every 3-5 days until callous formation is noted. Once full range of motion is obtained, limited weight bearing may be allowed. Healing is typically complete after 6-8 weeks. In women with amenorrhea, calcium supplementation and oral contraceptive use to induce regular menstrual cycles should be considered. Tension side fractures tend to be more unstable and warrant early referral to orthopedics for evaluation and treatment. Compression side fractures tend to have a better outcome and are less likely to require surgical intervention. Healing may take place after 6 to 8 weeks; however, full return to sport may take several more weeks.

Stress fractures are discussed in detail in Chapter 26.

The femoral shaft is not as susceptible to stress fractures because of the decreased stress forces as compared to the femoral neck. Femoral shaft stress fractures can occur, but they have an even lower incidence than stress fractures of the femoral neck.

Compression/Overuse Syndromes

Piriformis Syndrome

The piriformis muscle originates on the sacrum and inserts at the greater trochanter. Its function is to assist with external rotation and hip abduction. The sciatic nerve passes deep to the piriformis muscle (Figure 22-6). Minor trauma or prolonged compression (for example, a truck driver with a thick wallet) may lead to pain in the buttocks or hypesthesias and/or paresthesias in the sciatic nerve distribution. On physical examination, the patient holds the hip in external rotation due to spasm and tenderness in the buttock area over the piriformis. The patient may also demonstrate weakness of external rotation and abduction. Radiographs are usually not necessary. If the diagnosis is unclear, electromyography/nerve conduction velocity (EMG/NCV) may be used to distinguish sciatic nerve irritation caused by piriformis syndrome from nerve root impingement. Treatment, in addition to NSAIDs, includes stretching and strengthening exercises. A common piriformis stretch is to have the patient sit with the unaffected side leg straight. The patient takes the affected side foot and brings it to the lateral side of the unaffected side. The patient then grabs the affected side leg and

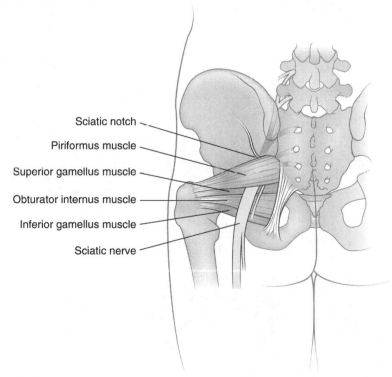

Sciatic notch
Piriformus muscle
Superior gamellus muscle
Obturator internus muscle
Inferior gamellus muscle
Sciatic nerve

Figure 22-6   Sciatic nerve as it passes through the sciatic notch and beneath the piriformis muscle—a site of possible nerve compression.

adducts it. If these measures fail, a radiologically guided injection of the piriformis with steroids may be performed. In unmanageable cases, referral for a surgical release may be considered.

Meralgia Paresthetica

Injury to the lateral femoral cutaneous nerve causes pain in the anterior and lateral proximal thigh area, which is known as meralgia paresthetica. This benign and self-limited disorder can sometimes be confused with hip joint pain. Anatomically, the lateral femoral cutaneous nerve passes superior to the hip joint, just below the anterior superior iliac spine (Figure 22-7). The pressure of the waist band may cause chronic compression of this nerve. Those at risk include women who wear tight-fitting pants, individuals who wear tight belts (including belts worn by weightlifters), individuals who have gained weight, and individuals who have sustained direct blunt trauma to the nerve. The patient presents with symptoms of pain or numbness and tingling along the nerve distribution, which is on the lateral thigh. The physical examination typically is normal. Reproduction of the symptoms can be accomplished by tapping over the ASIS with a hammer. Radiographs and nerve conduction tests are not indicated. The diagnosis of meralgia paresthetica is usually made on clinical grounds. Treatment for

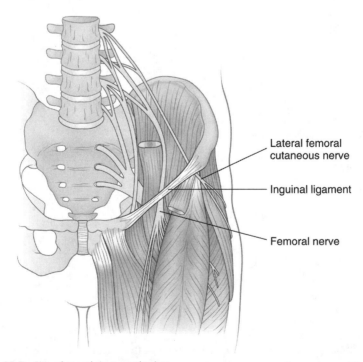

Lateral femoral cutaneous nerve

Inguinal ligament

Femoral nerve

Figure 22-7 Site of meralgia paresthetica.

this malady is to have the patient wear less constricting clothing. Other recommendations may be to avoid prolonged symptom-inducing positions. For example, patients who engage in activities which place them in a position where they are flexed at the hip for prolonged periods will benefit from standing and stretching. Very rarely, a steroid-lidocaine injection may be considered in stubborn cases.

"Snapping Hip"

"Snapping hip" is a palpable and/or audible symptom in which the patient describes a "snapping" or "popping" sound or sensation over the hip. There are several causes, the most common being the iliotibial band snapping over the greater trochanter. It can also be caused by snapping of the iliopsoas tendon over the iliopectineal line and the iliofemoral ligaments over the femoral head, as well as other places on the hip bone. Another symptom may be pain. The pathophysiology is an overuse problem initially precipitated by bursitis. In this disorder, the overlying tendon rubs against the inflamed bursal sac. In the case of the iliopsoas, the continual friction can lead to development of a nodule on the tendon. This nodule then gets caught as it travels over the pelvic brim. Clinically, the snapping may be reproduced when the affected area is taken through a range of motion. Initial treatment consists of ice, range-of-motion exercises, and NSAIDs. If symptoms persist, referral for corticosteroid injection under fluoroscopic guidance or for excision of the nodule is an option.

Osteitis Pubis

Originally associated with parturition, urinary tract infections, and arthritic disorders, osteitis pubis is now recognized as a common injury in athletes. This is a disorder of the symphysis pubis due to shear forces caused by cutting, twisting, or pivoting motions. This places stresses of the adductor muscles attached to the pubic rami, inciting an inflammatory response. The patient presents with cramping, burning, or stabbing pain emanating from the suprapubic, perineum, or groin. The physical exam may reveal tenderness to palpation over the suprapubic area. In addition, pain may be elicited with lateral compression over the iliac wing with the patient in the lateral decubitus position or with FAbER's test. A pelvic x-ray may reveal erosions of the symphysis pubis. A bone scan will reveal increased uptake in the symphysis pubis area. Treatment can include ice, limitation of activities, and NSAIDs. If these measures do not help, injection into the symphysis pubis with a corticosteroid/anesthetic combination under fluoroscopic guidance may be helpful.

Sportsman's Hernia

As with osteitis pubis, the sports hernia is a more recently identified problem in athletes. The pathophysiology is disruption of the posterior inguinal canal where the conjoined tendon, fascia tranversalis, and the common tendon of the internal oblique and transverses meet. It is similarly recognized in athletes who perform cutting, twisting, or pivoting motions. Patients present with groin pain that occurs suddenly or insidiously. The physical exam may be positive for a dilated tender inguinal ring, tenderness over the inguinal canal, and pain with resisted sit-up or resisted hip adduction. The physician needs to rule out indirect hernia. The diagnosis may be confused with adductor muscle strain or osteitis pubis. Pelvic x-rays are not helpful in diagnosis. Herniography is still not widely accepted or available, so diagnosis is by exclusion in many cases. Treatment is surgical repair of the posterior inguinal canal. The patient usually can return to activity in about 6-8 weeks.

Degenerative Joint Disease

Osteoarthritis is a degenerative joint problem that increases in prevalence with age. Approximately 16 million Americans are afflicted with this disorder. It is more common in patients over age 50 and is more common among females than males. Patients with a remote history of congenital or acquired disorders such as Legg-Calvé-Perthes disease, SCFE, or significant hip trauma are at greater risk for developing OA of the hip joint. Early in the course of the disease, the patient presents with symptoms of pain in the thigh or groin with activity. As the disease progresses, pain may occur even at rest. Patients may also have morning stiffness. On physical examination, the patient demonstrates a decreased range of motion at the hip joint. The patient may also have crepitus with joint motion, as well as tenderness to palpation, joint effusion, and joint deformity. In addition to hip pain, the American College of Rheumatology (ACR) diagnostic criteria for osteoarthritis include any two of the following three: 1) an erythrocyte sedimentation rate less than 20 mm/hr, 2) radiographic evidence of femoral and acetabular osteophytes, or 3) joint space narrowing. Radiographic findings should be approached with caution, since as many as 50% of adults may have radiographic evidence of osteoarthritis, but few of these patients are symptomatic. Patients benefit from regular exercise and should be encouraged to continue participating in their desired activity. Patients who are symptomatic should be treated similarly to those who are acutely injured. The recommendations should include a progressive program that starts with range-of-motion exercises and progresses to resistive exercises. Flexibility exercises should be included. NSAIDs may provide additional relief.

Adolescent-Specific Injuries

Because of the large muscle groups in the hip and pelvis, avulsion fractures are common in the skeletally immature patient whose secondary ossification centers are not completely fused. The five muscles with the corresponding apophysis are: 1) the sartorius (anterior superior iliac spine, ASIS), 2) rectus femoris (anterior inferior iliac spine, AIIS), 3) hamstring (ischial tuberosity), 4) transverse abdominis (iliac crest), and 5) iliopsoas (lesser trochanter). The mechanism of injury is a sudden forceful contraction that overcomes the weak cartilaginous connection at the apophysis. The affected site is activity- and sport-specific.

The iliac crest apophysis closes between the ages of 14 and 20. The transverse abdominis muscle may be separated from the iliac crest apophysis by direct trauma to that area (for example, helmet contact during a tackle in football). An increase in the amount or intensity of training may precipitate apophysitis of the iliac crest in long-distance runners. The patient presents with a dull pain that increases with activity. On physical examination, the patient is tender to palpation along the iliac crest. In addition to the routine anteroposterior and lateral radiographs, oblique views may be required to visualize the avulsion.

The anterior inferior iliac spine (AIIS) apophyseal center appears at age 13 and fuses between ages 16 and 18. Sprinting or jumping, with the act of hip extension and knee flexion, may cause avulsion of the rectus femoris from the AIIS. At presentation, the patient is usually limping and reports a history of sudden pain in the groin area. On physical examination, the patient has difficulty with passive extension of the knee and/or flexion of the hip. The patient may also demonstrate weak hip flexion on active range of motion and resistance testing. Palpation of the insertion site of the rectus femoris may reveal tenderness but may be difficult because of the depth of the apophysis.

The ischial tuberosity apophysis appears at age 13 and fuses between the ages of 16 and 18, similar to the AIIS. Runners and dancers may avulse the hamstring from the ischial tuberosity due to sudden deceleration or chronic stretching. Signs of an avulsion fracture include sudden localized pain and swelling, as well as pain radiation with contraction of the affected muscle (for example, with an eccentric contraction) or when the muscle is stretched. The patient reports inability to continue with activity. Tenderness is elicited by palpation over the insertion of the hamstrings at the ischial tuberosity. The diagnosis may be confirmed with plain radiographs, which show displacement of the avulsed apophysis; often, however, bilateral films are required to compare the injured and uninjured sides. Treatment for apophyseal injuries includes rest, ice, and compression. NSAIDs or narcotic analgesics may be used for pain control. Passive range of motion may be started within 24 hours of injury with progression as tolerated. In mildly symptomatic cases, patients may be able to return to play with protective padding. Other patients, especially those in whom weakness of the associated muscle occurs, may require cessation of the activity until full strength returns and there is no discomfort. This may be as long as 4-6 weeks.

SELECTED READING

Adkins SB, Figler RA. Hip pain in athletes. Am Fam Physician. 2000;61:2109-18.

Browning KH. Hip and pelvis injuries in runners: careful evaluation and tailored management. Phys Sportsmed. 2001;29(1):23-34.

Garrick GJ, Webb DR. Sports Injuries: Diagnosis and Management, 2nd ed. Philadelphia: WB Saunders; 1999.

Mellion MB. Sports Medicine Secrets. Philadelphia: Hanley & Belfus; 1994.

Mellion MB, Walsh WM, Madden C. Team Physician's Handbook, 3rd ed. Philadelphia: Hanley & Belfus; 2002.

Reider B. The Orthopaedic Physical Examination. Philadelphia: WB Saunders; 1999.

23

■　■　■

Knee Injuries

John P. Jamison, MD

David S. Ross, MD

K nee injuries present the treating physician with three distinct challenges. The first is to establish a complete and accurate diagnosis in
a timely manner in order to minimize time lost from work or athletic
activities. Second, the physician must present the pros and cons of various
treatment alternatives, taking into account the athlete's lifestyle, occupation, and commitment to rehabilitation. Finally, close communication must
be maintained between the physician, patient, and physical therapist
during the rehabilitation process.

Anatomy

The knee is one of the most flexible joints in the body and yet has very
little intrinsic stability as a result of its shape. For this reason, it is highly dependent on the integrity of its ligamentous structures (1).

The four major ligaments stabilizing the knee joint are the medial collateral ligament (MCL), the lateral collateral ligament (LCL), the anterior cruciate ligament (ACL), and the posterior cruciate ligament (PCL) (Figure
23-1). The MCL provides 55% to 71% of the valgus restraint to the knee (2).
The posteromedial capsule provides additional restraint when the knee is
near full extension. Structures on the lateral side of the knee include the
LCL complex, iliotibial band, biceps femoris, and popliteus complex. The
LCL complex provides 55% to 69% of resistance to varus loading, with additional support from the posterior lateral structures as the knee nears extension (2). The ACL and PCL also provide resistance to varus and valgus
stress when the knee is in full extension.

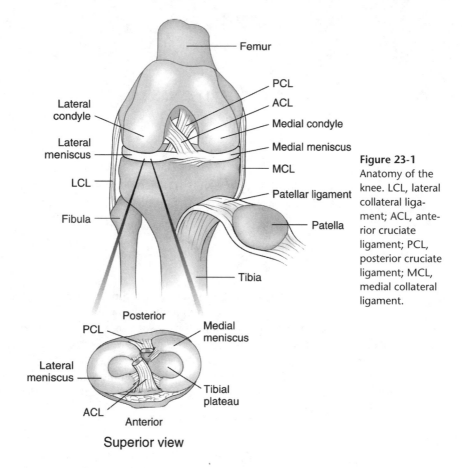

Figure 23-1
Anatomy of the knee. LCL, lateral collateral ligament; ACL, anterior cruciate ligament; PCL, posterior cruciate ligament; MCL, medial collateral ligament.

The ACL is the primary restraint to anterior translation of the tibia on the femur, providing approximately 85% of the resistance to that motion. The PCL provides approximately 95% of the resistance to posterior translation of the tibia on the femur and therefore is considered the primary posterior stabilizer.

The articular contact areas of the knee are usually divided into three compartments: medial, lateral, and patellofemoral. The menisci are two crescent-shaped cartilage structures that serve to deepen the articular surfaces of the medial and lateral compartments (see Figure 23-1). Each meniscus covers approximately two-thirds of the corresponding articular surface of the tibia (1). Recent studies have concluded that the menisci transmit at least 50% of the compressive load at the tibiofemoral joint between 0 degrees and 90 degrees of flexion. The patella has medial and lateral facets that articulate with the medial and lateral femoral condyles, respectively.

History

A complete and accurate history is essential to the establishment of a correct diagnosis. The mechanism of injury should be described in as much detail as possible. The majority of athletic knee injuries are noncontact in nature and involve cutting, decelerating, or landing from a jump. If contact is involved, the direction of force (medial, lateral, anterior) should be noted. Hearing or feeling a "pop," associated with rapid onset of effusion, is highly suggestive of an injury to the anterior cruciate ligament (ACL). The presence of mechanical symptoms such as popping, catching, clicking, locking, and buckling should also be recorded. Mechanical symptoms are generally nonspecific and may be associated with ligamentous, meniscal, extensor mechanism, or osteochondral injuries. Age, occupation, recreational interests, lifestyle, and past medical history may influence the recommended treatment once the diagnosis is made (3).

Physical Examination

Physical examination begins with documentation of height, weight, body habitus, and general laxity. Generalized ligamentous laxity is characterized by knee and elbow hyperextension beyond 10 degrees, hyperextension of the little finger metacarpalphalangeal joint beyond 90 degrees, and thumb abduction to touch the volar forearm with the wrist flexed. Neurovascular status must be evaluated and recorded. Active and passive range of motion, as well as overall leg alignment (varus, valgus), are noted. The extremity is checked for localized or generalized swelling and ecchymosis. The ability to bear weight and need for lateral support is documented. It is generally advisable to examine the uninjured extremity first, taking care not to cause additional pain and muscle spasm on the injured side. This provides baseline measurements of swelling, range of motion, and stability. The injured knee is then systematically palpated, and areas of point tenderness are recorded. Specific tests such as Lachman's, McMurray's, drawer, varus and valgus stress, and patellar apprehension are then carried out (3).

The *Lachman test* is performed with the patient supine and the knee flexed to 20 degrees to 30 degrees. The femur is grasped with one hand, while the other hand grasps the proximal tibia. The lower leg is then given a brisk forward tug. A positive test is one in which there is increased translation and no discrete end-point is felt, indicating an injury to the ACL (Figure 23-2, *A*) (3).

The *anterior drawer test* is performed with the knee flexed 90 degrees and the patient supine (Figure 23-2, *B*). The tibia is pulled forward, and a firm end-point should be felt if the ACL is intact.

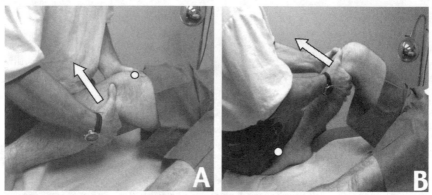

Figure 23-2   Tests of the anterior cruciate ligament. (A) Lachman test. (B) Anterior drawer test.

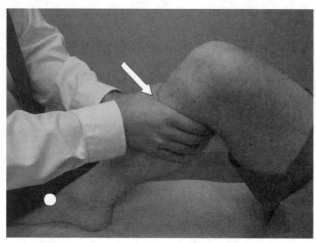

Figure 23-3   Posterior drawer test to assess the posterior cruciate ligament (PCL).

The *posterior drawer test* is performed with the knee at 90 degrees and the hip at 45 degrees of flexion (Figure 23-3). Posterior force is applied to the proximal tibia, and the extent of translation and quality of the end point are assessed. The relationship between the medial femoral condyle and medial tibial plateau should be palpated and compared with the contralateral knee. Normally, the medial tibial plateau lays one finger-breadth (1 to 1.5 cm.) anterior to the femoral condyle with the knee flexed to 90 degrees. With increasingly severe PCL injuries, the tibial plateau may be flush with, or even posterior to, the medial femoral condyle. Partial tears cause mild-to-moderate posterior translation of the tibia on the femur. In complete tears, the tibia can be pushed posterior to the femoral condyles. A "posterior sag" may be visible and palpable if the PCL is torn (Figure 23-4). Comparison with the contralateral extremity is very helpful.

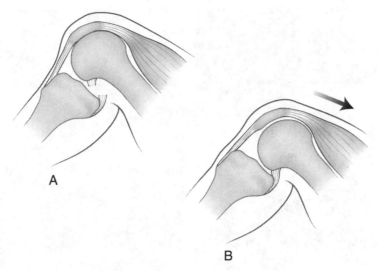

A

B

Figure 23-4   Posterior sag sign indicates deficiency of PCL. When the knee is flexed 90 degrees, the joint will exhibit a posterior tibial sag (A). The quadriceps active test will confirm PCL deficiency. Have the patient contract the quadriceps; the tibia will move from a posterior sag to a more normal position (B).

The medial and lateral collateral ligaments are tested with the patient supine and the leg over the side of the examining table (Figure 23-5). Both ligaments are tested in full extension and at 30 degrees of flexion. The femur is stabilized with one hand, while *varus* or *valgus stress* is applied. In full extension, the ACL and PCL contribute to varus and valgus stability. If the knee demonstrates varus or valgus instability in full extension, then one or both of the cruciate ligaments is torn in addition to the collateral ligament. If instability is present only at 30 degrees of flexion, then an isolated collateral ligament injury is present.

The status of the menisci is evaluated using the *McMurray test* (Figure 23-6), which is performed with the patient supine and the examiner standing to the side. The knee is extended from a fully flexed position with the foot externally rotated, while a valgus stress is applied to the knee. Pain or popping along the lateral joint line suggests a lateral meniscus tear. The medial compartment is loaded by extending the knee from a flexed position while internally rotating the foot and applying varus stress. Medial pain or popping with this maneuver is suggestive of medial meniscal tear (4).

The *patellar apprehension sign* is helpful in evaluation for patellar subluxation or patellar dislocation. The patient is in the supine position, and the leg is in extension. The examiner then gently pushes the patella laterally. If the patient becomes uncomfortable and senses that the patella is about to dislocate, the test is positive.

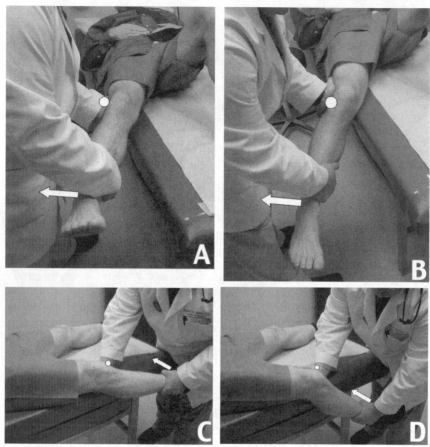

Figure 23-5   (A) Valgus stress in extension to test integrity of MCL. (B) Valgus stress in 30-deg flexion to test integrity of MCL. (C) Varus stress in extension to test integrity of LCL. (D) Varus stress in 30-deg flexion to test integrity of LCL. If laxity is noted in full extension, then one or both of the cruciate ligaments is torn in addition to the collateral ligament.

Radiography

Initial radiographic exam of the injured knee should include, at the minimum, anteroposterior, lateral, and patellar tangential views. A tunnel view may be added to clarify obscure lesions. The tunnel view is obtained with the knee flexed 60 degrees and the x-ray directed parallel to the tibia. It provides visualization of the posterior aspects of the medial and lateral femoral condyles, the intercondylar notch, and the tibial spines (Figure 23-7). If there is concern of an injury to the patella, a sunrise or Merchant's view may be of benefit (Figure 23-8). Comparison views of the contralateral knee are sometimes helpful, especially in skeletally immature patients. MRI is useful, if somewhat overused, to help delineate intra-articular

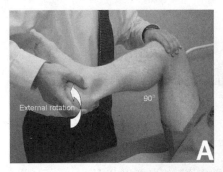
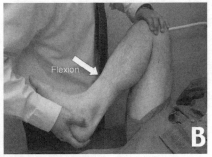
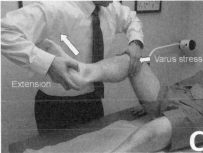

Figure 23-6   McMurray test to assess the medial meniscus. (A) With the patient supine, the knee is flexed to 90 degrees. To test the medial meniscus, the examiner grasps the patient's heel with one hand to hold the tibia in external rotation, with the thumb at the lateral joint line, the fingers at the medial joint line. (B) The examiner flexes the patient's knee maximally to impinge the posterior horn of the meniscus against the medial femoral condyle. (C) A varus stress is applied as the examiner extends the knee.

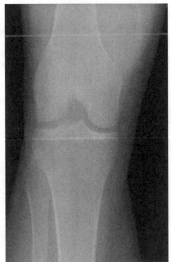

Figure 23-7   Tunnel view of the knee allows visualization of the posterior aspect of the medial and lateral femoral condyles, intercondylar notch, and the tibial spines.

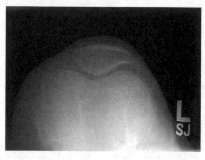

Figure 23-8   Sunrise view of the patella.

pathology that is not readily apparent after thorough history, exam, and routine x-rays. Arteriograms are required for suspected or documented knee dislocations.

Specific Disorders

Ligament Injuries

Anterior Cruciate Ligament Injuries

ACL instability is the most common cause of long-term disability of the knee. ACL injuries occur at a rate of about 1 in 3000 Americans per year. This results in approximately 95,000 injuries per year and about 50,000 ACL reconstructions per year (2). The ACL is the primary stabilizer to anterior tibial translation and hyperextension but also works as a secondary restraint to varus and valgus forces and limits excessive internal and external rotation.

A number of factors may predispose individuals to ACL injury. Individuals with femoral notch stenosis (defined by a notch width index < 0.2) appear to have a 60 times greater likelihood of noncontact ACL injury. Women athletes are also more susceptible than men to ACL tears, with a two-fold increase in ACL injuries in women collegiate soccer players and a four-fold increase in basketball players (2). Differences in limb alignment, joint laxity, skill, experience, and notch width have been suggested as possible causes of this discrepancy between male and female ACL injuries. Cleats with a majority of their grip on the periphery have the highest coefficient of friction on turf and are associated with a higher incidence of ACL tears.

Diagnosis of ACL tears can usually be accomplished by a thorough and a careful physical exam. Plain radiographs are routinely obtained to rule out concomitant fractures or avulsions, to evaluate preexisting degenerative changes, or to determine the status of the growth plates in younger patients. MRI is frequently unnecessary but may be helpful in patients who are unable to relax for examination, in patients for whom nonsurgical treatment is planned (to rule out meniscal pathology), for combined ligament injuries, and for suspected partial ACL tears. Partial ACL tears are relatively uncommon and may have a variable outcome. Partial ACL tears will present with a Lachman test that demonstrates only mild laxity and a definite end point.

The decision to proceed with surgical or nonsurgical ACL treatment can be complex. Certain individuals may function quite well with an ACL-deficient knee. Younger, more active patients, however, tend to have recurrent episodes of instability, leading to stretching of secondary restraints, meniscal tears, and ultimately osteoarthritis. The decision to proceed with surgical stabilization should be made based on the level and type of sport the athlete wishes to participate in rather than age or gender. The goal of treatment in the ACL-deficient knee is to prevent the recurrent episodes of instability, which lead to further knee damage and disability. Low-demand athletes not involved in cutting and pivoting sports can frequently accomplish this goal through rehabilitation and activity modification. Athletes involved in high-demand cutting and pivoting sports who are unwilling to alter their activities generally require ligament reconstruction.

Older, less active patients generally do well with nonoperative treatment of their ACL injuries, especially if they modify their activities and participate in a well-designed rehabilitation program emphasizing quadriceps and hamstring strengthening. Although their knees remain clinically unstable, they are usually satisfied with their function, rarely require later surgery, and the results do not appear to deteriorate over time. Functional bracing may help the low-demand patient participate in recreational activities but is typically not an adequate long-term solution for the aggressive athlete.

Surgical management of ACL deficiency is indicated in patients who wish to continue in high-demand cutting and pivoting sport activities and those with associated pathology. Surgery is usually delayed at least several weeks after injury to allow swelling to resolve and motion to return to normal. Direct repair of the ACL is generally not effective, and therefore reconstruction is the treatment of choice. The ACL can be reconstructed using donor grafts obtained from the patellar tendon, hamstring tendons, quadriceps tendon, or allograft tissue, and all have shown satisfactory results. With adherence to an aggressive rehabilitation program, the athlete can usually return to sports in 5 to 6 months (3,5,6).

Posterior Cruciate Ligament Injuries

The PCL is a primary stabilizer of the knee joint and is the major restraint to posterior translation of the tibia. PCL injuries were commonly overlooked in the past, but it is now believed that they may represent up to 30% of all knee injuries. Patients with acute, isolated PCL injuries may not present until the injury has become chronic. Improved awareness on the part of physicians and trainers has increased the recognition of isolated PCL injuries.

PCL tears are classified according to timing (acute or chronic), and according to severity (isolated or combined). Rapid recognition of combined injuries is extremely important because surgical treatment should be undertaken within the first 2 to 3 weeks for optimal results. PCL tears may be partial or complete. Partial tears can be treated nonoperatively with good results. Complete tears, especially those combined with other ligament injuries, require prompt referral to an orthopedic specialist. Many of these combined injuries require surgery in the acute phase in order to achieve optimal results. Combined ligament injuries carry a significant likelihood of bone or neurovascular injury. If both cruciates are injured, the physician must suspect knee dislocation and order an arteriogram, as the incidence of popliteal artery rupture with knee dislocation is approximately 33% (7,8).

A detailed history will often lead the physician to suspect an injury to the PCL. Athletic injuries involving hyperflexion of the knee with associated downward force on the thigh frequently lead to PCL tears. Hyperextension, sometimes associated with varus or valgus stress, is another common mechanism of injury. Patients usually do not report hearing or feeling a pop as they do when the ACL is injured. The most common nonathletic mechanism of PCL tear is the high-speed motor vehicle or "dashboard" injury in which there is a direct posterior force applied to the proximal tibia. Dashboard injuries frequently are associated with other ligament or bony injuries.

Physical examination begins with careful evaluation of neurovascular status followed by observation, palpation, measurement of range of motion, and instability testing. Routine plain radiographs are obtained, primarily to rule out avulsion fractures of the PCL in the acute setting and medial compartment degenerative changes in the chronic setting. Avulsion fractures can be repaired if recognized early and generally lead to excellent result. MRI is extremely helpful in evaluating PCL injuries and the extent of associated pathology. MRI accuracy in diagnosing PCL tears ranges from 96% to 100% (2).

In general, isolated PCL tears are treated nonoperatively and combined injuries (PCL plus ACL, MCL, or posterolateral corner) are treated surgically. Isolated PCL injuries are graded from 1 (minor) to 3 (more severe). Grade 1 injuries preserve some anterior position of the tibia relative to the femoral condyles with the knee flexed to 90 degrees; grade 2 injuries occur when the tibia is even with the femoral condyles; and grade 3 injuries allow the tibia to be displaced posterior to the femoral condyles (9). Grade 1 and 2 isolated PCL injuries require protected weight-bearing and quadriceps rehabilitation. Most of these patients can return to athletic activities within 2 to 4 weeks of injury. For grade 3 isolated PCL tears, a 4-week period of immobilization in full extension with partial weight-bearing is recommended to allow healing of the posterolateral structures. Quadriceps rehabilitation is started immediately. After 1 month, the patient can progress to full weight-bearing and begin range-of-motion exercises. Although the outcome of complete PCL injuries is less predictable than with lesser degrees of laxity, most athletes can return to their sports activities after approximately 3 months (7,8).

Medial Collateral Ligament Injuries

The primary function of the MCL complex is to prevent valgus instability and anteromedial translation of the tibia on the femur. It plays a secondary role in preventing anterior tibial translation in an ACL-deficient knee. Most MCL injuries are caused by valgus force applied to a flexed knee by either contact or noncontact means. Other mechanisms include external rotation pivoting injuries, blows to the anterolateral aspect of the knee, and knee dislocations.

MCL injuries are frequently suspected based on the patient's description of the mechanism of injury. Pain to palpation over the medial femoral condyle may indicate a tear of the proximal portion of the MCL. Pain over the joint line may indicate an injury of the medial meniscus in conjunction with a sprain of the midportion of the ligament. Severity of the MCL injury is assessed by applying valgus stress with the knee flexed 30 degrees (see Figure 23-5, B). The leg is placed over the side of the examining table and the fingers are placed over the medial joint line to evaluate the degree of opening and the presence of popping or crepitus. The presence of a "clunk" or crepitus would raise the likelihood of meniscal tear, chondral injury, or preexisting medial compartment arthritis. The amount of opening is graded according to the American Medical Association (AMA) guidelines: grade 1 injuries have less than 5 mm of joint line opening; grade 2 tears open 5 to 10 mm; grade 3 injuries open more than 10 mm and have no discernable end point, indicating a complete tear of the ligament. Frequently, patients with grade 1 or 2 tears will have significantly more pain than those with grade 3 injuries. Valgus stress is also applied at 0 degrees. A positive valgus stress test at 0 degrees indicates an injury to the MCL, as well as to the ACL, PCL, or both. It is important to compare stability of the injured knee with the uninjured knee. In the adolescent, stress radiographs should be obtained to make certain the injury involved the ligamentous structures, rather than the growth plate. MRI scans are not routinely necessary in the evaluation of MCL injuries but may be helpful when the diagnosis is in doubt.

Grade 1 and 2 MCL injuries are treated nonsurgically (10,11). The patient is allowed weight-bearing as tolerated, using crutches as needed. Ice is applied, and range-of-motion exercises are started within the first 24-48 hours. Quadriceps strengthening exercises are begun as soon as possible, progressing to an exercise bike early on. In general, isolated grade 3 injuries can be treated in the same manner as grade 1 and 2 tears. Casting has not shown to be helpful. Functional bracing is often used in the early recovery period, but benefits are inconclusive. Femoral-sided MCL injuries tend to respond better to nonoperative treatment than do tibial-sided tears. The location of the tear can usually be determined by careful palpation on initial physical exam. MRI may also be helpful in localizing the injury. Tibial-sided grade 3 tears should initially be treated nonsurgically, but if grade 3 instability remains after 4-6 weeks of treatment, surgery may be considered.

Lateral Collateral Ligament and Posterolateral Corner Injuries

Unlike the MCL, injuries to the lateral side of the knee are inherently unstable due to the convex surfaces of both the lateral femoral condyle and the lateral tibial plateau. Grade 3 injuries in this area therefore heal poorly with nonsurgical treatment. The most common mechanisms of injury include a blow to the anteromedial aspect of the knee, hyperextension injuries, and varus contact forces to a flexed knee. There is a 15% incidence of peroneal nerve injury with grade 3 injuries to the posterolateral structures of the knee. The grading scale for lateral-side injuries is similar to that of medial-side injuries, following AMA guidelines. The knee is tested in both 0 and 30 degrees of flexion (Figures 23-5, C and D). Plain radiographs should be obtained and may show a Segond fracture, which is a small flake of bone adjacent to the lateral tibial plateau, or fibular head avulsion. MRI is especially helpful in delineating the injury to individual components of the posterolateral corner of the knee.

Treatment of isolated grade 1 and 2 posterolateral knee injuries is nonsurgical. Casting in extension for 3 weeks is followed by a progressive functional rehabilitation similar to MCL injuries (2). Grade 3 injuries have been shown to do poorly with nonsurgical management, and anatomic repair of the torn structures is recommended within the first 1 to 2 weeks of injury. Grade 3 posterolateral injuries combined with ACL and/or PCL tears should be treated with repair or reconstruction of all injured structures within 2 weeks of the injury if at all possible. Repairs for chronic grade 3 posterolateral corner injuries are considerably less successful than acute repairs. For this reason, the physician must maintain a high level of suspicion for lateral-side injuries and be prepared to initiate appropriate treatment promptly.

Meniscal Injuries

The meniscus is one of the most frequently injured structures in the knee. The incidence of acute meniscal tears is 61/100,000. Degenerative meniscal tears are present in 60% of patients over the age of 65 (2). The meniscus performs numerous important functions in the knee, including lubrication, load transmission, shock absorption, and passive stabilization. The lateral meniscus is most commonly injured in association with acute ACL tears. The medial meniscus is most often found to be torn in stable knees or those with chronic ACL insuffiency. The primary function of the meniscus is to distribute loads transmitted across the knee joint. One study has shown that removal of the lateral meniscus resulted in a 235% to 335% increase in local contact pressures on the remaining articular cartilage (2).

This explains the more rapid development of arthritic changes in patients who have had previous menisectomy.

Case Study 23-1

A 17-year-old female high school volleyball player sustained a noncontact injury to her right knee. She went up to block an opponent's shot and, when she came down, she landed awkwardly on her right leg. She reported feeling her right knee pop and "go out of place." Several teammates standing on the sidelines also heard the pop. The player had rapid onset of swelling and pain but was able bear some weight on the knee.

Physical exam on the day after the injury revealed range of motion from -15 degrees to 90 degrees. Lachman test and anterior drawer tests were positive. All other stability tests were normal. The McMurray test could not be performed secondary to pain. An MRI revealed an acute tear of the ACL and a tear of the lateral meniscus. All other structures were normal

The player underwent rehabilitation in the high school training room for 4 weeks. She regained full range of motion and her effusion resolved. She then underwent a reconstruction of her anterior cruciate ligament using a graft obtained from her patellar tendon. Her lateral meniscus was repaired. She was started on an accelerated rehabilitation program with early range of motion and weight bearing. Four months after surgery, she was allowed to participate in limited volleyball drills, and 6 months after surgery, she was permitted to play competitively.

The diagnosis of meniscal injury can often be established by obtaining a detailed history, including the mechanism of injury, timing of the injury, presence of effusion, and symptoms. Most younger patients report a rapid change in direction or twisting injury. Tears in the central portion of the meniscus usually cause swelling the next day. Immediate onset of swelling should raise suspicion for a peripheral meniscus tear, ligament injury, or fracture. Bucket handle tears, in which a large fragment of meniscus becomes lodged in the center of the knee, most often cause locking of the knee. Degenerative tears typically present with recurrent effusions.

On physical examination, joint line tenderness is an accurate clinical sign, especially when present at the posteromedial or posterolateral joint line. If concomitant ligament injury is present, tenderness is less helpful. The McMurray test is also useful in detecting meniscal pathology.

Radiographic evaluation includes standard plain x-rays. MRI can be helpful in clarifying the diagnosis in appropriate patients. MRI accuracy ranges from 64% to 95% for medial meniscal lesions and from 83% to 94% for lateral meniscal lesions (2). False-positives are far more common with MRI than are false-negatives. MRI is not always indicated for the evaluation of meniscal pathology. For example, a young patient with an acutely locked knee will require arthroscopic evaluation, and the MRI will add little to the decision-making process. An elderly patient with moderate-to-severe arthritic changes will very likely have a degenerative meniscal tear on MRI, but, again, this will have little effect on the treatment plan.

Treatment of meniscal tears varies depending on the patient's age, activity level, chronicity of symptoms, type of tear, and associated pathology. Many tears less than 10 mm in length, if located in the peripheral vascular part of the meniscus, will either heal or become asymptomatic. Stable tears, degenerative tears in osteoarthritis, and partial thickness tears usually do not require surgical intervention and may be observed for a period of time. If the patient remains symptomatic after 3 months, surgery is recommended. Surgical treatment is aimed at preserving as much meniscal tissue as possible, resecting only the unstable portions of the cartilage. Meniscal tears in the vascular (peripheral) portion are repaired. Short-term results are rated excellent to good in 80% to 95% of patients after partial menisectomy (2). In the long term, some degree of degenerative arthritis is expected after menisectomy (2,12).

Patellofemoral Disorders

The patellofemoral joint is a common, if sometimes overlooked, source of pain and disability in the athlete. Differential diagnosis in these patients with anterior knee pain includes patellofemoral arthritis, patellar instability, patellar chondral defects, patellar tendinitis, medial plica syndrome, and meniscal tear. A careful history and physical exam will usually identify the source of the pathology. Patients with patellofemoral disorders may present with anterior knee pain, catching, popping, or grinding. They may have difficulties with squatting, kneeling, ascending or descending stairs, or getting up from a seated position. They may describe episodes of buckling or the knee "slipping out of place."

Patellofemoral problems are notorious for mimicking ligamentous or meniscal disorders. Peripatellar tenderness, patellofemoral crepitus, and a positive patellar apprehension test should raise the index of suspicion for patellofemoral disorders.

Clinical evaluation should include assessment of leg alignment, quadriceps function and atrophy, patellar mobility and stability, patellofemoral crepitus, as well as a knee exam. Radiographic evaluation must include a tangential view of the patella, such as a Merchant or sunrise view (see Figure 23-8). Tangential views allow assessment of patellar alignment and visualization of osteochondral lesions or fractures that may not be visible on routine anteroposterior and lateral films. MRI has limited usefulness in the evaluation of patellofemoral problems unless required to rule out other lesions such as meniscal tears.

Patellofemoral pain, without associated patellar instability, can usually be treated successfully by a directed exercise program. The program should include closed chain, pain-free resistance exercises, as well as quadriceps and hamstring flexibility exercises. Open-chain active knee extensions frequently exacerbate patellar symptoms and should be avoided. The patient should be thoroughly educated on activity modification. This may involve redesigning a workout program to avoid step aerobics, decreasing recreational basketball activities from 4 days a week to 2 days a week, or eliminating high-resistance quadriceps exercises from a weight-lifting program.

Case Study 23-2

A 32-year-old woman decided to "get back in shape" after the birth of her two children. In high school she played basketball and ran track, and she had never sustained a serious injury. She had not been athletically active during the past 5 years and was now about 15 lb overweight. She joined a health club and began working out with a personal trainer. Her workouts consisted of upper body strengthening, running on a treadmill, using a stair-stepper, and doing leg extensions, squats, and leg presses with weights.

One month after beginning her exercise program, she noted gradual onset of left anterior knee pain. The pain was particularly severe when she went up or down stairs, squatted, or arose from a chair. It was difficult for her to stand up when she had been seated for more than 10 or 15 minutes. She was unable to continue working with her personal trainer because of the pain.

Her physical exam revealed no effusion, and her range of motion was full. Her overall leg alignment was normal. Her knee was stable, and McMurray's test was negative. She had mild tenderness to palpation along the medial joint line and medial border of the patella. Patellar apprehension sign was negative. There was mild crepitus beneath the patellae bilaterally. X-rays of both knees, including standing anteroposterior, lateral, and Merchant views, were normal.

A diagnosis of patellofemoral pain was made, and the patient was started on NSAIDs. She resumed her upper body strengthening with her personal trainer, but her lower extremity strengthening program was modified under the supervision of a physical therapist. She was told to discontinue squats, leg extensions, leg presses, and stair-stepper. She was instructed on straight leg raises, hamstring and quadriceps stretches, and cycling. She was permitted to continue using the treadmill as long as it was not set at an incline. Six weeks later, she was pain-free and able to continue her modified exercise without further need for NSAIDs.

Most cases of patellar instability, including subluxation and dislocation, can also be treated with a well-designed exercise program. Acute dislocations are treated with a short period of immobilization and occasionally aspiration of the knee for pain control, followed by a rehabilitation program. Prolonged immobilization is contraindicated. A patellar stabilizing brace may be beneficial in some patients to prevent recurrence during sports activities. Studies have shown that patients with acute, first-time dislocations have a recurrence rate of 44% after an average of 13 years. Recurrent dislocations sometimes require surgical treatment to restore stability (2,13).

Miscellaneous Disorders

Patellar Tendinitis

Patellar tendinitis, or "jumper's knee," is characterized by pain localized to the distal pole of the patella, occasional localized swelling, and pain with strenuous quadriceps activity. It probably represents partial tearing of the tendon and is prevalent in athletes who play basketball, volleyball, football, and soccer. Weightlifters and triple, long, and high jumpers are also prone to patellar tendinitis.

Treatment consists of activity modification and quadriceps and hamstring stretching and strengthening, emphasizing eccentric exercises. Adjunctive treatments include NSAIDs, cryotherapy, and ultrasound. One may also consider the use of a patellar counterforce strap with activity. Steroid injection in the region of the patellar tendon is contraindicated, as it may lead to tendon rupture. Patients who fail to respond to nonsurgical treatment can generally be treated successfully with resection of the damaged portion of the tendon followed by rehabilitation.

Iliotibial Band Syndrome

Iliotibial band (ITB) syndrome is caused by excessive friction between the iliotibial band and the lateral femoral condyle. It most commonly occurs in cyclists and runners. Patients present with pain over the lateral side of the knee during activity. The pain is exacerbated by running on banked surfaces, hills, or stairs. On physical examination, pain is usually reproduced by compression over the lateral femoral condyle as the knee passes 30 degrees of flexion. Ober's test may indicate a tight iliotibial band (see Figure 22-2 in Chapter 22). The test is performed with the patient lying on the uninvolved side with the uninvolved knee flexed. The involved leg is then abducted and extended, then slowly lowered to the examining table. If the leg remains abducted, the test is positive, indicating a tight iliotibial band.

Treatment consists of correcting training errors and reducing inflammation. Training alterations may include stretching, limiting the duration of training, altering speed and stride length, and avoiding hills. Cyclists may benefit from changing seat height and cleat orientation. Symptomatic treatment includes rest, ice, NSAIDs, and ITB stretching. Steroid injections into the bursa are occasionally indicated. Surgery is rarely necessary.

Osteochondritis Dissecans

Osteochondritis dissecans is a condition found in both adults and children that involves fragmentation or separation of a portion of the articular surface of the knee. This most commonly occurs on the lateral side of the medial femoral condyle. The average age of presentation is between 5 and 15 years of age, with a 2:1 male predominance. Typical symptoms include vague pain, clicking, popping, and effusion. Plain radiographs, including tunnel view, will generally reveal the lesion, although the appearance is sometimes subtle. MRI is very helpful in evaluating the lesion. In children, nonoperative treatment (rest and/or immobilization) is often successful for stable fragments. In adults, the prognosis is considerably less favorable, and various surgical alternatives may be necessary.

REFERENCES

1. **Insall JN.** Anatomy of the knee. In: Insall Jn, ed. Surgery of the Knee. New York: Churchill Livingstone; 1984:1-20.

2. **Arendt EA, ed.** Orthopedic Knowledge Update Sports Medicine 2. Rosemont, IL: American Academy of Orthopedic Surgeons; 1999:291-364.

3. **Ivey FM.** Acute knee injuries. In: Griffin L, ed. Orthopedic Knowledge Update—Sports Medicine. Rosemont, IL: American Academy of Orthopedic Surgeons; 1994: 255-60.

4. **Solomon DH, Simel DL, Bates DW, et al.** Does this patient have a torn meniscus or ligament of the knee? JAMA. 2001;286(13):1610-20.

5. **Daniel DM, Stone ML, Dobson BE, et al.** Fate of the ACL-injured patient: a prospective outcome study. Am J Sports Med. 1994;22:632-44.

6. **Shelbourne KD, Porter DA.** Anterior cruciate ligament-medial collateral ligament injury: nonoperative management of medial collateral ligament tears with anterior cruciate ligament reconstruction. Am J Sports Med. 1992;20:283-6.

7. **Harner CD, Hoher J.** Evaluation and treatment of posterior cruciate ligament injuries. Am J Sports Med. 1998;26:471-82.

8. **Miller MD, Harner CD, Koshiwaguchi S.** Acute posterior cruciate ligament injuries. In: Knee Surgery. Baltimore: Williams & Wilkins; 1994:749-67.

9. **Koral KJ.** Orthopedic Knowledge—Update 7. Rosemont, IL: American Academy of Orthopedic Surgeons; 2002:489-512.

10 **Kannus P.** Long-term results of conservatively treated medial collateral ligament injuries of the knee joint. Clin Orthop. 1988;226:103-12.

11. **Lundberg M, Messner K.** Long-term prognosis of isolated partial medial collateral ligament ruptures: a ten-year clinical and radiographic evaluation of a prospectively observed group of patients. Am J Sports Med. 1996;24:160-3.

12. **Bolano LE, Grana WA.** Isolated arthroscopic partial menisectomy: functional radiographic evaluation at five years. Am J Sports Med. 1993;21:432-7.

13. **Sallay PI, Poggi J, Speer KP, Garrett WE.** Acute dislocation of the patella: a correlative pathoanatomic study. Am J Sports Med. 1996;24:52-60.

24

■ ■ ■

Leg and Ankle Injuries

Kyle J. Cassas, MD

ower extremity and ankle injuries are some of the most common musculoskeletal complaints encountered daily in the primary care physician's office. Up to 1 million physician visits per year are secondary to acute ankle injuries, with approximately 27,000 ankle sprains occurring daily in the United States. The majority of ankle injuries are secondary to acute ankle sprains, which can account for up to 30% of all injuries in sports such as basketball, volleyball, football, and soccer. Although most athletes recover quickly from these injuries with little disability, it must be appreciated that without proper diagnosis, management, and rehabilitation, there is the potential for these injuries to lead to lost playing time and chronic disability in up to 40% of cases (1-3).

This chapter reviews leg and ankle injuries encountered in both the elite and recreational athlete, including acute lateral ankle sprains, syndesmotic ankle sprain ("high" ankle sprain), Achilles' tendinitis and rupture, medial tibial stress syndrome (shin splints, or traction periostitis), posterior tibialis tendinitis, and acute and chronic compartment syndrome.

Anatomy

The articulation of the talus with the distal tibia (medial malleolus) and fibula (lateral malleolus) compose the ankle joint (talocrural joint) (4). The lateral complex is composed of three ankle ligaments: the anterior talofibular ligament (ATFL), the calcaneofibular ligament (CFL), and the posterior talofibular ligament (PTFL) (Figure 24-1). On the medial aspect of the ankle, the deltoid ligament forms a strong, fan-shaped structure (superficial and deep fibers) (Figure 24-2). The ATFL is the weakest of the lateral ankle ligaments (most taut in plantarflexion) and therefore the one most commonly injured (up to two-thirds of cases). The PTFL (most taut only in

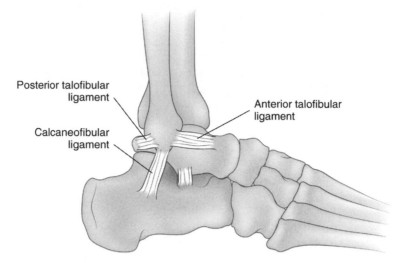

Posterior talofibular ligament

Anterior talofibular ligament

Calcaneofibular ligament

Figure 24-1   Lateral aspect of ankle.

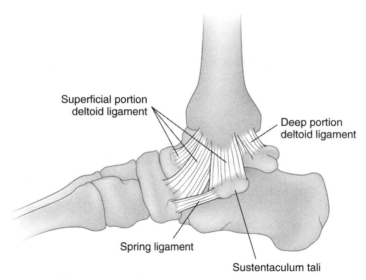

Superficial portion deltoid ligament

Deep portion deltoid ligament

Spring ligament

Sustentaculum tali

Figure 24-2   Medial aspect of ankle.

severe dorsiflexion) is the strongest and least likely injured of the three lateral ligaments (approximately 10% of cases) (2).

The Achilles' tendon is formed from the distal portions of the gastrocnemius and soleus muscles and contributes to ankle plantarflexion. The anatomy of the syndesmosis includes the following ligaments: anterior inferior tibiofibular ligament (most commonly injured), the posterior inferior tibiofibular ligament, the transverse tibiofibular ligament, and the interosseous ligament and membrane.

Finally, the ankle is surrounded by dynamic stabilizers, including the peroneal tendons (peroneal longus and peroneal brevis), which assist with ankle eversion and plantarflexion, and the tibialis posterior tendon, which assists with ankle inversion and plantarflexion.

History

It is important to determine the mechanism of injury by asking the athlete if he or she sustained an inversion ("I rolled my ankle") or eversion type of injury. The athlete may describe feeling or hearing a "popping" sensation, followed by immediate pain, swelling, and difficulty ambulating or continuing the sport. Other important issues to ask about include previous ankle injuries, the ability of the athlete to continue play or ambulate, the use of ankle support devices (orthosis or taping), and any previous rehabilitation exercises.

Physical Examination

The physical examination should begin with the observation of the patient's gait and ability to ambulate. Inspection should be performed from all sides to determine the amount of swelling and ecchymosis, along with looking for any scars, calluses, masses, or deformities. Standing alignment should be performed to allow the examiner to determine if the athlete has a pes planus (flat arch) or pes cavus (high arch) foot deformity. Range of motion (dorsiflexion, plantarflexion, inversion, and eversion) should be assessed and comparison made to the uninjured side. The examination should continue with palpation of bony structures, strength and stability testing, and assessment of neurovascular status.

Commonly used ankle stability tests include the anterior drawer and the talar tilt. The anterior drawer test, which assesses the integrity and stability of the ATFL, is performed with the knee flexed. The foot is in either the neutral or slightly plantarflexed position to avoid contraction of the gastrocnemius. The examiner then stabilizes the lower extremity with one hand while cupping the heel with the other and provides an anterior translational force (Figure 24-3). The examiner must note the quality of the ligamentous end point, along with the amount of anterior translation. The talar tilt or inversion stress test determines the integrity and stability of the CFL. The test is performed by again stabilizing the patient's lower extremity with one hand while the other hand provides an inversion force on the ankle (Figure 24-4).

Comparison of any abnormal findings should be done with the uninjured extremity, which may allow the examiner to detect any generalized ligamentous laxity, which may be normal for that patient. It may not be always possible or necessary to perform the anterior drawer or talar tilt test

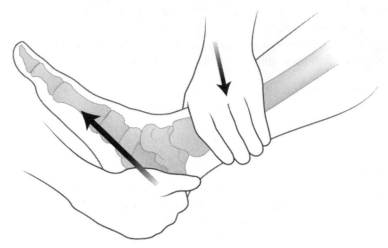

Figure 24-3   Anterior drawer test to assess anterior talofibular ligament.

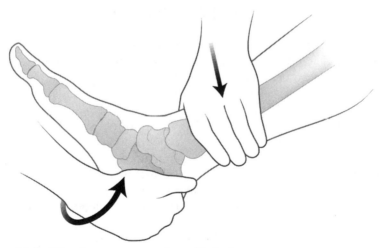

Figure 24-4   Talar tilt test to assess calcaneofibular ligament.

in the acute setting secondary to patient pain and discomfort. Often, these tests can be performed on close follow-up to provide insight into the severity and grading of injury.

To evaluate the syndesmosis, a squeeze test is performed by squeezing the tibia and fibula together at the midcalf (Figure 24-5). A positive test will refer pain to the syndesmosis region (Figure 24-6). The Thompson test is performed to evaluate for a possible Achilles' tendon rupture by squeezing the midportion of the calf while assessing for passive ankle plantarflexion (Figure 24-7).

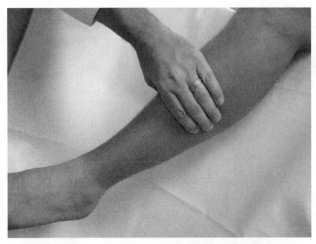

Figure 24-5 Squeeze test to evaluate for syndesmosis injury. A gentle force is applied by squeezing the tibia and fibula together at the midcalf. A positive test elicits pain in the syndesmosis region.

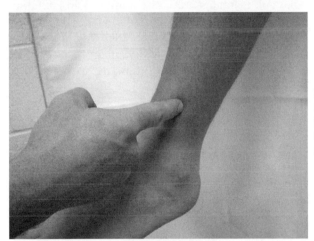

Figure 24-6 Tenderness over the anterior tibiofibular ligament and lower interosseous membrane.

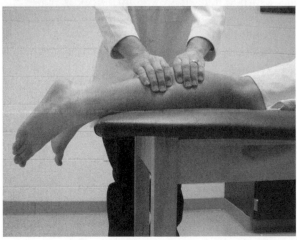

Figure 24-7 The Thompson test is performed by squeezing the gastrocnemius and soleus muscle complex at the midcalf. A test is considered positive when there is absence of passive ankle plantarflexion. A negative test is shown here.

Table 24-1   Ankle Sprain Classification

- *Grade I (mild):* Stretching of the ATF with or without involvement of the CF
- *Grade II (moderate):* Partial tear of the ATF with stretching of the CF
- *Grade III (severe):* ATF and CF ligament rupture, with partial tearing of the PTF

ATF, anterior talofibular ligament; CF, calcaneofibular ligament; PTF, posterior talofibular ligament.
Adapted with permission from O'Donoghue DH. The Treatment of Injuries to Athletes, 4th ed.
Philadelphia: WB Saunders; 1984.

Lateral Ankle Sprain

Lateral ankle sprains are common injuries encountered in sporting activities. The mechanism of injury usually involves an inversion force with the foot in slight plantarflexion. This inversion injury may occur during landing on an uneven surface or on an opponent's foot. The majority (85%) of ankle sprains occur on the outer aspect of the ankle involving the lateral ligament complex. Medial ankle sprains are less common than lateral injuries because of the inherent strength and stability of the deltoid ligament.

Risk factors often believed to be associated with ankle injuries include prior ankle sprains, generalized ligamentous laxity, inappropriate shoe wear, uneven playing surfaces, and cutting and jumping sports such as soccer, football, and basketball (4).

Ankle Sprain Classification

The acute ankle sprain can be classified in severity from grade I to grade III (I, mild; II, moderate; III, severe) (Table 24-1). The athlete with a grade I, or mild, ankle sprain will usually be able to bear weight without pain or a limp. The patient will display a minimal amount of ankle tenderness and swelling on the lateral aspect, with no mechanical instability or loss of function. These athletes will usually return to full activity within 1 week of injury.

The grade II ankle injury will cause a moderate amount of pain, swelling, and ecchymosis, with difficulty in ambulation. The patient will display a mild-to-moderate amount of ligamentous instability on examination and should be able to return to full activity within 2 weeks of injury.

The grade III ankle injury will cause a severe amount of pain, swelling, and ecchymosis, and the patient is unable to ambulate. These patients also display a greater amount of ligamentous instability during stability testing (anterior drawer, talar tilt). These patients may require up to 3 weeks until return to full sporting activities.

Case Study 24-1

A 22-year-old male soccer player presented to clinic after sustaining an inversion injury to the right ankle the day before. The patient complained of pain, swelling, and decreased motion; however, he was able to bear weight both immediately and on initial presentation with minimal discomfort. He denied any prior ankle injuries.

Upon examination, he demonstrated minimal soft tissue swelling of the lateral ankle without ecchymosis. Range of motion was limited secondary to pain. Tenderness was elicited over the ATF and CF without involvement of the PTF, syndesmosis, or deltoid ligament. The anterior drawer and talar tilt tests were not performed because of pain. The Thompson test and squeeze test were normal with a normal neurovascular exam. There was no tenderness over the malleoli, midfoot region, navicular, or base of the fifth metatarsal.

The patient was diagnosed with a grade I ankle sprain and was instructed in the PRICE principles. A compression wrap was prescribed to control swelling along with acetaminophen for pain. He was encouraged to begin early range-of-motion exercises once pain was controlled along with instruction for ankle rehabilitation exercises. The patient was allowed to return to play once full function of the ankle had returned approximately 10 days postinjury.

Radiology

The use of plain radiographs may not be always indicated in the management of the acute ankle sprain unless there is suspicion for fracture or growth plate injury based on a careful history and physical examination.

The Ottawa ankle rules (Figure 24-8) may be implemented in those patients over 18 years of age as a guide to determine the necessity of plain radiographs. With the implementation of these rules, the physician can not only reduce the number of unnecessary radiographs but also approach a sensitivity of 100% for the exclusion of significant ankle fractures. Radiographs should be considered for any patient who cannot bear weight (ambulate for four steps) both immediately and on presentation or has point tenderness over the distal aspect of medial or lateral malleolus (posterior edge or inferior tip) or midfoot zone.

Patients with chronic ankle complaints (pain up to 6 weeks postinjury) despite appropriate treatment and rehabilitation should undergo plain radiographs for further evaluation.

Initial ankle radiographs should include anteroposterior (AP), lateral, and mortise (20-degree internal oblique) views (3,5). Comparison views should be considered in adolescent athletes with open growth plates to determine if a subtle growth plate injury is present.

Patients with abnormal plain radiographs (fracture, talar dome lesion, and so forth) should be referred to a sports medicine specialist or orthopedic surgeon as indicated for further workup and evaluation (Table 24-2).

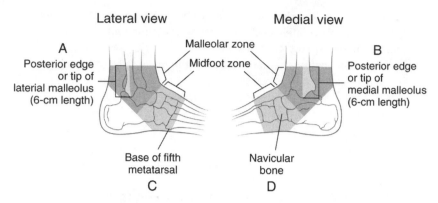

Figure 24-8   Ottawa ankle and foot rules. An ankle radiographic series is indicated if a patient has pain in the malleolar zone and any of these findings: bone tenderness at *A*, bone tenderness at *B*, or inability to bear weight immediately and in the emergency department (or physician's office). A foot radiographic series is indicated if a patient has pain in the midfoot zone and any of these findings: bone tenderness at *C*, bone tenderness at *D*, or inability to bear weight immediately and in the emergency department (or physician's office).

Table 24-2   Indications for Referral for Ankle Injury

• Fracture	• Neurovascular injury
• Dislocation	• Peroneal tendon subluxation/dislocation
• Syndesmosis injury	• Mechanical symptoms (locking, popping, catching)
• Osteochondral injury	

Treatment and Rehabilitation

The treatment of the acutely injured ankle includes the incorporation of the PRICE (protection, rest, ice, compression, and elevation) principles.

Protection can be obtained with the use of splinting devices or a semi-rigid pneumatic ankle brace (Airstirrup-type brace) for moderate-to-severe ankle injuries, with the avoidance of cast immobilization. The athlete should undergo relative rest, with the use of crutches for those patients unable to ambulate or those with a significant amount of pain. Icing of the injured extremity (approximately 15 minutes, 3-4 times daily) is an easy, inexpensive, and effective way to reduce pain and control swelling. Medications such as acetaminophen can be safely used in the first 24-48 hours, with the avoidance of nonsteroidal anti-inflammatory medications, which may lead to increased bleeding and soft tissue swelling. After the first few days postinjury, a nonsteroidal anti-inflammatory may then be used to control further pain and inflammation. A compressive wrap or elastic bandage can provide pain relief, as well as the prevention of swelling in the dependent portion of the ankle. Elevation of the injured extremity above the heart is also useful for the early reduction of swelling. Prolonged immobilization and/or a non-weight-bearing status is felt to have a detrimental effect on recovery and return to sport; therefore early range-of-motion exercises while continuing to protect the ligamentous structures is imperative (6). Joint range-of-motion exercises promote collagen healing and bundle reorientation, allowing athletes to recover more quickly (7).

The rehabilitative process is a gradual, step by step program designed to restore range of motion and function, improve performance, and prevent repeat ankle injuries. When possible, the athlete should undergo a supervised program with either a certified athletic trainer or physical therapist. This program may begin with range-of-motion exercises (alphabet exercises), stretching and strengthening of the gastrocnemius and soleus muscles, with progression to activities such as marble pickups, towel scrunches, and proprioceptive exercises (wobble board) as tolerated. Once motion is improved, the athlete can begin further strength and flexibility exercises, as well as brisk walking or light jogging, stationary bike, and swimming. The final stage of rehabilitation will include sport-specific drills and conditioning exercises (figure 8s, sprints, and so forth) designed to test the stability and strength of the athlete in a controlled environment. Consideration should be made for the use of prophylactic athletic taping or support devices (nonrigid functional ankle brace) to prevent further ankle injuries, along with proper warm-up, stretching, and conditioning programs (1,2,4).

Syndesmosis Injury

Injury to the syndesmosis, or "high" ankle sprain, accounts for 10–20% (2) of all ankle sprains encountered in sports such as football, rugby, soccer, and basketball. The term *high ankle sprain* comes from the fact that this injury occurs above the ankle joint and is usually a more severe injury, requiring a longer recovery time and rehabilitative process. The mechanism of injury involves an eversion or external rotation force on the ankle.

The examination will reveal minimal soft tissue swelling and ecchymosis over the upper aspect of the ankle or lower leg. Tenderness to palpation will be located over the anterior portion of the syndesmosis (Figure 24-6). It is important to palpate over the region of the deltoid ligament along with the fibula to evaluate for a possible Maisonneuve fracture (high fibular fracture associated with a medial ankle injury). To evaluate the syndesmosis, a squeeze test is performed as previously described. A positive test will refer pain to the syndesmosis region. Other maneuvers include the external rotation test performed by external rotation of the foot and ankle while the knee is flexed to 90 degrees. Again, pain will be referred to the syndesmosis region during a positive test.

Radiographs of the foot, ankle, and fibula should be performed for those patients with syndesmosis injury, to evaluate the extent of injury and to rule out an associated fracture. Particular attention should focus on the ankle mortise to evaluate for any abnormal widening, which may signify an associated deltoid ligament injury. Those patients with tenderness over the fibula should also have radiographs performed to evaluate for a Maisonneuve fracture. Those patients with significant widening of the mortise on radiographs should be referred to an orthopedic surgeon for possible surgical fixation using a syndesmosis screw. Because of the severity of injury associated with a high ankle sprain, the treatment course is longer than the typical ankle sprain and may require 4-6 weeks for complete recovery.

Treatment options of high ankle sprain (without mortise widening) include the use of a fracture walker or boot with crutches for up to 2 weeks. The athlete should be evaluated on a weekly basis and may begin weight bearing once the area of injury is nontender and the patient is able to stand without pain. The athlete may be placed in a functional ankle brace for further support and allowed to ambulate as tolerated. A rehabilitation program should begin early on during the treatment course to improve range of motion, decrease pain, and strengthen the surrounding structures. Athletes are allowed to return to play after completion of a rehabilitation program in a gradual, stepwise approach.

Achilles' Tendon Disorders

Achilles' Tendinitis

Tendinitis of the Achilles' tendon is a common condition in runners, gymnasts, tennis players, dancers, and basketball players (8). This overuse injury occurs at the terminal portions of the gastrocnemius and soleus muscles fibers at the insertion upon the calcaneus. Athletes with Achilles' tendinitis will have posterior leg and foot pain or tightness of the calf. The athlete may demonstrate soft tissue swelling and tenderness to palpation at either the insertion or midportion of the tendon. Treatment includes relative rest, icing, anti-inflammatory medication, heel lifts, and physical therapy. Corticosteroid injections and oral steroids should be avoided in this condition because of the possibility of, and association with, Achilles' tendon rupture as described below (8). To maintain cardiovascular fitness, the athlete may cross-train using activities such as swimming or an elliptical trainer. Most athletes with Achilles' tendinitis are able to return to full activity in 10-14 days.

Achilles' Tendon Rupture

The Achilles' tendon is the strongest and largest tendon in the body (2,8), therefore requiring a significant force to cause rupture. Rupture of the

Achilles' tendon is a condition often overlooked on initial presentation in up to 25% of cases (8). This condition occurs in the "weekend warrior" or athlete in the 30-50 year age group (often because of lack of flexibility) involved in running or jumping sports. The usual site of rupture is in the area of poor blood supply approximately 2-6 cm from the insertion upon the calcaneus. A common history includes the athlete attempting a jump or rapid movement who reports hearing or feeling a "pop" or sensation of someone kicking them in the heel. The athlete is usually unable to continue their sport or activity. Risk factors for this injury include systemic use of medications such as corticosteroids and fluroquinolones (9,10), prior tendinitis, or previous tendon rupture.

On examination, the patient will have soft tissue swelling and ecchymosis of the posterior foot and ankle and may be unable to ambulate because of pain. Tenderness to palpation is located along the course of the tendon. A palpable defect may be present but can often be misleading because of surrounding soft tissue swelling. The Thompson test is performed to confirm the diagnosis (absence of passive ankle plantarflexion on squeezing of the midportion of the calf) (see Figure 24-7). The patient may also have weak active plantarflexion and/or inability to perform a single toe raise. Radiographs are not necessary for diagnosis unless there is suspicion for other associated injuries. MRI can be used to confirm the diagnosis or be of additional benefit in equivocal cases.

Treatment for active individuals includes surgical repair of the tendon. For those who are poor surgical candidates or who elect conservative treatment, cast immobilization for up to 12 weeks is an option. A supervised physical therapy and rehabilitation program should be completed in either treatment option with full return to activity in 4-6 months.

Case Study 24-2

A 30-year-old male presented to clinic after suffering a left foot injury during a basketball game. He reports coming down from a lay-up and felt that someone may have "kicked" him in the heel. He had immediate swelling of the posterior foot and ankle and was unable to continue activity because of pain. He initially presented to the local emergency room where x rays were performed, which were negative for fracture. He was told he had an ankle sprain and was sent for follow up and further evaluation.

Upon examination, the patient had moderate swelling and ecchymosis of the posterior foot and ankle. The patient was nontender over the ATF, CF, PTF, syndesmosis, deltoid ligament, and was without focal bony tenderness. He was tender over the distal Achilles' region and was unable to bear weight without pain. A squeeze test was negative, with no passive ankle plantarflexion during the Thompson test. Distal neurovascular findings were within normal limits. The patient was diagnosed with an acute Achilles' tendon rupture.

Treatment options included surgical management and serial casting. The patient elected for surgical repair and was evaluated by an orthopedic surgeon. Surgery was performed without complication, and the patient began a postoperative rehabilitation program. He returned to full activity 5 months post-injury.

Medial Tibial Stress Syndrome

Medial tibial stress syndrome (MTSS), previously termed *shin splints* or *traction periostits*, is a common cause of activity-related lower leg pain and accounts for 13% of all running injuries (11). MTSS was first described in 1982 by Drez and Muharek to replace the term *shin splints*. Other disorders leading to activity-related leg pain include stress fracture, exertional compartment syndrome, vascular or peripheral nerve entrapment, muscle strain, and fascial herniation (12).

The patient with MTSS will present with diffuse leg pain or a dull ache along the medial border of the tibia. A patient with a stress fracture will have focal symptoms, whereas the athlete with exertional compartment syndrome will experience calf tightness and pain during exercise. Risk factors for MTSS include training errors such as an abrupt change in intensity or duration, improper footwear or running surface, and excessive foot pronation (12).

The most widely accepted cause of MTSS includes increased stress on the medial soleus insertion on the tibia during the stance phase of running (12). This stress reaction of the posteromedial leg may lead to the development of a stress fracture if not treated early and properly. During evaluation, the athlete with this condition will demonstrate diffuse tenderness to palpation along the posteromedial middle and distal third of the tibia.

Radiographs in patients with MTSS are usually normal. A triple phase bone scan may be used to confirm the diagnosis, which will reveal a diffuse longitudinal uptake along the posteromedial tibia during the delayed portion of the scan (12). Some authors prefer MRI in the evaluation of leg pain in athletes (11); however, this is usually not necessary when the history and physical examination are consistent with MTSS.

Treatment of this condition includes relative rest, activity modification, icing, anti-inflammatory medication, correction of training errors, and orthotics in those athletes with a pes cavus or pes planus foot deformity. Cross-training activities such as water running may be performed while pain-free to maintain cardiovascular fitness during the recovery period. Surgery is only considered in recalcitrant cases (12).

Posterior Tibialis Tendinitis

Tendinitis of the posterior tibialis tendon is usually encountered in dancers and in soccer, basketball, and tennis players. The posterior tibialis tendon is located behind the medial malleolus and attaches to the tarsonavicular region. A common pneumonic used to remember the structures behind the medial malleolus is "Tom, Dick, ANd Harry": posterior Tibialis tendon, flexor Digitorum longus tendon, posterior tibial Artery and Nerve, and flexor Hallucis longus tendon. Athletes may report posteromedial ankle pain and demonstrate swelling and tenderness to palpation along the course of the tendon. Patients may also have weakness or pain with resisted foot inversion.

Treatment includes relative rest, icing, NSAIDs, and physical therapy. In severe cases, a short period of immobilization in either a cast or a removable boot may be indicated. Arch supports are considered for those athletes with excessive foot hyperpronation. Patients are usually able to return to full activity in 4-6 weeks.

Compartment Syndrome

The term *compartment syndrome* refers to a condition either acute or chronic in nature, leading to elevated pressures within the tissues of the lower extremity. This elevation in tissue pressure may lead to alterations in perfusion and/or injury to the muscle and neurovascular structures. Acute compartment syndrome is usually secondary to lower extremity trauma such as fracture or crush injury. This condition may also occur with tight-fitting casts. Chronic compartment syndrome or exertional compartment syndrome is often related to exercise and seen in runners or endurance athletes. These athletes may present with leg pain, swelling, and paresthesias associated with activity. The most common compartment involved is the anterior and deep posterior compartments in up to 80% of chronic cases (13).

The fascial compartments of the leg include the anterior, lateral, and superficial posterior, and deep posterior. Important structures within these compartments include the sural nerve (superficial posterior compartment), tibial nerve (deep posterior), superficial (lateral compartment), and deep peroneal nerves (superficial compartment).

The diagnosis of acute compartment syndrome should be considered in those athletes with pain out of proportion to exam with history of recent trauma. Tense swelling may be noted within the affected compartment along with paresthesias or sensory disturbances. Palpable pulses may be present in those with acute compartment syndrome and is often unreliable in ruling out the diagnosis.

To diagnose compartment syndrome, intracompartmental pressures must be evaluated via slit/wick catheter techniques or other pressure monitoring devices. Normal resting pressures within the compartment are usually less than 10 mm Hg (14). In acute compartment syndrome, intra-compartmental pressures greater than 30 mm Hg confirm the diagnosis. The diagnostic criteria for chronic exertional compartment syndrome include pre-exercise compartmental pressures greater that 15 mm Hg or a 1-minute postexercise pressure greater than 30 mm Hg; and/or a 5-minute postexercise pressure in excess of 20 mm Hg (13,14).

Treatment for acute and chronic compartment syndrome is surgical; fasciotomies performed on the involved compartments have a success rate greater than 90% (13). Return to sporting activity may be considered once the athlete has completely recovered from surgery and is able to demonstrate full functional return.

REFERENCES

1. **Wolfe MW, Uhl TL, Mattacola CG, McCluskey LC.** Management of ankle sprains. Am Fam Physician. 2001;63:93-104.
2. **Title CI, Katchis SD.** Traumatic foot and ankle injuries in the athlete: acute athletic trauma. Orthop Clin North Am. 2002;33:587-98.
3. **Dunfee WR, Dalinka MK, Kneeland JB.** Imaging of athletic injuries to the ankle and foot. Radiol Clin North Am. 2002;40:289-312.
4. **Casillas MM.** Ligament injuries of the foot and ankle in adult athletes. In: Delee JC, Drez D, Miller MD, eds. Delee and Drez's Orthopaedic Sports Medicine: Principles and Practice, 2nd ed. Philadelphia: WB Saunders; 2003:2324-58.
5. **Stiell IG, McKnight RD, Greenberg GH, et al.** Implementation of the Ottawa ankle rules. JAMA. 1994;271:827-32.
6. **Hockenbury RT, Sammarco GJ.** Evaluation and treatment of ankle sprains. Phys Sportsmed. 2001;29:57-64.
7. **Anderson SJ.** Acute ankle sprains. Phys Sportsmed. 2002;30:29-35.
8. **Mazzone MF, McCue T.** Common conditions of the Achilles tendon. Am Fam Physician. 2002;65:1805-10.
9. **Hersh BL, Heath NS.** Achilles tendon rupture as a result of oral steroid therapy. J Am Podiatr Med Assoc. 2002;92:355-8.
10. **Huston KA.** Achilles tendonitis and tendon rupture due to fluroquinolone antibiotics. N Engl J Med. 1994;331:748.
11. **Andrish JT.** The leg. In: Delee JC, Drez D, Miller MD, eds. Delee and Drez's Orthopaedic Sports Medicine: Principles and Practice, 2nd ed. Philadelphia: WB Saunders; 2003:2155-9.
12. **Kortebein PM, Kaufman KR, Basford JR, Stuart MJ.** Medial tibial stress syndrome. Med Sci Sports Exerc. 2000;32:S27-33.
13. **Andrish JT.** The leg. In: Delee JC, Drez D, Miller MD, eds. Delee and Drez's Orthopaedic Sports Medicine: Principles and Practice, 2nd ed. Philadelphia: WB Saunders; 2003:2163-70.
14. **Hutchinson MR, Ireland ML, Roberts WO.** Chronic exertional compartment syndrome. Phys Sportsmed. 1999;27:101-2.

SUGGESTED READINGS

Casillas MM. Ligament injuries of the foot and ankle in adult athletes. In: Delee JC, Drez D, Miller MD, eds. Delee and Drez's Orthopaedic Sports Medicine: Principles and Practice, 2nd ed. Philadelphia: WB Saunders; 2003:2324-58.

Kortebein PM, Kaufman KR, Basford JR, Stuart MJ. Medial tibial stress syndrome. Med Sci Sports Exerc. 2000;32:S27-33.

Mazzone MF, McCue T. Common conditions of the Achilles tendon. Am Fam Physician. 2002;65:1805-10.

Wolfe MW, Uhl TL, Mattacola CG, McCluskey LC. Management of ankle sprains. Am Fam Physician. 2001;63:93-104.

25

■　■　■

Foot Disorders

Peter F. Davis, MD

F oot injuries are common in sports that involve running and jumping. Injuries are closely linked with the ankle and can range from fractures to corns and calluses.

Anatomy

The foot is composed of three main areas: the hindfoot, the midfoot, and the forefoot (Table 25-1). The hindfoot composes one-third the length of the foot and is the link between the ankle and the foot. The bones of the hindfoot are the calcaneus and talus (Figure 25-1). The talus has a broad front and has a large dome superiorly that articulates with the fibula and tibia. The calcaneous is where the Achilles' tendon inserts and the plantar fascia originates. The subtalar joint is the joint between these two bones and allows the foot to invert and evert (about 5 degrees in each direction). The tarsal tunnel exists in the region of the hindfoot. The posterior tibialis nerve and the posterior tibialis artery pass here.

The midfoot composes one-sixth the length of the foot. Bony structures here include the cuboid, medial, mid and lateral cuneiforms, and the navicular. The tibialis posterior inserts on the navicular, which helps maintain the arch and plantarflex and inverts the foot. The Lisfranc joint is the articulation between the forefoot and midfoot. It is the articulation between the cuboid, cuneiforms, and metatarsals. The sinus tarsi, also known as the talocalcaneal sulcus, is also found here. It is an anatomical space between the inferior neck of the talus and the superior aspect of the calcaneus. Patients who have persistent ankle pain after an inversion sprain may have injured the ligaments in this area. The midfoot also contains the spring ligament, which supports the talus. The peroneal longus and brevis cross the

Table 25-1   Foot Anatomy

Region	Bones	Notable Soft Tissues
Hindfoot	Calcaneus, talus	Achilles' insertion, plantar fascia origination, tarsal tunnel
Midfoot	Navicular, cuneiforms (medial, mid, lateral), cuboid	Tibialis posterior insertion, spring ligament, Lisfranc joint, sinus tarsi
Forefoot	Metatarsals (1-5), phalanges (14 total), MTP joint sesamoids	First MTP capsule complex, posterior tibial nerve and branches

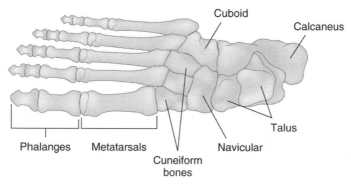

Figure 25-1   Anatomy of the foot.

midfoot and help to evert the foot. The tibialis anterior helps to dorsiflex the foot.

The medial longitudinal arch is formed by the calcaneous, talus, navicular, three cuneiforms, and metatarsals 1-3. It is supported by the calcaneneonavicular ligament (spring ligament). When this ligament weakens, the foot tends to pronate, which may put additional stress on ligaments that function within the medial arch such as the tibialis posterior. The entire arch of the foot aids in balance and absorbing shock loads.

The bony structures of the forefoot are the 5 metatarsals and 14 phalanges. Important to the forefoot is the first metatarsal phalangeal joint, which contains sesamoids. The sesamoids help to increase the fulcrum and force of the flexor hallicus brevis. Sesamoids may be multipartate. The medial sesamoid is more often multipartate. The first metatarsal phylangeal joint is surrounded by a capsuloligamentous complex, which provides restraint to forceful stresses. It is composed of the collateral ligaments, abductor and adductor tendons, short flexor and extensors, sesamoids, and the plantar plate. Hyperextension injuries may damage this complex. The posterior tibial nerve branches at the forefoot into the medial and lateral plantar nerves, which innnervate small muscles in the sole of the foot and supply sensation to the medial and lateral plantar surface of the foot.

Physical Examination

Basic Examination

The basic exam of the foot differs little from any other extremity. The clinician should develop a systematic method for evaluation. Inspection should involve looking at both feet with proper exposure. The foot should be examined in both a non-weight-bearing position and standing (if pain allows). One should observe for pes planus (flat feet) and may identify deformities of the heel while observing the patient from behind. In patients with chronic foot pain, the examiner should look for calcaneal inversion or eversion or forefoot valgus or varus. These types of disorders may be amendable to correction with orthotics. The presence of calluses should also be noted. Calluses may indicate improper footwear or anatomic disorders causing improper biomechanics of the foot. Again, the unaffected side should be used for comparison. Excessive medial callus formation may indicate excessive pronation, which, again, may be amendable to correction with medial foot orthotics. The inspection may also include gait evaluation.

Palpation should proceed in an organized way. Tenderness over bony landmarks such as the navicular and metatarsals should be noted. The plantar fascia should also be palpated along its length. Tinel's testing may be performed over areas of suspected involvement such as the cubital tunnel (see below). Palpation of interdigital spaces that elicits pain may give clues to the existence of neuromas.

Range of motion of the foot is limited to evaluating the subtalar joint, motion of the forefoot, and motion of the metatarsal-phylangeal (MTP) joint. One should carefully compare the first MTP joint motion if pathology is suspected in this area. Athletes with turf toe, for example, may have limited MTP joint motion.

Gait Examination

The gait cycle begins at heel strike and ends at the next heel strike of the same foot. There are two phases: the stance and swing phase (Table 25-2). The stance phase is further divided into three stages. Contact is characterized by subtalar pronation. Midstance follows where there is subtalar

---

Table 25-2   Gait Phases

1. Stance
   - *a)* Contact
   - *b)* Midstance
   - *c)* Propulsion
2. Swing

---

supination. Propulsion causes further subtalar supination. The clinician should observe gait abnormalities when examining a patient with foot complaints. Excessive pronation in an athlete may cause midfoot or ankle dysfunction, which in turn may lead to knee or hip pain. One should note antalgic gait, any rotational abnormalities (for example, forefoot valgus), and observe the medial arch for proper function.

Conditions of the Foot

Hindfoot Conditions

Pes planus is common in children and found in up to 15% of adults (1). Pes planus itself is not pathologic, but, as mentioned, it may lead to dysfunction in other areas such as the ankle or knee. It is usually asymptomatic in children. Adults may acquire this deformity with weakening of the medial longitudinal arch or with tibialis posterior dysfunction. Unilateral pes planus usually indicates an acquired deformity or arch dysfunction. Individuals with arch dysfunction will not be able to invert their calcaneous fully. An observer may ask the patient to stand on their "tip toes" and observe for calcaneal inversion. If the calcaneus does not invert, one should look for things such as tibialis posterior dysfunction, rigid tarsal coalition, or an accessory navicular. If pes planus is symptomatic, treatment may involve relative rest. Orthotics or arch supports may provide some benefit in mild cases, whereas surgical intervention may be warranted for adults with traumatic disruptions of the medial arch.

Rigid tarsal coalition is a congenital deformity found in 1% of the general population. Another name for this disorder is peroneal spastic flat foot. The cause is a bony bar or cartilaginous bridge between osseous structures in the foot. A talocalcaneal bridge is found more commonly in individuals aged 8-12, whereas a calcaneal navicular bridge is more commonly discovered in patients aged 12-16. A common reason for presentation to the clinician is recurrent inversion ankle sprains in a young athlete. Physical exam will reveal a rigid flat foot. The calcaneous will not invert with the "tip toe" test, and first toe dorsiflexion will fail to increase the medial foot arch. If suspected, plain radiographs may reveal a bridge; however, CT may be needed to confirm the diagnosis. Treatment involves casting for 4 to 6 weeks to reduce inflammation and pain. Orthotics may be useful for less severe cases. Severe cases require surgical referral to resect the bar.

Plantar fasciitis is found in up to 10% of runners and is common in other sports such as basketball, tennis, soccer, and gymnastics (2). It is caused by damage to the plantar fascia at its medial origin, producing a tendinosis. Typically, patients will experience heel pain that is at its worst with the first few steps of the morning. Physical exam will reveal pain with palpation over the medial calcaneal tuberosity. Gait may reveal overpronation. Toe jumping may also produce pain in the heel, in contrast to fat pad syndrome where no pain is produced. Radiographs are rarely useful and may show only a heel spur. The importance of heel spurs in plantar fasciitis is debatable; however, current data suggest that the significance of spurs is probably negligible (2). Treatment involves relative rest and anti-inflammatory medications. A stretching program should be prescribed that involves stretching the Achilles' tendon and the gastroc-soleus complex. Night splinting has been used whereby the patient sleeps with a splint that places the foot in a slightly dorsiflexed position. Localized corticosteroid injections have been used to effectively treat this condition as well. For recalcitrant cases, extracorporeal shock wave therapy is a newer approach that has been shown to have beneficial effects, although its exact mechanisms are not clear.

Case Study 25-1

A 32-year-old female runner presented to the office with a complaint of right heel pain. She noted that the pain had increased with hill training and was worse at the beginning of the day. Physical exam revealed tenderness to palpation over the medial calcaneus on the plantar surface. The patient was diagnosed with plantar fasciitis, instructed on Achilles' tendon stretching exercises and local icing techniques, and told to limit hill running. She was able to resume full activity in 6 weeks.

Fat pad syndrome is characterized by heel pain due to thinning of the fat pad at the plantar aspect of the calcaneous. This may happen due to age-related atrophy or repetitive trauma and is more commonly seen in older athletes or those who participate in sports with bare feet. Heel pain is typically worse with progression of activity in contrast to plantar fasciitis. There are few treatment options for this syndrome. Heel cups or cushion inserts can be used. Steroid injections should be avoided in patients with this condition.

Sever disease is an apophysitis of the calcaneous at the insertion site of the Achilles' tendon. It is typically seen in active children and adolescents ages 7-15 and is often associated with individuals who have rigid high arches. Individuals who sprint in cleated shoes may be more likely to develop this disorder due to an increased force in the ankle flexors. Physical exam will reveal tenderness at the posterior portion of the calcaneous to palpation with decreased dorsiflexion of the ankle. Radiographs are generally not necessary. Like most forms of apophysitis, it is self-limited, and parents should be reassured. Treatment consists of a program of relative rest, stretching of the gatroc-soleus complex, localized ice, and heel lifts to functionally shorten the Achilles' tendon.

Haglund disease has been referred to as "pump bump" or retrocalcaneal exostosis. It is a prominence that develops in the posterior/superior calcaneous, and its cause is unknown. Patients may present with posterior heel

pain, and the exam may reveal a bony prominence over the posterior portion of the calcaneous. It is more common in females. Shoewear should be
inspected, and the clinician should suggest heel counters that fit properly if
excessive pressure is noted. Padding to the area may be useful, or notching
of the shoe may be required. Only extreme cases require surgical referral.

Os trigonum syndrome is a cause of posterior ankle and foot pain. The
os trigonum is an accessory bone in the posterolateral area of the foot and
is found in 3-13% of the population (Figure 25-2) (3). Injuries that involve a
mechanism of foot hyperplantar flexion can damage the os triguonum,
which is typically asymptomatic. Physical exam may reveal tenderness in
the region of the posterior calcaneous and Achilles' tendon. Treatment of
this condition involves relative rest. Occasionally, this injury may require
surgical referral for excision in cases where symptoms persist.

Tarsal tunnel syndrome is an entrapment neuropathy involving compression of the posterior tibial nerve within the tarsal tunnel (Figure 25-3).
Patients may have medial foot pain or paresthesia, which may radiate to the
forefoot. Patients who overpronate or whose feet are chronically everted
may be predisposed to this condition due to excessive stress over the tarsal
tunnel. Severe ankle sprains may also damage the tarsal tunnel resulting in
subacute or chronic ankle and foot pain. Individuals with diabetes, alcoholism, or who have lower extremity varicosities may be at increased risk.

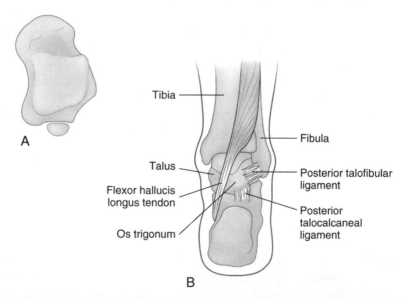

Figure 25-2 An os trigonum forms when the talar lateral posterior tubercle fails to fuse
with the body of the talus (A), as shown in this superior view. Repetitive plantar flexion, as
in soccer or football, can cause impingement of the os trigonum between the calcaneus
and the distal tibia, leading to pain. This syndrome can also lead to inflammation of the
flexor hallucis longus tendon and to avulsion injuries of the posterior talofibular and posterior talocalcaneal ligaments (B).

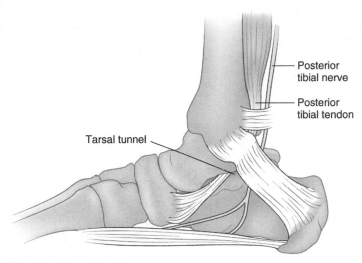

Figure 25-3   Tarsal tunnel syndrome.

Physical exam may reveal a positive tinnel's sign at the tarsal tunnel. Electromyelography (EMG) or nerve conduction velocity (NCV) testing may be useful to confirm the diagnosis. Treatment involves stretching and strengthening of the gastroc-soleus complex and foot arch. Foot orthotics may he helpful for those individuals with pes planus. Localized corticosteroid injections may also be beneficial. Surgery to release the nerve may be required for severe, prolonged cases.

Lateral plantar nerve syndrome is an entrapment neuropathy of the foot. In this syndrome, a branch of the posterior tibial nerve becomes entrapped between the abductor hallicus and quadratus plantae. Patients may present with heel and foot pain, which may be mistaken for plantar fasciitis. The patient may also have pain that radiates to the ankle. It may be seen in runners, dancers, and soccer players. Physical exam does not typically reveal sensory changes. Treatment consists of relative rest and using properly fitted footwear once activity resumes.

Fractures of the hindfoot are uncommon in athletics. Traumatic calcaneous fractures typically require surgical referral. Stress fractures may be encountered in endurance athletes who experience vague heel pain with insidious onset. An athlete may have pain with compression of the calcaneous on physical exam. Bone scanning or computed tomography is usually required to identify these fractures. Treatment involves relative rest, and return to play may take up to 3 months once clinical and radiographic healing has taken place. Athletes should be encouraged to use an ankle support brace once they return to their sport.

Acute talus fractures should be referred to an orthopedist for evaluation. Stress fractures of this bone are rare. The athlete may complain of diffuse

Table 25-3   Hindfoot Conditions in Athletes

• Pes planus	• Sever's disease
• Rigid tarsal coalition	• Haglund's disease
• Plantar fasciitis	• Os trigonum syndrome
• Fat pad syndrome	• Tarsal tunnel syndrome

midfoot pain and may have tenderness with subtalar motion (inversion and eversion). These types of fractures should be immobilized in a cast or immobilizing boot. Healing time can be prolonged, in some cases up to 6 months (4).

Hindfoot conditions are listed in Table 25-3.

Midfoot Conditions

The *Lisfranc sprain* or *fracture* is a midfoot injury that requires a high degree of suspicion to diagnose. This is a midfoot injury of the tarsal metatarsal junction involving the cuneiforms with the base of the first and second metatarsals. The patient will typically present with a painful midfoot and will describe an injury that involves the foot in a forced plantar flexed position. Physical exam will reveal pain at the tarsal-metatarsal joint. Standard foot radiographs should also include a weight-bearing view to better determine any avulsion fracture. More advanced imaging (that is, CT or MRI) may be required in high-level athletes where injury to this joint is suspected and plain radiographs are unrevealing. Injuries to the Lisfranc joint without fracture should be treated with 3 to 6 weeks of non-weight-bearing immobilization in a cast or cam type boot (5). Full recovery can take as long as 4 months. Lisfranc fractures should be referred for surgical intervention. Typical recovery time after surgery is 10-12 weeks.

Case Study 25-2

A 20-year-old male recreational soccer player presented to the office with foot pain. He reported falling to the ground when another player fell on his heel. Radiographs in the emergency department the day of injury were unrevealing, and the patient was given crutches to use as needed.

Examination 5 days later revealed foot swelling and tenderness over the dorsal midfoot. Repeat radiographs, which included a weight-bearing anteroposterior view, revealed a separation of the first and second metatarsals with a small bony fragment in the Lisfranc joint (Figure 25-4). The athlete was referred for open reduction and internal screw fixation and returned to competition the following season.

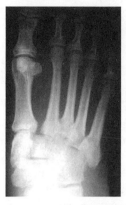

Figure 25-4 Separation of first and second metatarsals with small bony fragment in Lisfranc joint.

Kohler disease is found typically in boys aged 5-10 years and may present as a painful lump. It is characterized by an idiopathic necrosis of the navicular. The patient may have pain to palpation of the navicular, and radiographs will reveal sclerosis of the bone. Treatment involves a weight-bearing short leg cast for 6 weeks followed by arch supports that may be used in the shoes used for athletics.

When a patient presents with midfoot pain after an inversion ankle sprain, one should examine for any tenderness over the cuboid. *Cuboid syndrome* involves subluxation of the cuboid dorsally and laterally due to traction from the peroneal tendon. This injury, while poorly understood, may be more prevalent in dancers. Physical exam may reveal tenderness over the peroneal groove on the plantar aspect of the calcaneus. Radiographs usually add little to aid in the diagnosis, which is typically one of exclusion. Treatment involves addressing the ankle sprain and bracing (see Chapter 28). Some clinicians have used manipulation in successfully treating this disorder (6).

Younger athletes may present with midfoot pain related to an accessory navicular that is present in 10% of normal individuals (7). Also referred to as *os tibiale externum*, this pain may be caused by overpronation of the foot, which results in irritation to the ossicle, especially in young athletes. Physical exam may reveal tenderness over the navicular, and radiographs show what appears to be an avulsion of the navicular. X-rays of the contralateral side should be obtained to confirm the diagnosis. This disorder should be treated as an overuse injury with rest. Orthotics to help with arch support may be useful.

Midfoot fractures are uncommon in athletes. If seen, these types of fractures usually involve high-velocity trauma. Cuneiform fractures are rare and even more so in isolation. If the clinician detects this type of fracture, especially if dislocation is noted, the patient should be referred to an orthopedist for wire fixation. Cuboid fractures may occur with trauma. A "nutcracker" fracture is a fracture of the cuboid as a result of compression of the cuboid between the calcaneous and fourth and fifth metatarsals. Fractures without comminution may be treated with a short leg cast for 6 weeks. Displaced or comminuted fractures should be referred for surgical repair.

Navicular fractures of the foot are more common in athletes than cuneiform or cuboid fractures. Traumatic injuries that result in nondisplaced fractures may be treated with a short leg weight-bearing cast for 6 weeks. Displaced fractures require referral. An avulsion fracture may also be treated with a short leg cast for 6 weeks. The clinician should rule out an accessory navicular by obtaining contralateral foot radiographs. Occasionally, an endurance athlete may present with vague medial midfoot pain with tenderness at the navicular. The clinician should consider a navicular stress fracture in this population. Plain film radiographs may be unrevealing, and therefore bone scanning or computed tomography can be useful in making this diagnosis. These injuries are rare. Treatment involves non-weight-bearing in a cast or removable type boot for 6 to 8 weeks followed by progressive return to activity. Further details on treatment of these injuries are given in Chapter 26.

Midfoot conditions are shown in Table 25-4.

Forefoot Conditions

Many forefoot conditions are seen in athletes (Table 25-5). Patients who present with vague pain over the plantar aspect of the metatarsal head without a history of trauma may have *metatarsalgia*. This is a common cause of forefoot pain that athletes may describe as a burning sensation. Physical exam may reveal poorly localized pain in the forefoot to palpation. Causes vary but include overuse, improperly fitted shoes, an elongated metatarsal, or overpronation. Radiographs will typically be

---

Table 25-4   Midfoot Conditions in Athletes

• Lisfranc sprain or fracture	• Os tibiale externum (accessory navicular)
• Kohler's disease	• Navicular fracture
• Cuboid syndrome	• Medial longitudinal arch injury

Table 25-5   Forefoot Conditions in Athletes

• Metatarsalgia	• Turf toe
• Freiberg's infarction	• Hallux valgus
• Morton's neuroma (interdigital neuroma)	• Hallux rigidus
• Sesamoiditis	

unrevealing. Treatment for this disorder involves changing footwear to accommodate the width of the foot or metatarsal pads, which act to splay the metatarsals apart (Figure 25-5).

If an adolescent athlete presents with pain at the head of the metatarsals, one should consider *Freiberg infarction*. This is an avascular necrosis of the metatarsal head, typically the second or third. This disorder occurs in the second decade of life and is more common in females than in males (8). Physical exam will reveal tenderness of the forefoot, and radiographs will show osteosclerosis of the distal metatarsal. If detected early, treament involves a short leg walking cast until symptoms have abated. If radiographs reveal metatarsal collapse (sclerosis and destruction of the metatarsal head), orthopedic referral is required. Conservative treatment may require 4 weeks to 4 months of recovery before return to activity.

Morton's neuroma or *interdigital neuroma* is an entrapment neuropathy or perineural fibrosis of the forefoot first described in the 1800s. It involves the interdigital nerve, and patients with this disorder may have pain or dysesthesias of the foot or web space. The most common area is the web space between the third and fourth digits, and palpation in this interspace may illicit pain or a click. Athletes with pes cavus tend to have a higher incidence of this disorder. Treatment involves using footwear with a wide toe box or using a metatarsal arch pad in the athletes' shoe (see

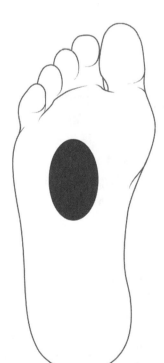

Figure 25-5   Metatarsal pad designed to be worn in the shoe.

Figure 25-5). Localized corticosteroid injection may provide relief of pain. Referral for surgical excision may be required for severe, recalcitrant cases.

The sesamoids of the forefoot lie within the flexor hallucis brevis tendon and aid in increasing the force at the first MTP joint. These may become inflamed by direct trauma or repetitive microtrama, such as is seen in dance, causing symptoms of pain at the base of the first phalynx. Physical exam will reveal pain at the plantar aspect of the MTP joint, and active flexion of the joint may also elicit pain. Radiographs are typically unrevealing, although one may detect a bipartite sesamoid or fracture. The medial sesamoid is more commonly involved. *Sesamoiditis* should be treated with shoes with a wide toe box and a stiff sole to prevent MTP joint motion. A "dancer's pad" may be useful to insert in the shoe (Figure 25-6). Fractures of the sesamoid require a short leg cast without weight bearing for 6 weeks. Sesamoids are not typically removed and operative treatment is rare.

Another injury of the first MTP joint is *turf toe*, which is a sprain of the joint. The name is derived from the association of this injury with athletic play on artificial turf. The capsule that surrounds this joint, including the plantar plate, is forced into a position of hyperextension resulting in injury. Injuries may be graded on a scale of I to III with grade I representing stretch injury and grade III representing complete tearing of the capuloligametnous complex (9). Athletes will present with pain at the MTP joint with

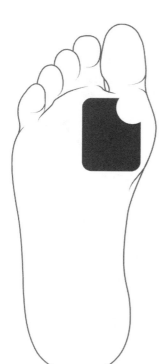

Figure 25-6   Dancer's pad. Note the C-shaped cut-out over the sesamoids at the first MTP joint.

possible swelling and ecchymosis. Loss of motion will be noted, and intoeing gait may be seen. Radiographs may be useful in acute injuries if a fracture is considered. Return to play can be accomplished by using rigid footwear or rigid inserts in grade I injuries. Grade III injuries usually require immobilization for several days with limited weight-bearing and progressive return to activity once range of motion is restored.

Hallux valgus is a lateral deviation of the big toe that causes the development of exostosis on the medial side of the first metatarsal (bunion). Athletes with this disorder should be encouraged to use footwear with a wide toe box, and hyperpronation should be corrected with arch supports or orthotics to relieve stress in this area. Surgery may be indicated for cases in which extended conservative treatment care fails.

Halux rigidus is a loss of mobility of the first MTP joint. Causes include trauma, osteoarthritis, or post-traumatic fracture. This can be particularly problematic in athletes because dorsiflexion of this joint followed by forceful push-off is essential for running. Using rigid orthotics to limit motion of the MTP joint may be helpful. If an osteophyte is present on the dorsal surface of the joint, surgical referral may be useful.

Metatarsal fractures may be encountered in traumatic athletic injuries. Nondisplaced fractures that involve digits 2, 3, or 4 may be casted without weight bearing for 3-4 weeks followed by placing the patient in an oversized shoe for comfort. Return to play is based on symptoms. Displaced fractures require orthopedic referral. One should be alert for first metatarsal fractures. These types of fractures, particularly if they involve any portion of the MTP joint space, should be referred for surgical evaluation. Stress fractures (Chapter 26) may be treated conservatively. *Phalynx fractures* can be treated with simple splinting or buddy taping. The patient may use a hard-soled shoe for comfort. If there is no significant displacement and if the athlete has minimal pain, immediate return to play is acceptable. Typical recovery time is 4-6 weeks.

Fractures of the fifth metatarsal deserve special attention because these types of injuries are common in sports. There are several patterns of fractures of this bone (Table 25-6 and Figure 25-7).

Table 25-6   Fifth Metatarsal Fracture Patterns

- Tuberosity avulsion
- Proximal fifth metatarsal fracture (Jones' fracture)
- Stress fracture
- Spiral fracture ("dancer's" fracture)
- Apophysitis of the tuberosity (not a true fracture)

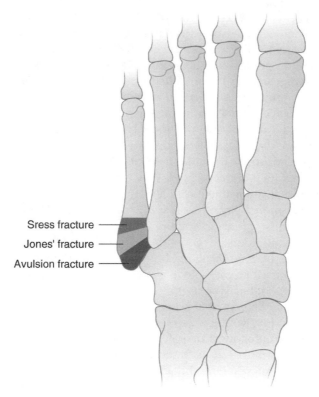

Sress fracture

Jones' fracture

Avulsion fracture

Figure 25-7   Fractures of the fifth metatarsal.

Tuberosity avulsion fractures may occur when there is an inversion of the foot and ankle causing the peroneus brevis to pull a bone fragment from the metatarsal. Physical exam will reveal tenderness at the tuberosity. These types of fractures, if minimally displaced, can be treated with a short leg cast or walking type boot.

Proximal fifth metatarsal fractures, which occur distal to the tuberosity but proximal to the metaphyseal-diphyseal junction, are referred to as *Jones' fractures*. Conservative treatment of this type of fracture may have unacceptable results in athletes given the possibility of nonunion. The mechanism that causes this injury may involve inversion to the foot while the ankle is plantarflexed. On exam, tenderness will be elicited over the fifth metatarsal base or shaft. Radiographs should be examined for significant fracture displacement. Conservative treatment is an option for those athletes wishing to defer surgical intervention. Non-weight-bearing in a short leg cast for 6 to 8 weeks is recommended if nonoperative treatment is to be attempted. Fractures may take as long as 21 weeks to heal, and the nonunion rate may be as high as 28% (4). Up to one-third of these fractures may refracture on returning to competition. Given these data, surgical referral should be considered for elite-level athletes. Once fixation is accomplished, the athlete should wear modified footwear, including flexible steel inserts.

Stress fractures of the fifth metatarsal may present as pain with a history of prodromal symptoms several weeks before the acute injury. Treatment of this type of injury is discussed in Chapter 26.

Spiral fractures of the fifth metatarsal are sometimes referred to as *"dancer's" fractures*. Foot plantarflexion and inversion are typical mechanisms of injury, and the patient will be tender over the midshaft of the metatarsal. If no there is no significant displacement, the patient may be placed in a short leg cast or removable walking boot. Treatment endpoints focus on patient comfort. The patient may bear weight once pain-free, typically 2 weeks after injury. Typically, athletes will require 4 more weeks of immobilization, which can be followed by a program of physical therapy focusing on increasing ankle and foot strength. Individuals involved in ballet will usually require 12 total weeks of recovery before dancing on pointe.

REFERENCES

1. **Staheli LT**. Fundamentals of Pediatric Orthopedics. New York: Raven Press; 1992.
2. **Shea M, Fields KB.** Plantar fasciitis; prescribing effective treatments. Phys Sportsmed. 2002;30:473-82.
3. **Cooper ME, Wolin PM.** Os trigonum syndrome with flexor hallucis longus tenosynovitis in a professional football referee. Med Sci Sports Exerc. 1999;31: S493-S496.
4. **Hunter SC, Deloach JG, McLean RB**. Foot problems. In: Team Physician's Handbook, 3rd ed. Philadelphia: Hanley & Belfus; 2002:535-46.
5. **Burroughs KE, Reimer CD, Fields KB.** Lisfranc injury of the foot: a commonly missed diagnosis. Am Fam Physician. 1998;58:118-24.
6. **Marshall P, Hamilton WG**. Cuboid subluxation in ballet dancers. Am J Sports Med. 1992;20:169-75.
7. **Gregg JR, Das M**. Foot and ankle problems in the preadolescent and adolescent athlete. Clin Sports Med. 1982;1:131-47.
8. **Sullivan AJ**. Ankle and foot injuries in the pediatric athlete. In: Pediatric and Adolescent Sports Medicine. Philadelphia: WB Saunders; 1994:453.
9. **Title CI, Katchis SD.** Traumatic foot and ankle injuries in the athlete. Orthopedic Clin North Am. 2002;33:587-98.

SUGGESTED READING

Baxter DE, Zingas C. The foot in running. J Am Acad Orthop Surg. 1995;3:136-45.

Early JS. Fractures and dislocations of the midfoot and forefoot. In: Bucholz RW, Heckman JD, eds. Rockwood and Green's Fractures in Adults, 5th ed. Philadelphia: Lippincott Williams & Wilkins; 2001:2181-246.

McCluskey LC. Functional anatomy of the foot and ankle. In: CL Baker, ed. The Hughston Clinic Sports Medicine Book. Baltimore: Williams and Wilkins; 1995:559-64.

Omey ML, Micheli IJ. Foot and ankle problems in the young athlete. Med Sci Sports Exerc. 1999:31:S470-86.

van Wyngarden TM. The painful foot, Part I: common forefoot deformities. Am Fam Physician. 1997;55:1866-76.

26

■ ■ ■

Stress Fractures

David M. Harsha, MD

S. Craig Veatch, MD

S tress fractures are a common problem in active individuals, especially military personnel and athletes. They have been recognized as a consequence of physical activity for more than a century. In 1855, a Prussian army physician named Breihaupt reported painful swollen feet in recruits after long marches (1). These fractures are often coined "march" fractures due to their relationship to military training. Stress fractures occur most frequently in the lower extremities but may occur in the upper extremities as well. As more people become physically active to improve health and treat disease, these injuries are increasing in frequency. Stress fracture type and incidence vary depending on the specific sport and demands imposed on the athlete. Much of the literature about stress fractures has come from military studies. Recently, however, athletes have been studied in greater detail.

Stress injury to bone appears to occur on a continuum. "Bone strain" and "stress reaction" are terms used to describe the progression of bone injury from normal bone remodeling to obvious cortical fracture (2,3). Stress injuries to bone are believed to involve interactions between mechanical, hormonal, and nutritional environmental factors, as well as genetic predisposition (3). Stress fractures are further defined as "fatigue fractures" that occur when abnormal stress is applied to normal bone (4,5). These fractures occur as a result of repeated application of a stress lower than that required to fracture the bone in a single loading situation (6). In contrast, insufficiency fractures occur in bone more susceptible to fatigue failure as a result of underlying conditions such as osteoporosis, diabetic or idiopathic neuropathy, smoking, alcoholism, anorexia nervosa, and rheumatoid arthritis (4).

Epidemiology

Stress fractures occur most frequently in running and jumping sports. Due to a lack of sound epidemiological data, it is difficult to estimate the risk of developing a stress fracture in any specific sport (7). However, many case series report that stress fractures comprise 0.7% to 15.6% of all injuries sustained by athletic populations (7). Studies reporting stress fracture incidence in athletic populations have noted incidences from 1.9% to 6.9% per year (2,3). Bennell and colleagues reported an overall stress fracture rate of 0.70 fractures per 1000 training hours in track and field athletes. In the same study, 60% of athletes that sustained a stress fracture had a previous stress fracture history (8). This study highlights the importance of identifying underlying risk factors in susceptible individuals.

Stress fractures occur in areas of the body subjected to the mechanical stress of a particular sport (Table 26-1). The most common sites appear to be the tibia, metatarsals, and fibula. Other sites include the femur, tarsal navicular, and pars interarticularis of the lumbar spine. They may also occur in the ribs, upper limbs, and pelvis. Runners and ballet dancers seem to have the highest risk of tibial stress fractures. Tarsal navicular stress fractures occur more frequently in older athletes and those participating in track and field. Pars interarticularis fractures are related to participation in sports that cause hyperextension of the lumbar spine. These include gymnastics, ballet, diving, racquet sports, and field events. Upper extremity and rib fractures occur more commonly in baseball and crew athletes.

In military recruits, a difference exists between stress fracture incidence in men and women. The risk of stress fracture in female recruits ranges from 1.2 to 10 times that of men (9). However, in athletes this difference has not been as evident. Studies show either no difference or a slightly increased risk for women (7,9). It is surmised that this lack of difference between male and female athletes is due to female athletes being more conditioned to exercise than their military counterparts. Overall, however, stress fractures appear to comprise a higher proportion of women's total injuries in sport as compared to men.

Table 26-1   Stress Fractures Associated with Sports Events

Fracture Location	Sports
Metatarsal	Running, ballet, basketball, marching
Navicular	Running, track and field, football
Tibia	Running, ballet
Femur	Distance running, ballet
Pars interarticularis	Gymnastics, diving, golf, football, volleyball

Risk Factors

Training errors are one of the most common extrinsic risk factors for stress fractures (2-5,7). Abrupt changes in the frequency, intensity, and duration of athletic activity are the most common errors athletes make. "Too much, too fast" frequently overloads a bone's ability to repair. Worn out and improperly fitting shoes also place the athlete at risk. Shock absorption is lost in worn-out shoes. In general, athletes should get new shoes every 300 to 400 miles or every 6 months.

Numerous studies have found an association between menstrual irregularities and stress fractures (9). Up to 50% of female runners have menstrual irregularity (5). Even moderate menstrual irregularities may have a negative effect on bone mineral density. Menstrual irregularities may be part of the "Female Athlete Triad." This triad includes disordered eating, amenorrhea, and osteoporosis. It is important to search for this triad in female athletes suffering from stress fractures (5). In a prospective study of risk factors in track and field athletes by Bennell, female athletes found to be at risk of stress fractures included those with lower bone density, history of menstrual disturbance, less lean mass in the lower limb, discrepancy in leg length, and lower fat diet (10). Risk of stress fracture increased significantly with a later age of menarche and smaller calf girth.

Other risk factors for the development of stress fractures include genetic predisposition, low initial fitness level, white ethnicity, lack of weight-bearing exercise, inadequate calcium and caloric intake, and low body weight (3). Some studies have indicated advancing age may be a risk factor. However, other studies have refuted this finding. Biomechanical factors may play a significant role. Varus alignment in the ankle and forefoot, pronated feet, leg length discrepancy, a high longitudinal arch of the foot, and a narrow tibia are reported as factors contributing to stress fractures of the lower extremity (11).

Differential Diagnosis

Overuse injuries such as tendinitis, tendinosis, and muscle injuries (hematoma, strain, or delayed-onset muscle soreness) can present similarly to stress fractures. In addition, compartment syndromes in the lower leg cause exertional leg pain and require careful consideration. Compartment syndromes typically cause paresthesia and paresis with activity. Formerly known as shin splints, traction periostitis presents with leg pain along the posteromedial border of the tibia. In this common entity, however, pain is relatively diffuse and often bilateral. Bone scan may help in differentiation from stress fracture. Finally, bone tumor and infection may mimic findings seen in stress reactions.

History and Physical Examination

In the history and physical exam, three questions are useful in making the diagnosis of stress fracture (5):

1. Is the pain of bony origin?
2. If so, which bone is involved?
3. At what stage in the continuum of bone stress is this injury?

The typical athlete will present with insidious onset of deep, aching pain during activity. Rest quickly relieves the pain. Pain is usually localized to the site of the suspected fracture. Occasionally, pain is referred, as may be the case with femoral neck fractures referring pain to the anterior thigh or knee. Night pain and antalgic gait may be noted. It is likely that the athlete will have significantly increased the intensity, frequency, or duration of their recent training schedule. Symptoms usually present about 4 to 5 weeks after a change in training regimen (2). Many athletes ignore the warning signs and continue to participate until their pain becomes severe enough to limit their sports participation. It is at this point that athletes usually seek medical attention (12).

A detailed menstrual history should be obtained in female athletes. Previous stress fracture history, dietary history focused on calcium and caloric intake, and screening for disordered eating should be done. It is important to ask athletes the age and fit of their shoes and whether they have changed to new training surfaces. It is helpful to determine how serious the athlete is in regard to his or her sport and to obtain the competition schedule. Medications should be reviewed including OCP use and any medications that could affect bone density.

Physical examination usually reveals tenderness over the bone involved. Erythema and swelling may also be present. Percussion at a distance from the fracture may reproduce pain at the fracture site. Range of motion is usually normal but may be painful when a fracture is near a joint. Examination should ideally include a biomechanical analysis for underlying risk factors such as leg length discrepancy, malalignment (especially overpronation in the foot), flexibility deficits, and muscle weakness (13). Provocative maneuvers may prove helpful in identifying fractures. Walking or running down the hall, walking on toes (base of second metatarsal fracture), hopping on the affected leg (femur, tibia fractures), or using a fulcrum test (femoral shaft fracture) may elicit pain in the affected bone (2,12). The fulcrum test is performed on a seated patient by gently placing pressure on the anterior thigh while using the other forearm as a fulcrum under the posterior thigh.

Imaging Studies

Plain films remain the initial test of choice in identifying stress reactions. They have poor sensitivity but high specificity (13). Abnormalities on plain radiographs may not be evident for 2-3 weeks after the onset of symptoms. In those athletes with positive findings noted on plain films, no further radiological study is necessary. In a significant percentage of patients, plain films may not become positive for up to 3 months or may never become positive. Findings on plain films include endosteal and periosteal thickening. Osteoclastic activity may result in a cortical lucency, frequently on tension areas of bone such as the anterior tibia or the superior femur.

If the plain film is negative yet there is still strong suspicion of fracture, a *three-phase radionuclide bone scan* is usually performed. The three phases of a bone scan include the blood flow (angiogram) phase, blood pool phase, and delayed images 1 to 1.5 hours after radionuclide injection. Patients should avoid applying ice within 2 to 4 hours of a bone scan due to its ability to decrease blood flow and affect tracer uptake on the scan (14). The bone scan is usually positive within 48-72 hours after the onset of symptoms. Bone scans are 100% sensitive but are not specific. They reflect osteoblastic activity and may be positive in atraumatic conditions such as osteomyelitis or bone tumor. They may be positive in sites not in question based on history and physical exam. As such, positive sites on bone scan may reflect "bone strain" and represent areas of bone undergoing normal remodeling in response to stress (13). Therefore, it is important to correlate positive findings on bone scan to the clinical exam of the affected area. Stress fractures characteristically appear as a fusiform or sharply marginated area of increased uptake in all three phases of the scan. Shin splints, now known as traction periostitis, typically show a patchy, fairly linear uptake along the medial border of the tibia. The blood flow and blood pool phases of the bone scan are normal in traction periostitis.

CT scanning may be useful in confirming a fracture or in differentiating a fracture from conditions that mimic stress fracture (13,15). It is most frequently used in certain fractures to define fracture location, morphology, and state of healing. Typical fractures where CT is frequently useful include the tarsal navicular and lumbar pars interarticularis fractures.

MRI is increasingly being recommended as the confirmatory test of choice in stress fractures (16). Like bone scans, it has a high sensitivity. Unlike bone scans, however, MRI is more specific due to its ability to evaluate other causes of the athlete's pain. Differentiating lesions such as osteomyelitis, soft tissue tumor, and infection from stress fractures is possible with MRI. T_1-weighted and bone edema sequences are necessary to assess stress injuries adequately (13). Specific details of MRI scans have been used to grade stress injuries and guide treatment and return to activity (17). The downside to MRI is its cost. Limited MRI scans using dedicated extremity scanners may make the cost more reasonable, but they are not yet widely available.

DEXA scanning is recommended for those with amenorrhea or oligomenorrhea (> 6-12 months), disordered eating and low body weight, repeated stress fractures, and in individuals reluctant to modify activity or undergo treatment (3). DEXA also may be useful in assessing the effectiveness of treatment in those with low bone density. Marx and colleagues found a high percentage of osteopenia in women sustaining a fracture in cancellous bone. Based on this evidence, they have recommended the use of DEXA in all women under 40 who have a stress fracture involving cancellous bone (18).

General Treatment Principles

Most stress fractures can be successfully managed using conservative treatment. The most important principle in the treatment of stress fractures is activity modification. Rest from offending activities allows repair processes to dominate resorption. Most fractures heal in 6-8 weeks (15). Crutches are used for those with a significant limp or severe pain. They are seldom needed beyond 7-10 days. Pain control is best achieved with NSAIDs and physical therapy modalities such as ice and electrical stimulation. Relative rest through cross-training to maintain cardiovascular fitness is extremely important to athletically active individuals. Activities that do not load the involved bone are chosen. Biking, stair-stepper, swimming, or pool running in a flotation vest are excellent choices in this regard. Maintenance of muscular fitness may be accomplished by using upper and lower body weight-lifting programs, usually without risk (15). It is important to educate the patient that activity must be pain-free. Once ambulating pain-free, patients may begin a graduated activity program. A gradual increase in training volume and intensity is allowed. If the athlete experiences pain, activity should be discontinued, followed by several days of rest with cross-training. The athlete should then restart the graduated activity program at a lower intensity and duration and proceed as pain allows. Many authors use specific protocols for return to activity (15). These protocols involve a gradual progress from pain-free activities of daily living, to aggressive walking, then running at a normal pace. Each step in the process must be pain-free.

Women with menstrual disorders should undergo evaluation and treatment to restore normal menses and attempt to preserve normal bone mineral density (BMD) (5). Reducing the amount and intensity of activity or increasing body fat may allow normal menses to return (13). If the athlete is resistant to these options, hormonal treatment in the form of oral contraceptive pills is commonly used to resume menstrual cycles. BMD assessment is frequently recommended, but one must be mindful that BMD is frequently higher in female athletes than their inactive counterparts.

Because BMD assessments compare each individual to the "average," it is not clear how to interpret this in any one person (13). BMD measurement in this case may be useful to establish a baseline and to aid the clinician in treatment of those athletes hesitant to undergo therapy.

Identifying individual factors that lead to an athlete sustaining a stress fracture is an important piece in the treatment and prevention of recurrent injury. Training errors should be sought and corrected. Coaches may need education on the need to individualize programs in athletes with stress fractures resulting from overtraining. Excessive pronation or supination of the feet and varus alignment should be evaluated and corrected when possible. Shock-absorbing footwear should be used for those with pes cavus.

High-Risk Fractures

Certain fractures are at higher risk of complications such as delayed union, nonunion, or fracture displacement. These fractures usually occur in areas of tension stress and relatively decreased vascular supply. They include the femoral neck, patella, anterior cortex of the tibia, medial malleolus, talus, tarsal navicular, fifth metatarsal proximal diaphysis, and great toe sesamoids (5).

Specific Stress Fractures

Metatarsals

Stress fractures may involve any of the metatarsals. They usually involve the shaft, most commonly of the second or third metatarsal. Like most stress fractures, they occur after an abrupt increase in activity or a change in shoewear. Swelling, point tenderness, and pain with ambulating may occur. X-rays will usually be negative in the first 3 weeks after the onset of symptoms. X-ray findings may include endosteal thickening, periosteal callus formation, or a faint lucency. A bone scan is not usually necessary but may be helpful if the diagnosis is in question. Most cases are successfully treated with a wooden shoe and by avoiding the offending activity. Crutches with partial weight-bearing may be helpful if walking is difficult. If ambulating is particularly painful, a walking boot or cast may be applied for 7-10 days followed by gradual progression to sporting activities, with pain guiding the level of activity. Setbacks occur with too rapid an advancement of activity. Follow-up x-rays should be done to document healing (19). Stress fractures of the proximal second metatarsal occur more frequently in ballet dancers and may require prolonged treatment.

Case Study 26-1

A 22-year-old white female presented to the office complaining of a 3-week history of pain in the dorsum of her right foot. She ran on a regular basis but recently began training for a half-marathon coming up in 2 months. She was running more on roads to increase her mileage. Her physical exam was remarkable for mild swelling over the dorsal midfoot. She was point tender on the midshaft of the third metatarsal. A plain x-ray was ordered (Figure 26-1). A diagnosis of metatarsal stress fracture was made. She was advised to wear a hard shoe and cross-train with pool running or stationary cycling. When she became pain-free, she was guided through gradually increasing her mileage with pain as her guide. She returned to her prior level of activity about 6 weeks after diagnosis. A review of her risk factors was performed as part of her care. She had normal periods and ate a healthy diet. Her caloric and calcium intakes were adequate. No biomechanical risk factors were noted on exam.

Special consideration is necessary in stress fractures of the fifth metatarsal. Acute Jones' fractures involve the metaphyseal-diaphyseal junction and may extend into the fourth and fifth intermetatarsal articulation (Figure 26-2). These fractures are at risk of delayed union or nonunion, even with ideal treatment. This is due to a relatively poor blood supply that may compromise healing (20). An acute Jones' fracture usually occurs due to a sudden force being applied to the proximal fifth metatarsal. Treatment is with a short leg non-weight-bearing cast for 6-8 weeks followed by short leg walking cast treatment for 4 weeks if still symptomatic. Lack of radiographic healing by 3 months is an indication for orthopedic referral unless the primary care clinician is familiar with managing these fractures. Stress

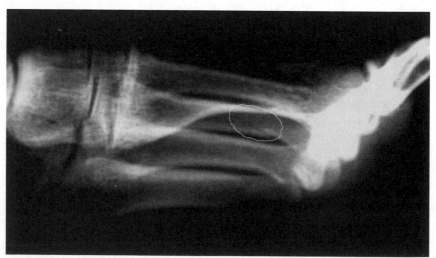

Figure 26-1   Stress fracture of third metatarsal with linear lucency midshaft. The patient's pain correlated with the site of fracture on the x-ray.

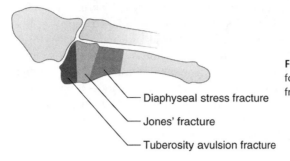

Diaphyseal stress fracture

Jones' fracture

Tuberosity avulsion fracture

Figure 26-2   Fracture zones for proximal fifth metatarsal fractures.

fractures of the proximal diaphysis of the fifth metatarsal are different from Jones' fractures in that patients with the former usually have prodromal symptoms of pain in the lateral foot. X-rays should be performed, and bone scans are indicated if the x-ray is negative. Type I fractures are those with normal x-rays and those with a clear fracture line. Type II injuries show delayed union as evidenced by widened fracture line and medullary sclerosis. Type III fractures show obliteration of the medullary canal and are representative of nonunion. Type I fractures have a high success rate for healing with conservative therapy. Non-weight-bearing immobilization for 4-6 weeks followed by 2-4 weeks of weight-bearing casting is successful in most cases. Lack of healing by 3 months and type II or II fractures require orthopedic referral. Many practitioners advocate surgical treatment of athletic individuals in all types of fracture. Therefore, referral should be considered in all cases of this injury (19).

Navicular Stress Fractures

Tarsal navicular stress fractures most frequently occur in track and field athletes. Presentation is that of a vague ache in the dorsum of the midfoot. Pain may radiate to the medial arch. Athletes may ignore the pain or try short periods of rest to relieve it. Unfortunately, only 26% of navicular stress fractures will heal correctly with activity modification alone. Frequently, patients present after several months of symptoms (2,21). On examination, tenderness is noted at the dorsal navicular. Inverting or everting the forefoot allows identification of the "N" spot (the proximal dorsal aspect of the navicular), which is tender in 81% of these fractures (21). Pain may be reproduced with hopping and standing on toes. Plain radiographs are frequently negative, and bone scan is the next step in the evaluation. If the bone scan is positive, CT scanning of the talonavicular joint is indicated to guide classification of the fracture and plan treatment.

Type I fractures involve a dorsal cortical break. Type II lesions involve propagation of the fracture into the body of the navicular. Type II fractures involve extension of the fracture into another cortex. Nondisplaced fractures are treated with a well-fitted short leg non-weight-bearing cast for 6 weeks. If the patient is still tender after 6 weeks, additional non-weight-bearing casting is recommended until he or she is pain-free. Successful treatment occurs in 86% of cases, with an average return to normal activity of 5-6 months (21). A graduated return to athletic activity is then allowed. Patients with displaced fractures and those exhibiting delayed or nonunion should be referred to an orthopedic surgeon. Consideration for referral should be given to all highly active individuals desiring the earliest possible return to sport.

Tibial Stress Fractures

The tibia is the most common location of lower extremity stress fracture. Tibial stress fractures usually occur in running sports such as distance running, soccer, ballet, and basketball. Runners tend to have shaft fractures at the junction of the middle and distal thirds of the tibia. Jumping sports are associated with proximal tibial stress fractures, whereas midshaft fractures occur most frequently in ballet dancers. Insidious onset of pain relieved by rest is characteristic of these injuries. Pain initially occurs at the end of activity but without appropriate rest occurs progressively earlier. Eventually, the athlete will be unable to complete a workout.

Examination reveals point tenderness and occasionally swelling. Percussion at a site distant from the fracture may cause pain at the involved site. Lower extremity range of motion and neurovascular exam are usually normal. The hop test (patient jumping on injured extremity) may elicit pain in patients with stress fracture. Initial x-rays will frequently be negative and should be followed by three-phase bone scan with or without MRI. A special case involving plain films is that of an anterior cortical lucency in the midshaft. This is known as the "dreaded black line," and these fractures are at high risk of delayed union, nonunion, and complete fracture as they are in an area of high tension stress (2,4,5,12,13,15). Bone scan may be negative in these fractures. This finding should prompt referral to a provider skilled in treating these injuries.

Case Study 26-2

A 34-year-old female runner presented to the office complaining of distal leg pain and swelling for the past 4 weeks. Her pain was severe, and she had stopped all athletic activity. She limped into the office. Her exam was remarkable for point tenderness in the distal third of the tibia. There was mild swelling of the distal leg and ankle, but knee and ankle exams were normal. Hop test was positive, and percussion away from the site of the fracture caused pain at the site of point tenderness. X-rays were normal. An MRI revealed a distal tibial fracture. Treatment was instituted with relative rest and crutches with partial weight-bearing. A pneumatic leg brace was prescribed. Pain-free ambulating occurred in 1 week, and return to normal activities occurred in 3 weeks. Gradual return to running was allowed, and she was fully active in 6 weeks. Follow-up x-rays showed a fracture line and excellent healing of the fracture.

Tibial stress fractures need differentiation from tibial periostitis (shin splints) and exertional compartment syndromes. Rest from athletic activity, pain control with ice, NSAIDs and therapeutic modalities, and a graduated return to activity with pain as a guide is appropriate treatment. Algorithms for graduated return to play have been published (13,22). Consideration should also be given to bracing. Swenson and colleagues reported on the use of a pneumatic ankle brace (22). In this prospective, randomized study, the bracing group returned to sport in 21 ± 2 days, whereas the usual treatment group returned in 77 ± 7 days. The authors propose that the brace shifts load-bearing from the tibia to the soft tissues of the leg.

Femoral Stress Fractures

Femoral neck stress fractures are four times more frequent in female versus male runners (5). There are two types to consider. Compression fractures occur on the inferior aspect of the femoral neck, whereas tension-type fractures occur on the superior aspect of the femoral neck. Tension side fractures are at risk for displacement (23). Clinical presentation is that of a deep, achy pain in the groin of the affected athlete. Pain may radiate to the anterior thigh or knee. Pain to palpation may be present in the inguinal region, and pain may be noted at end range of motion at the hip. Plain films may show a cortical defect or sclerosis. If plain films are negative, three-phase bone scan or MRI should be ordered. Treatment depends on location of the fracture. Tension-type fractures are potentially unstable and require referral for operative stabilization. Compression side stress fractures may be treated with rest and protected weight-bearing while following plain x-rays to evaluate for displacement. Once pain-free, a graduated return to activity is allowed. Return to sport may take 7.5 to 11.5 weeks (2).

Femoral shaft stress fractures are much less common than those of the femoral neck. They generally present with pain in the groin or thigh. The junction of the proximal and middle thirds is particularly susceptible to injury. A fulcrum test may be helpful in identifying these fractures. In a seated patient, applying pressure to the dorsal knee while using the other arm as a fulcrum beneath the posterior thigh elicits pain as the fulcrum arm is moved proximal to the fracture site (2,24). These fractures are successfully treated with relative rest with protected weight-bearing and a gradual return to activity. Return to sport usually occurs in 8-16 weeks (24).

Pars Interarticularis Stress Injuries

Spondylolysis is a defect in the pars interarticularis (Figure 26-3). It is usually unilateral but may be bilateral. Bilateral stress fractures are at risk of

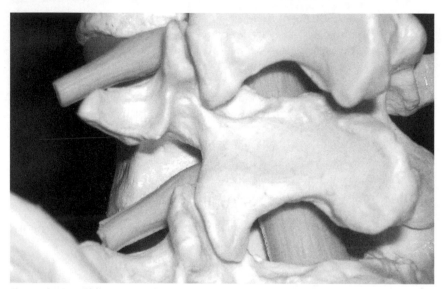

Figure 26-3   Oblique view of the lower lumbar spine showing the pars interarticularis as the neck of the "Scottie dog."

vertebral slip, or spondylolisthesis. This, however, is uncommon after the early teen years. Spondylolytic fractures are at risk of nonunion, but overall prognosis is good, even with continued sporting activity (19). Spondylolysis most frequently occurs in adolescent athletes. Repetitive hyperextension and rotation of the lumbar spine are felt to be underlying causes. Characteristic sports loading the spine in this fashion include gymnastics, golf, tennis, diving, volleyball, and football (linemen).

Athletes usually present with low back pain that may radiate into the buttocks and posterior thigh(s). Recent increases in activity level are often noted. Physical exam is remarkable for normal range of motion with painful extension. Tight hamstrings are frequently noted. The one-leg hyperextension test should be performed in all adolescent athletes who report low back pain. Having the athlete stand on the leg of the painful side and hyperextend the lumbar spine augments pain in the affected athlete. Neurovascular exam is typically normal.

In athletes with a positive one-leg hyperextension test, oblique lumbar plain films and a bone single photon emission computed tomography (SPECT) scan are used to properly evaluate for fracture of the pars interarticularis. Several situations evolve from this testing. Negative plain films and a negative bone scan suggest non-bony causes of the athlete's pain and should prompt evaluation for other causes. A positive plain film and negative bone SPECT scan suggest either a congenital defect in the pars or an old fracture of the pars interarticularis healed by fibrous union.

Athletes with lumbar pars injuries benefit from core strengthening of the lumbar extensors and abdominal musculature and stretching of the hamstrings. Activity modification is imperative to allow healing to occur. Athletes should ideally be pain-free before starting a rehabilitation program. There is little evidence to suggest that a fracture evident on plain film with a negative bone scan will heal with bracing. Therefore, physical therapy and activity modification is the mainstay of treatment. (Rehabilitative strategies are discussed in Chapter 27.) Individuals with a stress reaction are treated with activity modification and physical therapy. Once pain-free, activity may begin and be advanced with pain as a guide. Stress fracture treatment includes 0-degree antilordotic bracing for 3 6 months. The brace is worn 23 hours per day during this time period. After the bracing period, rehabilitation and gradual return to activity is allowed. Return to sports usually takes 3-6 months (19). Once again, if the primary care physician is unfamiliar or uncomfortable with the care of this injury, consultation with an orthopedic spine surgeon should be considered.

REFERENCES

1. **Breihaupt MD.** Zur pathologie des mensch lichen fussess. Medizin Zeitung. 1855; 24:169-77.
2. **Monteleone GP.** Stress fractures in the athlete. Orthop Clin North Am. 1995;26(3): 423-32.
3. **Nattiv A, Armsey TD.** Stress injury to bone in the female athlete. Clin Sports Med.1997;16(2):197-224.
4. **Eisele SA, Sammarco FJ.** Fatigue fractures of the foot and ankle in the athlete. J Bone Joint Surg. 1993;75-A:290-8.
5. **McBryde AM, Barfield WR.** The Female Athlete. Philadelphia: WB Saunders; 2002:299-316.
6. **Martin AD, McCulloch RG.** Bone dynamics: stress, strain and fracture. J Sports Sci. 1987;5:155-63.
7. **Bennell KL, Bruckner PD.** Epidemiology and site specificity for stress fractures. Clin Sports Med. 1997;16(2):179-96.
8. **Bennell KL, Malcolm SA, Thomas SA, et al.** The incidence and distribution of stress fractures in competitive track and field athletes. Am J Sports Med. 1996; 24:211 7.
9. **Brukner PD, Bennell KL.** Stress to fractures in female athletes: diagnosis, management and rehabilitation. Sports Med. 1997;24(6):419-29.
10. **Bennell KL, Malcolm SA, Thomas SA, et al.** Risk factors for stress fractures in track and field athletes: a twelve-month prospective study. Am J Sports Med. 1996:24:810-8.
11. **Korpelainen R, Orava S, Karpakka J, et al.** Risk factors for recurrent stress fractures in athletes. Am J Sports Med. 2001;29(3):304-10.
12. **Maitra RS, Johnson DL.** Stress fractures: clinical history and physical examination. Clin Sports Med. 1997;16(2):259-74.

13. **Brukner PD.** Exercise-related lower leg pain: bone. Med Sci Sports Exer. 2000; 32(3):S15-S26.

14. **Deutsch AL, Coel MN, Mink JH.** Imaging of stress injuries to bone: radiography, scintigraphy and MR imaging. Clin Sports Med. 1997;16(2):275-90.

15. **Knapp TP, Garrett WE.** Stress fractures: general concepts. Clin Sports Med. 1997; 16(2):339-56.

16. **Ishibashi Y, Okamura Y, Otsuka H, et al.** Comparison of scintigraphy and magnetic resonance imaging for stress injuries of bone. Clin J Sport Med. 2002;12:79-84.

17. **Arendt EA, Griffiths HJ.** The use of MR imaging in the assessment and clinical management of stress reactions of bone in high-performance athletes. Clin Sports Med. 1997;16(2):291-306.

18. **Marx RG, Saint-Phard D, Callahan LR, et al.** Stress fracture sites related to underlying bone health in athletic females. Clin J Sport Med. 2001;11:73-6.

19. **Eiff MP, Hatch RL, Calmbach WL, et al.** Fracture Management for Primary Care, 2nd ed. Philadelphia: WB Saunders; 2002:239-44.

20. **Nunley JA.** Fractures of the base of the fifth metatarsal: the Jones fracture. Orthop Clin North Am. 2001;32(1):171-80.

21. **Coris EE, Lombardo JA.** Tarsal navicular stress fractures. Am Fam Physician. 2003;67:85-90.

22. **Swenson JE, DeHaven KE, Sebastianelli WJ, et al.**The effect of a pneumatic leg brace on return to play in athletes with tibial stress fractures. Am J Sports Med. 1997;25(3):322-8.

23. **Egol KA, Koval KJ, Kummer F, Frankel VH.** Stress fractures of the femoral neck. Clin Ortho Rel Res. 1998;348:72-8.

24. **Boden BP, Speer KP.** Femoral stress fractures. Clin Sports Med. 1997;16(2):307-17.

27

■ ■ ■

Principles of Rehabilitation in Orthopedic and Sports Physical Therapy

Michael Lucido, PT, OCS, COMT

hysical therapy has been an essential part of the health care delivery system since the First World War and is a profession with an established theoretical and scientific basis that is used to treat more than 750,000 people a day in the United States (1). The physical therapy profession, while taking the lead in the rehabilitation of individuals with varying diagnoses and physical impairments, has followed the medical model in its recognition of specialties and subspecialties. The central theme that brings this diversified profession into focus and describes the overall goal of the physical therapist intervention is to "normalize movement."

The information in this chapter is designed to introduce the primary care physician to the principles and theoretical bases of orthopedic physical therapy.

Physical Therapist Evaluation

The responsibility of the primary care physician is to rule out serious pathology and provide a differential medical diagnosis before referring the patient to a physical therapist. The purpose of the physical therapist evaluation is to clarify the medical diagnosis in regard to severity, irritability, and nature of the diagnosis so that a reasonable expectation can be made that a person can improve with an appropriate course of physical therapy. The physical therapist's evaluation consists of a history, observation, active/passive and resistive testing, neurology, special testing, and an assessment of joint function. The physical therapist is well trained in the movement sciences, so the examination is typically directed to the

443

recognition of movement dysfunction in certain regions of the body or a specific joint and its related structures. For example, the primary care physician may refer a person to a physical therapist with the diagnosis of "impingement syndrome" of the shoulder. In an attempt to clarify the diagnosis, the physical therapy examination should be able to reproduce the "impingements signs" during the examination with an additional finding of a tight posterior glenohumeral joint capsule. This finding, though not part of the medical diagnosis, is incorporated in the physical therapy treatment program because of its cause-and-effect relationship to the medical diagnosis. Another important part of the physical therapy examination is to assess how the individual's condition has changed since seen by the primary care physician. Many times, the physical therapist is monitoring a neurological condition that changes in the course of treatment over several days or weeks, and the physical therapist must ethically report a progressive medical condition back to the referring physician (2).

Physical Therapy Treatment Plan

The physical therapy treatment plan is based on the information provided by the referring physician along subjective and objective findings in the physical therapist's evaluation and assessment. This information is presented to the patient, and the patient's goals and understanding of treatment are discussed, in order to obtain patient consent for treatment. The treatment plan is based on the stage of healing (inflammatory, fibroblastic, and maturation) of the specific affected tissue or region of the body. Many times, the tissue healing curve is related to its mechanical properties, vascularity, and metabolism. For example, a tear of the medial collateral ligament of the knee repairs itself without surgical intervention and moves through all three stages quickly (4-6 weeks), whereas the same injury to the Achilles' tendon can take 6 months to a year postsurgery to restore its full mechanical properties.

Soft-tissue healing is typically recognized as occurring in three phases: inflammatory, fibroblastic, and maturation.

Inflammatory Phase

Definition
Inflammation, the body's response to injurious agents, is almost always the same regardless of the location of the injury or nature of the injury (3). The inflammatory phase represents cellular changes in the injured tissue that initiates the healing process by removing damaged cells and debris. The therapeutic goal in this phase is to control the pain and assist in the cellular changes by applying various therapeutic modalities.

Therapeutic Modalities

Cryotherapy and various types of electrotherapeutic modalities such as direct current assist in controlling the amount of pain and edema that is present. The therapeutic application of ice has been used for years in the acute phase of injury management. Therapeutic cold has been seen in clinical research to decrease swelling and modulate pain due to the slowing of axon conduction velocity (4). The therapeutic use of direct current—also known as galvanic stimulation or high voltage stimulation—has the electrical properties of small-pulse duration with relatively small amplitude, which makes the treatment more comfortable for the patient. Direct current also has unique properties that allow it to carry a positive or negative charge, which can be used therapeutically to deliver selected ions to a small area of tissue for treatment of inflammation, calcium deposits, and pain. Griffin and Karselis state that other forms of electrotherapeutic devices (for example, transcutaneous electrical nerve stimulators, or TENS) fall into the category of medium- or low-frequency currents, which work theoretically on the "gate control" mechanism of neuromodulation theorized by Melzak and Wall (4). This theory states that the electrical stimulation is picked up in the periphery by large afferent sensory receptors/nerves and travels to the spinal cord faster than the nociceptive impulses, thus blocking pain signals. The benefit to the patient is muscle relaxation and decreased pain with an increase in function.

In addition to therapeutic modalities, it is imperative to educate the patient about minimizing mechanical forces that could prolong the inflammatory process, thus delaying healing. Placing the involved joint or tissue at rest with appropriate splinting, taping, and other supports is an integral part of the physical therapy treatment in the inflammatory phase. Toward the very end of the inflammatory phase, specialized cells known has fibroblasts are present at the wound site, thus marking the transition to the next phase of healing—the fibroblastic phase.

Fibroblastic Phase

Definition

The fibroblastic phase is crucial to the repair and the functional rehabilitation of an individual or athlete who suffers an injury. The fibroblastic phase starts around the fifth day postinjury and can last up to 10 weeks (5). This phase represents the laying down of collagen fibrils, which quickly form into collagen aggregates and begin to increase the ability of the new collagen to restore its mechanical properties. This "neocollagen" formation takes place in the connective tissue fibroblasts, which have been reported to be activated by different forms of energy including biomechanical stresses (6).

Therapeutic Modalities

Therapeutic ultrasound (acoustic energy) is used in the fibroblastic phase by the physical therapist because of its unique quality of deep penetration, unlike forms of electromagnetic energy (electrotherapy) and its thermal and nonthermal physiological effects (4). Most of the thermal effects of ultrasound are secondary to its capacity to raise the tissue temperature, resulting in hyperemia to the area being treated. The nonthermal effects of ultrasound are primarily mechanical in that exposure to ultrasonic energy has been seen to aid in protein synthesis in the fibroblast, thus affecting collagen proliferation and organization (7). Therapeutic ultrasound has widespread clinical usage from osteoarthritis to softening hypertrophic scarring but is traditionally used in the orthopedic physical therapy setting for strains and sprains of skeletal muscle and connective tissue.

Manual Physical Therapy. Manual therapy, one of the oldest forms of therapeutic intervention for musculoskeletal pain, dates back to Hippocrates in 400 BC. Manual therapy techniques are commonly used in the fibroblastic phase by physical therapists and are defined as a broad group of skilled hand movements used to mobilize or manipulate soft tissues and joints for the purpose of modulating pain, increasing range of motion, and reducing swelling (1). The physiological effects of manual therapy have been reported to vary from pain modulation to mechanical effects on connective tissue (8). For example, a patient that is referred to a physical therapist with a diagnosis of "frozen shoulder" will undergo different grades of manual therapy depending on the stage of healing and clinical signs and symptoms the patient is presenting. In the early phase of treatment, when the frozen shoulder is very painful, the physical therapist will use grade I techniques that are designed to stimulate mechanoreceptors and thus modulate pain. For a patient who has more stiffness than pain, the technique will change to grade III, designed to increase motion.

Therapeutic Exercise. For the sake of this chapter, principles of therapeutic exercise fall into two categories: functional exercise (active, passive, and resistive) and proprioceptive neuromuscular facilitation techniques. The benefits of movement in the form of therapeutic exercise to the injured tissue and the musculoskeletal system are numerous. Salter's classic work in the 1970s on the biological effects of movement to various tissues of the musculoskeletal system caused a shift in the way soft tissue injuries were managed (9). The clinical application of Salter's work emphasized "early and frequent" motion during the crucial fibroblastic phase, which allowed the physical therapist to initiate therapeutic exercise earlier than was thought to be appropriate. Functional exercise in the form of active, passive, and resistive exercise are necessary to assist in the formation of collagen and protein synthesis of contractile structures (10). Active and active-assistive exercise are forms of therapeutic exercise that involve the patient, to some degree, taking the extremity through its physiological range of motion. Passive exercise is when little or no patient involvement takes place and another force is moving the extremity into its physiological range. Resistive exercise in physical therapy can range from very small resistance given by the physical therapist to heavier weights in sports-specific type training. Specific sets of repetitions and weight are given to the patient once the physical therapist decides what functional goal is trying to be achieved (joint nutrition, strength, pain inhibition). For example, the postural muscles of the spine are considered tonic in nature, and when exercising this muscle, group exercises are typically done in 3 sets of 30-40 repetitions several times a day. The theory is to exercise the muscle group according to its muscle fiber type and what that muscle is asked to do during a typical day or athletic endeavor.

Another form of resistance exercise used by the physical therapist is proprioceptive neuromuscular facilitation (PNF). PNF is an approach to therapeutic exercise that was developed in the late 1940s by Herman Kabat, later joined by Margaret Knott, who assisted in the refinement and instruction to physical therapists worldwide. The underlying theory of PNF is to enhance the movement patterns of the patient with appropriate manual contacts and verbal instructions (11). For example a physical therapist may use PNF of the shoulder girdle to ensure that the patient is moving in the correct plane of shoulder elevation with the proper recruitment of muscle before placing the patient on resistive exercise equipment.

Maturation Phase

This phase represents no new collagen development but its reorganization and maturation in order to improve the tensile properties of the repair, which can last up to 12 months. It is in this phase that the physical therapist begins sport-specific training and more functional exercise programs in preparation of the athlete's return to his or her event. Independent exercises or a "home program" is imperative so that what has been gained in the form of restoring normal movement can be maintained and progressed with varied forms of resistance in order to continue motor recruitment so as to avoid reinjury.

Case Study 27-1

A 29-year-old female was referred to an outpatient physical therapy facility with the medical diagnosis of lumbar herniated nucleus pulposus by her primary care physician. The patient was a recreational water skier but had not been able to participate in this activity recently. Approximately 3 weeks earlier, she was doing gymnastics when she felt something in her low back "pop." Within hours, she had an onset of left-sided low back pain. In the next several days, the pain changed from dull to more sharp and radiated into her buttocks. Her physician took x-rays, gave her a prescription, and recommended physical therapy. Her present complaint was left-sided low back pain with radiation into left posterior thigh and shooting electrical-like sensations to the left lateral aspect of her lower leg with tingling on the top of her left foot. Sitting and driving made the pain worse, as did riding her road bicycle. Walking or lying down on either side eased symptoms. Day pattern indicated morning pain and stiffness on rising and a return of this later in the day. She denied saddle paresthesia and bowel or bladder difficulties. She rated her pain as an 8/10.

Goals of Treatment
- Reduce neurological signs/decrease pain
- Improve normal movement patterns by increasing lumbar flexion
- Educate patient on home treatments and disk pathology
- Restore normal activity level
- Return to water skiing (patient's goal)

Treatment One (Inflammatory Phase)

Initial treatment was designed to decrease the inflammation of the spinal nerve root and the periarticlar structures that are involved and to decrease the muscle hypertonicity secondary to the underlying chemo-mechanical dysfunction. The patient was placed on ice and direct current with the active electrodes being negative for 20 minutes followed by soft-tissue mobilization of the left erector spinae and deep spinal myofascial system for 7 minutes. The patient was then placed on her left side for a grade I segmental traction technique to modulate pain through the type one mechanoreceptors found in the zygapophyseal joints of the lumbar spine. The patient was also taught a home exercise with the goal of recruiting the deep segmental muscles in her spine (multifidus, transverse abdominus) to prevent further atrophy and inhibition (12). She was to repeat this exercise 3 times a day for 25-30 repetitions each (holding for 5 seconds).

Treatment Two (Inflammatory Phase)

The patient explained that she now had fewer shooting episodes into her left lower leg than before but still had the tingling on the top of her foot. She rated her low back/left posterior leg pain as a 6/10. She continued to state that sitting/driving were the most painful activities, though the pain was still relieved by walking. Treatment in this session consisted of ice and direct current to the lumbar spine followed by soft-tissue techniques. A soft-tissue manual therapy technique designed to modulate pain was used. The patient was told to continue the home program as instructed on the first day.

Treatment Three (Fibroblastic Phase)

The patient stated that she slept extremely well last night. The tingling on top of her foot was less constant, but her low back and posterior thigh were about the same. It was decided that at this session lumbar traction would be used in the prone position for 20 minutes. The positioning (prone) was due to the particular pattern that was seen in the exam and her history of extension being more comfortable than flexion.

Treatment Four (Fibroblastic Phase)

The patient returned stating that her leg now felt the best it had since she developed this problem. Re-evaluation showed an increase in lumbar range of motion (ROM) in flexion and left-side bending with no improvement of extension. Traction was applied again followed by instruction in extension exercises to be done every 3 hours 15 to 20 times.

Treatment Five (Fibroblastic Phase)

The patient returned stating that she had not felt tingling sensations in her foot or leg for 3 days and rating her left-sided low back pain as a 3/10. Upon reassessment of her ROM, she had gained lumbar extension to about normal. Intermittent traction was implemented again for 20 minutes at 50 pounds in the prone position. She was then progressed to supine stabilization exercises with movement of the lower extremities in the form of a modified bicycle. The patient was also given a videotape on proper lifting and basic spine self-care techniques.

Summary

Physical therapists possess a unique scientific and theoretical basis that allows them to assess and treat a wide range of physical impairments. The clinical decision-making by the physical therapist is a constellation of the medical information from the referring physician and information obtained from an examination that looks for movement dysfunctions. The stage of healing of the individual (inflammatory, fibroblastic, maturation) dictates what type of treatment is implemented. The overall goal of treatment is to normalize movement by decreasing pain, improving function, and returning the individual to his or her preinjury level of activity.

REFERENCES

1. Guide to Physical Therapy Practice, 2nd ed. rev. Alexandria, VA: American Physical Therapy Association; 2003:13.

2. **Meadows JT.** Orthopedic Differential Diagnosis in Physical Therapy; A Case Study Approach. New York: McGraw-Hill; 1999.

3. **Gould LA.** Orthopaedic and Sports Physical Therapy, 2nd ed. St. Louis: CV Mosby; 1990:88.

4. **Griffin JE, Karselis TC.** Physical Agents for Physical Therapists, 2nd ed. Springfield, IL: Charles C Thomas; 1982:242-3.

5. **Lee D.** The Pelvic Girdle, 2nd ed. New York: Churchill-Livingstone; 1999:75.

6. **Cantu RI, Grodin AJ.** Myofascial Manipulation; Theory and Clinical Application. Gaithersburg, MD: Aspen; 1992:34

7. **Dyson M, Suckling J.** Stimulation of tissue repair by ultrasound: a survey of mechanisms involved. Physiotherapy. 1978;64:105-8.

8. **Threlkeld JA.** The effects of manual therapy on connective tissue. Phys Ther. 1992;72(12):893-902.

9. **Salter RB.** Continuous Passive Motion; A Biological Concept for the Healing and Regeneration of Articular Cartilage, Ligaments, and Tendons. Philadelphia: Williams & Wilkins; 1993.

10. **Buckwalter JA, Woo SL.** Injury and Repair of the Musculoskeletal Soft Tissues. American Academy of Orthopaedic Surgeons; 1988.

11. Course notes from PNF 1: The Functional Approach to Proprioceptive Neuromuscular Facilitation. Houston, 21-24 August 2003.

12. **Richardson C, Jull G, Hodges P, Hides J.** Therapeutic Exercise for Spinal Segmental Stabilization in Low Back Pain. New York: Churchill-Livingstone; 1999.

28

■ ■ ■

Taping, Wrapping, and Bracing

T. Ross Bailey, MEd, ATC, LAT

Athletic trainers and coaches have all heard injured athletes plea, "Tape it, wrap it up, and let me get back in there!" Athletic trainers and other allied health professionals use adhesive tape and other materials to help support joints and muscles that are stressed, strained, and in need of a little supportive help. Although many think that this is a "new" and modern practice associated with athletics and sports medicine, its historical origins are ancient.

One of the first books on taping was published by Johnson and Johnson in 1944. They state, "Available evidence suggests that the use of adhesive masses and plasters can be traced from the beginnings of recorded medical history, as early, possibly, as *circa* 3000 B.C. in Egypt. From later antiquity there is ample evidence of the use of adhesive, or at least sticky, mixtures as healing preparations, applied directly to local lesions, and the Greeks are known to have used for this purpose a paste consisting of olive oil, lead oxide, and water" (1). Today, the practitioner has many choices in materials, adhesives, and techniques for applying both prophylactic and treatment taping or wrapping.

Types of Tape

The most prevalent tape is a cotton, zinc oxide adhesive mass that is known throughout most of the world as "white tape," zinc oxide tape, or "athletic tape." Elastic tapes made from various materials and a new line of tapes that are cohesive are now on the market. Cohesive tapes stick to themselves and not to the patient. Because these tapes do not stick to the hair, they are very helpful when dealing with both human and animal patients where body hair is present. "Pre-wrap" was introduced to the athletic training world in various forms starting in the late 1960s. These products along with tape adherents have lessened the skin irritation often associated with earlier tape jobs.

Taping versus Bracing

Taping, strapping, and/or wrapping can be done both prophylactically as well as after an injury. Strapping, taping, or bracing is done when the practitioner needs to support an injured joint or when the biomechanical forces of the activity are high enough that some prophylactic support is desired. Taping is also a very good way to determine if bracing might be helpful to the patient. Taping, when applied correctly and with skill, becomes a "custom" brace of sorts that can be used when a patient does not fit into the normal sizing of an off-the-shelf brace. Taping can also be used on a temporary basis so that a brace does not need to be purchased immediately. Tape can also be a short-term addition to care for a patient that might not need long-term bracing.

There has been much debate recently about the use of taping verses bracing. Taping will loosen up over the course of a practice or contest, and it is affected by water and/or sweat. The brace can be removed, laced back up, and reapplied if necessary, but it is only effective if it fits and is worn correctly. Wrapping continues to be a standard first aid practice to help with compression of an area to help decrease localized edema and in many cases to hold a bandage or other treatment item in place.

Three different kinds of braces are found in the sports medicine marketplace. *Prophylactic braces* are commonly used for ankle bracing as well as in collision sports for medial knee protection. Ankle braces have improved dramatically in recent years in both biomechanical design as well as materials. Knee braces are thought to provide lateral impact protection for individuals participating in collision sports. The protection result is still open for more research. Many football linemen will wear braces to help provide some level of lateral knee impact protection. Down lineman is the most injured position in collegiate Division 1 football, and knee injuries occur at a higher percentage than ankle injuries (2).

The primary questions surround the amount of protection and the mechanism of protection. Does the brace lessen the kinetic forces placed on the joint? Does the brace provide the millisecond of time required for athletes to tighten their muscles and resist the force themselves? Unfortunately, because much of the research has been conducted on cadavers, the testing methods do not adequately reproduce real-life situations!

Rehabilitation braces are used to limit excessive range of motion, to limit range of motion to a particular range, or to protect a joint from side-to-side movements during the healing process. One of the best examples of a rehab-type brace with everyday practical application is a short leg walking boot. These boots many times will allow a patient to be able to weight-bear fully, yet provide the necessary protection for the ankle or foot injury to heal adequately. Post-op joint braces are used to provide a safe but protected range of motion after injury with or without surgical intervention. Although taping is a common application in protecting the ankle joint after lateral ankle sprains, it is also used to help limit range of motion with finger and thumb injuries as well as to support a sprained longitudinal arch in the foot.

Functional braces are primarily seen in knee applications for use with ACL protection after surgical reconstruction. One of the most common types of functional bracing is a counter-force strap for lateral epicondylitis (tennis elbow).

Although many people throughout the years have worn elastic or neoprene sleeves over joints, these types of braces do little to provide structural support. However, they may provide benefit in helping to increase joint proprioception as well as in providing a mechanism to help keep a joint warmer. They may not provide the structural support of a functional brace, but if they provide an increased level of comfort and warmth to a joint, they possibly serve a function.

This chapter is by no means a complete listing or description of all styles and techniques. Each patient needs, and each injury will require, the practitioner to be creative and use sound principles as well as anatomical knowledge to "construct" the next taping or strapping job.

Before taping, it is necessary to establish 1) what you want to accomplish by applying the tape or wrap, and 2) what anatomical structures are going to be supported and/or protected. Taping is more than picking up a book and following the diagram; like many items related to sports, a good, solid plan is required before starting. If the practitioner does not have a solid plan, then it is time to rethink the taping application. Likewise, not every joint, injury, or ailment is going to respond to taping. Taping, wrapping, or even bracing will not make up for excessive joint laxity due to ligament injury. The area to be supported should be evaluated and assessed by the properly trained medical or allied health practitioner if the goal is to support a previously injured structure. Functional testing should be performed before return to physical activity regardless of taping, wrapping, or bracing.

Taping Precautions

It is important that the tape, wrap, or brace should not aggravate the anatomical structure to be supported. The application of the tape should not impede normal circulation to the anatomical structures distal to the area taped nor should the tape job contain wrinkles, rolls, or bind the skin. The application of the tape job should follow the contours of the limb (if applicable). Under no circumstances should any tape not originally designed for humans be used. Duct tape has a million uses, but it is not to be applied directly to the skin of the athlete!

Taping Basics

The skin of the patient should be prepared before the application of the tape; various products help the practitioner with this task. Pre-wrap, as previously discussed, has replaced roller gauze to protect the skin before the application of the tape. Skin irritation and friction blistering may occur as the result of some of the tape adhesives and the direct application of tape to the skin if the area is not first protected by a "pre-wrap" product. Tincture of benzoin was one of the first tape adherents that was used to provide skin protection and to aid in the adherence of the tape application. Today, there are several different products and manufacturers for pre-wrap and taping adherents.

Tape removal is as important as proper tape application. Tape should be removed with the correct bandage scissors or tape cutters. Do not attempt to remove tape from a limb with standard sharp-tipped scissors or a knife. Once cut, the tape should be slowly removed from the skin while holding down any loose skin. Do not jerk or rip the tape off the skin. This "technique" might result in tissue damage from the attempted rapid removal of the tape pulling off some of the epithelial tissue.

Ankle Taping

The pre-wrap should be applied with slight tension in a circular pattern to completely cover the area to be taped. The tension is not intended for any support but rather keeps the product taut and in place (Figure 28-1).

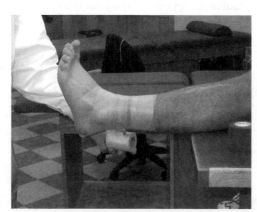

Figure 28-1   Pre-wrap application.

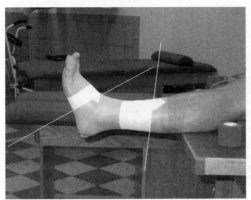

Figure 28-2   Anchor application.

The anchors of the white tape are applied so that they will fit the contour of the leg. They should be taut in tension but not too tight: the limb will expand when under a load as in weight bearing. If the practitioner desires more strength and wants to decrease the chance of slippage, the anchors should be applied directly to the skin. The present author suggests that a full width of tape be applied over a shaved area. If too little skin is used for the tape application, chaffing or blistering can occur (Figure 28-2).

The metatarsal anchor should be applied with minimal tightness. The reference point is the base of the fifth metatarsal. The foot will spread out approximately two widths when weight-bearing, thus the need to apply with minimal tension. Some patients will report aching, pain, or a loss of distal circulation if the tape is applied too tightly. Another solution to this problem is to apply an anchor out of 3-inch elastic tape.

The tape should always overlap the previous strap by approximately one-half the tape width. Always work in a proximal to distal pattern. Place the first strip at the highest point and work distally down the limb (Figure 28-3).

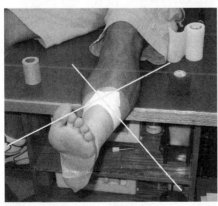

Figure 28-3   Tape overlapping.

The ankle stirrups typically start on the medial side of the ankle and are pulled with tension to the lateral side. The majority of ankle sprains are of the inversion nature, thus the need for tension to the lateral side of the ankle. The first stirrup should begin on the backside of the ankle near the rear of the medial malleolus and calcaneus. The next strip is applied toward the front of the ankle while overlapping approximately half the previous strip. Care must be taken to keep all of the stirrups out of the arch area and over the calcaneus in order to stay over a bony structure and out of the soft tissue of the arch (Figure 28-4).

Figure 28-5 shows the progression of the stirrups and their relationship over the lateral malleolus and the lateral ligament complex. Notice how the tape fans out at the top of the ankle and tapers near the calcaneus. This

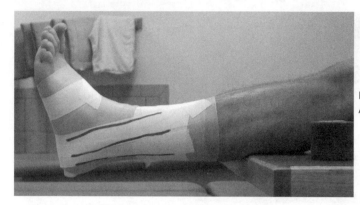

Figure 28-4
Ankle stirrups.

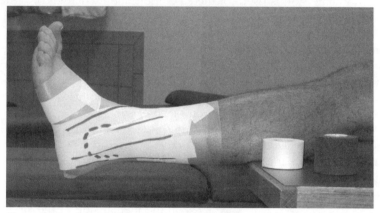

Figure 28-5   Stirrups fanned out over malleolus.

fanning of the tape allows for good coverage and support over the lateral ligamentous complex.

Figure 28-6 shows the stirrups in place and the cover strips or anchors applied to hold down the supporting stirrups. These strips are applied with moderate tension. Once again, they overlap the previous piece of tape and are angled to fit the contour of the leg. The basket-weave tape job, also known as the Gibney, has been used by athletic training professionals since the mid-1920s. Many practitioners have modified the standard basket weave. They no longer alternate stirrups and anchor strips; rather, they apply all of the stirrups and then apply the anchors. This method is not only quicker but much more consistent in tension.

Figure 28-7 shows a completed tape job with the cover strips and anchors in place. The angles are highlighted, and the overlapping of the tape is visible.

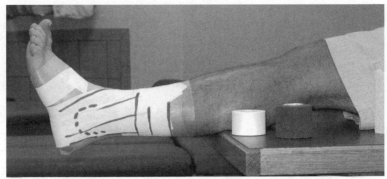

Figure 28-6   Anchors over stirrups.

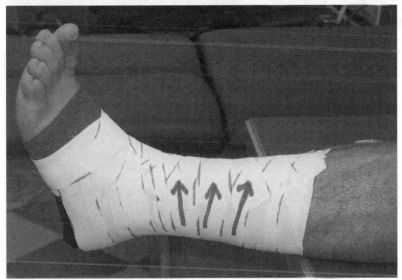

Figure 28-7   Anchors and cover strips.

The heel locks are intended to lock the talus in place within the ankle mortise (Figure 28-8). The stirrups and anchors have addressed forces to the ankle joint from linear angles but not from rotational forces; the figure-of-8 and the heel locks help to reduce the rotational stresses placed on the joint during activity.

The tape is started from the proximal to the distal along a 45-degree angle to the tibia. The tape goes behind the ankle, over the Achilles, under the calcaneus, back up over the front of the ankle mortise, and then either torn or continued for the other side. This step will take some practice, but it is important to master so that no wrinkles are located over the Achilles' tendon or the instep.

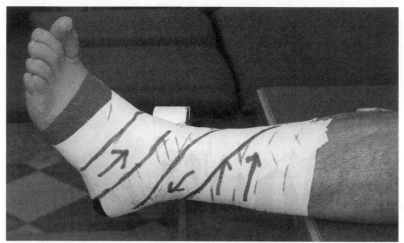

Figure 28-8   Heel locks.

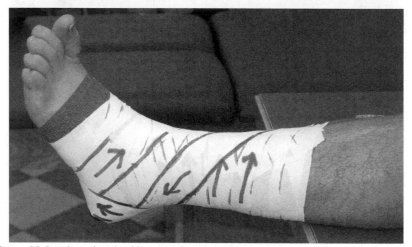

Figure 28-9   Completed ankle tape job with heel locks in place.

Figure 28-9 shows the completed heel locks to both the medial and lateral sides. The heel locks and figure-of-8 are the most difficult portion of the tape job to apply for the novice. If they are the last applied, they are easier to get off and re-do if there is excessive wrinkling of the tape or the positioning has not been correct.

Taping for Patellar Tendinitis and Tennis Elbow

The taping concept is the same for patellar tendinitis (jumper's knee) and tennis elbow.

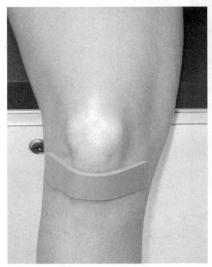
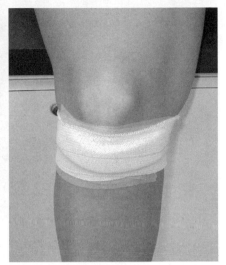

Figure 28-10   Patellar tendinitis strap.   **Figure 28-11**   Patellar tendinitis strap.

Patellar Tendinitis Strap

The counter-force strap and pad work to effectively shorten the pull of the patellar tendon (resulting in a functional shortening) and thus take the stress off of the insertion site (Figures 28-10 and 28-11). The foam pad is used to provide extra compression over the tendon. The area is then wrapped with elastic tape to provide compression. If this works in the office and is tried in a functional setting with good result (that is, a reduction in pain), then the practitioner knows that a semipermanent brace or strap will be effective for the patient. Counter-force bracing is very effective for use with knee patellar tendinitis as well as elbow lateral epicondylitis. The tape is a good trial to see if such an application would be appropriate, but for the patient, a commercially available counter-force strap (tennis elbow strap, Cho-Pat knee strap) is much easier to apply on a daily basis.

Tennis Elbow Strap

For tennis elbow, the elastic tape is applied over the pad and the insertion of the extensor, supinator muscle attachments (Figure 28-12). This effectively changes the pull on the tendinous insertion and is a good, readily available technique that can be used to see if a Velcro or similar elastic band will be effective for daily use in treating tennis elbow.

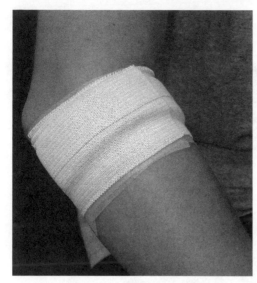

Figure 28-12   Tennis elbow strap.

Knee Compression Wrap

The knee compression wrap is used to provide compression and support for an acutely injured knee (Figure 28-13). The wrap is a 6-inch elastic bandage with a Velcro closure attached. The strip is a piece of white tape that has been folded over to help keep the elastic wrap from sliding. The wrap is started from the inferior position and applied with an upward circular motion. Wrapping from inferior to superior keeps the patient's pants from rolling up the wrap as they are pulled up. The wrap should not be left on during the night because it may cause some distal edema due to limiting venous return.

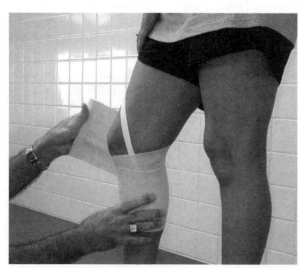

Figure 28-13   Knee compression wrap.

REFERENCES

1. Professional Uses of Adhesive Tape, 3rd ed. New Brunswick, NJ: Johnson & Johnson; 1972.
2. Statistics available at www.ncaa.org/membership/ed_outreach/health-safety/index.html.

Index

calcium, 26
  blood pressure and, 217
  osteoporosis, 71
calcium channel blockers, 224
callosities, 179
calories. *See* nutrition
Canadian C-Spine Rule, 274
cancer
  benefits of exercise, 82
  clearance-to-play decisions, 13
  testicular, 156
carbohydrates, 22-23
  diabetic patients, 192
  fluids and hydration, 21, 23
cardioselective beta-blockers, 223
cardiovascular system. *See also*
    bleeding; blood
  altitude-related illnesses, 57-59
  anemia, responses to, 135
  athletic heart syndrome (AHS),
      199-209
    identification of, 200-208
    natural history of, 208-209
  benefits of exercise, 82
  blood flow, gastrointestinal, 117-
      118, 121
  cardiac remodeling, 199-200
  eating disorders, 68
  fitness testing, 93
  focal cold injuries, 53-55
  hazards of exercise, 40-42, 84
  hypertension, 213-226
    clinical evaluation, 214-216
    exercise and, 225-226
    treatment, 216-225
  hypothermia, 50-53
  intensity of exercise, 97
  iron deficiencies, 26
  lightning injuries, 60, 61
  preparticipation screening, 6, 209-
      210
  pulmonary function testing, 86-87
  thermal regulation, 46
carpal tunnel syndrome, 334-335
central alpha-agonists, 223
central nervous system. *See*
    neurologic conditions
certirizine, 244

cervical cord neurapraxia, 277-279
cervical osteoarthritis, 352-353
cervical spine injury, 252, 350. *See
    also* neck and head
CFL (calcaneofigular ligament), 397-
    398
chilblain, 55
children
  discitis, 352
  elbow injuries, 315-317
  exercise performance, 83
  hip and pelvic injuries, 376-377
  osteochondritis dissecans, 312, 395
  spondylosis, 347
Chlamydia trachomatis, 155-156
chlorpromazine, 48
chronic fatigue. *See* overtraining and
    overuse syndromes
circulatory system. *See* cardiovascular
    system
civil liability, 16-17
clearance to play
  brachial plexus injuries, 275
  concussion, 253-255
  gastrointestinal system, 128-130
  neck and spinal injuries, 275, 278-
      280
  preparticipation, 13-16
  renal injuries, 152
  wrist injuries, 327
clenbuterol, 74-75
cluneal nerves, 355-356
Cobb angle, 346
cocaine, 74
cognitive-behavioral therapy, 78
cold-related illnesses and injuries,
    50-56
  frostbite, 53-54
  hypothermia, 50-53
collagenous nodules, 180
collapse, exercise-associated, 40-42
Colles' fractures, 328-329
colonic motility, 121-122
communicable disease. *See* infectious
    diseases
communications at mass-
    participation events, 33, 38
compartment syndrome, 409-410